EXTRAORDINARY ACCL
FASTING GIRLS

(For more outstanding praise, please turn page . . .)

JOAN JACOBS BRUMBERG teaches American women's history, family history, and the social history of medicine at Cornell University. She has published *Mission For Life: The Judson Family and American Evangelical Culture*, as well as numerous articles on the changing historical experience of female adolescence.

"A unique and probing fusion of history, cultural, and psychological observations."—*The Bookwatch*

"Accomplishes the rare feat of weaving social history with science in a manner that satisfies the reader on both accounts. Appropriate for a wide variety of audiences, this book is a 'must read.' "—*Science Books and Films*

"Informative, fascinating, and well-written . . . required reading for anyone who deals professionally with any disorder having medical, psychological, and cultural components."—*The Ithaca Journal*

"Concise, penetrating, compassionate!"
—*Times Literary Supplement*

"Lively and compassionate . . . a helpful sense of historical perspective."—*Feminist Bookstore Review*

"A compassionate, engrossing account."
—Susie Orbach, author of
Fat Is A Feminist Issue

Fasting Girls

The History of
Anorexia Nervosa

Joan Jacobs Brumberg

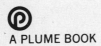

A PLUME BOOK

PLUME
Published by the Penguin Group
Penguin Books USA Inc., 375 Hudson Street, New York, New York 10014,
U.S.A.
Penguin Books Ltd, 27 Wrights Lane, London W8 5TZ, England
Penguin Books Australia Ltd, Ringwood, Victoria, Australia
Penguin Books Canada Ltd, 2801 John Street, Markham, Ontario, Canada L3R
1B4
Penguin Books (N.Z.) Ltd, 182-190 Wairau Road, Auckland 10, New Zealand

Penguin Books Ltd, Registered Offices: Harmondsworth, Middlesex, England

Published by Plume, an imprint of New American Library, a division of Penguin
Books USA Inc.

BOOKS ARE AVAILABLE AT QUANTITY DISCOUNTS WHEN USED TO PROMOTE PRODUCTS
OR SERVICES. FOR INFORMATION PLEASE WRITE TO PREMIUM MARKETING DIVISION,
PENGUIN BOOKS USA INC., 375 HUDSON STREET, NEW YORK, NEW YORK 10014.

REGISTERED TRADEMARK—MARCA REGISTRADA

Library of Congress Cataloging-in-Publication Data

Brumberg, Joan Jacobs.
    Fasting girls : The history of anorexia nervosa / Joan Jacobs Brumberg.
        p.   cm.
    Reprint. Originally published: Cambridge, Mass. : Harvard University
Press, 1988.
    Bibliography: p.
    Includes index.
    ISBN 0-452-26327-1
    1. Anorexia nervosa—History.   2. Anorexia nervosa—Social aspects.
3. Teenage girls—History.   I. Title.
RC552.A5B784   1989
616.85'262—dc20
                                                              89-9414
                                                              CIP

First Plume Printing, October, 1989

3 4 5 6 7 8 9 10 11

PRINTED IN THE UNITED STATES OF AMERICA

For Sidney Jacobs and
Frances Storck Jacobs
with love and appreciation

Illustrations

Following page 188

Saint Catherine of Siena, one of the religious women of the Middle Ages for whom fasting was part of a larger penitential program

1812 broadside on the subject of Ann Moore, the fasting woman of Tutbury

Mollie Fancher, a fasting girl from Brooklyn in the 1860s who claimed to be clairvoyant as well as abstemious

Sir William Withey Gull, who named and identified anorexia nervosa in 1873

Several of William Gull's early anorexic patients

Charles Lasègue, the French physician who identified and described *l'anorexie hystérique* a few months before William Gull's report

The sixteen-year-old British schoolgirl who in 1895 was the first reported death from anorexia nervosa

Thomas Eakins' *Portrait of a Lady with a Setter Dog*, the epitome of Victorian femininity

Fading Away, by Henry Peach Robinson, which depicts the alarm of the Victorian family when a daughter became emaciated

Annette Kellerman, a strong advocate of female athleticism and the primacy of the body in the 1920s

One of the advertisements that promoted cigarettes as a way of helping women become or remain slim

The dinner table, centerpiece of the problems and pleasures of family life in the early twentieth century

The first published photograph, in 1932, of an anorectic in an American medical journal

Karen Carpenter, popular singer who died in 1983 from complications of anorexia nervosa

One of the eating-disorder clinics that in the 1980s provide comprehensive medical and psychiatric treatment

Ms. cartoon that captures the thinking of most American women of today's middle and upper classes

Contents

Fasting Girls

Introduction

I am not a recovered anorectic nor am I the mother of an anorexic daughter.[1] I make this point at the outset so that my readers will understand the perspective of this book. I am a historian and my interest in anorexia nervosa stems, in part, from observation of social change within my own lifetime.

In 1965, while a senior at the University of Rochester, I tutored patients in the pediatrics section of Strong Memorial Hospital. One of my students, a young woman named Sherry, was so emaciated and withdrawn that I found it painful to be with her. Although she looked like twelve or thirteen years old, Sherry was actually fifteen and the nurse told me that she suffered from anorexia nervosa. I learned that Sherry would not eat and that some anorectics actually starve to death. When I carried this disturbing information back to my friends in the dormitory, my news was met with both shock and skepticism. None of us had ever heard of anorexia nervosa before.

By 1985, I was a faculty member at Cornell University teaching large undergraduate courses in the history of American women and the family. In this role, I met and listened to many undergraduate women. What I heard was a surprising amount of sophisticated talk about anorexia nervosa, talk that revealed a real familiarity with the disorder and its symptoms. I also discovered, as a member of the admissions committee, that some female students applying to Cornell related their choice of major to experience with anorexia nervosa during high school: "The field of psychology has begun to intrigue me," wrote one applicant, "[because] my best friend is anorexic. I provide as much support as I can but I feel helpless." Eventually I realized that it was nearly impossible to find a young middle-class woman who did *not* know about anorexia nervosa. This situation provided a sharp contrast to my own experience twenty years earlier when my friends and I marveled at the mystery of the exotic "starving disease." As a historian, I had to ponder the new "popularity" of anorexia nervosa.

Why does a disease become more prominent in one time period than another? This question has enormous relevance for American life in the 1990s. As a society, we are preoccupied with medical discourse and with the discovery and conquest of disease. Acquired immune deficiency syndrome (AIDS), Alzheimer's, herpes and chlamydia, osteoporosis, premenstrual syndrome, and anorexia nervosa all seem to be "new" diseases, unknown or unnoticed in prior generations.

Anorexia nervosa became the focus of my professional research when I joined the Department of Human Development and Family Studies at Cornell as its resident historian. I had already demonstrated a particular interest in the changing historical experience of female adolescence in the United States; now I was drawn into the world of the behavioral sciences and a range of issues having to do with adolescent physical, social, and cognitive development—with family relations, education, and sexuality. As the sole spokesperson for history in a department of psychologists and sociologists, I was repeatedly challenged by my colleagues to explain the origins of contemporary social problems, especially those that affect adolescent girls in our society.

Inevitably, I had to confront the issue of anorexia nervosa and eating disorders since both were gaining attention and momentum. My curiosity, provoked by personal experience over two decades ago, prompted me to ask a set of basic questions: what is the history of anorexia nervosa? Which historical forces account for its emergence as a modern disease? Why is there so much anorexia nervosa *now*?

Today's anorectic is one of a long line of women and girls throughout history who have used control of appetite, food, and the body as a focus of their symbolic language. Although anorexia nervosa is a relatively modern disease, female fasting is assuredly not a new behavior. In fact, there is a long history of food-refusing behavior and appetite control in women dating back, at least, to the medieval world. Anorexia nervosa implies important continuities in female experience across time and place.

Historical, anthropological, and psychological studies suggest that women use appetite as a form of expression more often than men, a tendency confirmed by scholars as well as clinicians.[2] Work by the historian Caroline Walker Bynum, for example, demonstrates that in the High Middle Ages (the thirteenth through sixteenth centuries) the lives of women such as Catherine of Siena were characterized by extensive fasting and passionate devotion to the eucharist (taking only the wafer and wine, symbols of the body and blood of Christ).[3] Moreover, where writings by these women survive, we find the same pervasive images of eating, drinking, and food that appear later in the thought of the twentieth-century anorectic who is food obsessed, constantly counts calories, and structures her life around the avoidance of food. Medieval scholarship unambiguously demonstrates that there have been moments in time, other than our own, when large numbers of women and girls refused to eat regularly or practiced extraordinary forms of appetite control.[4]

Despite this pattern, we should avoid easy generalizations about the existence in past times of the modern disease entity anorexia nervosa or about "women's nature." Although the fasting and food preoccupations of medieval women suggest anorexia nervosa, the symptomatic continuities can be misleading. Just because a behavior occurs across cultures or time does not necessarily mean that it has the same cause or that it is biologically based. I address this issue by presenting a tableau of women fasters, one that demonstrates that there are not only changing interpretations of food-refusing behavior but also varying reasons for female control of the appetite. Even as basic a human instinct as appetite is transformed by cultural and social systems and given new meaning in different historical epochs.

The story of anorexia nervosa lays bare the extent to which disease is a cultural artifact, defined and redefined over time, and therefore illustrative of fundamental historical transformations. Consequently, my response to the frequent question, Is anorexia nervosa a new disease? must be somewhat ambiguous: anorexia nervosa is a historically specific disease that emerged from the distinctive economic and social environment of the late nineteenth century. Thus the modern clinical term "anorexia nervosa" should be used to designate only a disease of modernity.

Anorexia nervosa was named and identified in the 1870s, almost simultaneously by professional medical men in England,

France, and the United States. The "birth" of the disease in the Victorian era was related not only to the new authority of medicine but also to changes in the larger society that had consequences for young women. Anorexia nervosa emerged during the throes of industrial capitalist development and was nurtured by central aspects of bourgeois life: intimacy and material comfort, parental love and expectation, the sexual division of labor, and popular ideas about gender and class. An early and distinctive psychopathology of middle-class family life, the disease itself preceded the familiar body-image imperatives usually associated with it. A historical perspective shows that anorexia nervosa existed before there was a mass cultural preoccupation with dieting and a slim female body.

It is the task of the social and cultural historian to maintain connection with a particular historical moment in order to understand people and their behavior on their own terms.[5] For this reason I choose to avoid psychohistory in its most traditional form: I do not apply modern psychological or psychoanalytic theory to cases of female fasting in the past. To my mind, the effort to produce congruence between a current psychological model and fragmentary historical evidence, garnered from "the world we have lost," is relatively empty in the case of anorexia nervosa. I do recognize certain transhistorical emotional features—such as denial and anger—in medieval religious asceticism and present-day anorexia nervosa. But as a historian I am usually unable to make pronouncements about the psychogenesis of individual cases. The documentary record is simply inadequate and the patient too distant for psychoanalysis.

Rather than follow a "presentist" line of interpretation, I emphasize the distinctive social and cultural contexts in which young women have chosen to refuse food, and I focus on how they understand their own behavior. Instead of insisting that anorexia nervosa is an absolutely consistent psychological experience throughout history, I suggest that we place this specific syndrome on a wide and multifaceted continuum that represents the variety of human, especially female, eating behaviors. As we look at that broad spectrum of eating behaviors we need to ask, Why is it that women and girls in certain cultural systems and historical epochs become susceptible to particular forms of exaggerated behavior centering on food?

By putting the question in this way we can decode the changing meaning of the refusal of food. But to do so, food itself must be a central concern. In thinking about anorexia nervosa and its relation to food, we need to explore more than questions of availability or nutritional value. Because food functions as a system of signs and symbols with multiple meanings, we must consider the symbolic value of what is rejected.[6] Simply put, we need to comprehend what food has meant to women at different points in time and how the food vocabulary of one historical period differs from that of another.

Changing ideas about food and its meaning are only a key to a larger historical issue. In essence this book charts the transition from sainthood to patienthood, a process that historians describe with two familiar words, secularization and medicalization. Secularization refers to the long and uneven process by which a society moves from a religious to a nonreligious world view; medicalization suggests a parallel process whereby the language and ideology of scientific medicine come to predominate in explanations of human behavior.[7] Using cases drawn from the sixteenth through nineteenth centuries, I show how the understanding of food-refusing behavior evolved in response to new developments in religion and medicine. By the nineteenth century a general decline in faith and the rise of scientific authority had, for the most part, transformed refusal of food from a religious act into a pathological state. Yet even in the last years of the century, and despite the protests of prominent physicians, the so-called fasting girls were still considered by many to have miraculous powers. The public discussion of these cases revealed the staying power of traditional piety and belief. Throughout the nineteenth century women who refused their food were a focal point in the great debate between priests and physicians over who should be the prime interpreter of human behavior. Even after the issue was settled and anorexia nervosa became a working diagnosis, the medical profession debated the cause or etiology of the new disease and how it should be treated. In truth, neither secularization nor medicalization occurred in short order or with much precision.

To examine the responsiveness of disease to cultural settings, we must look beyond the doctors, diagnoses, and therapies to the patients themselves. People express both physical pain and psychic discomfort in myriad ways, depending on their gender and age, their class, their ethnic origins, their world view, and a host of other cultural variables. Expressions of physical anguish and mental stress are selected quite unconsciously from a repertoire of symptoms that we learn simply by being part of a culture. Put another way, even when an illness is organic, being sick is a social act.[8]

For these reasons we should expect to see anorexia nervosa "present" differently, in terms of both predisposing psychological factors and actual physical symptoms. The chapters that follow explain how and why the symptomatology in anorexia nervosa changed in response to a different social and cultural environment. Although the modern anorectic's claims ("I am full," "I am not hungry," or "I eat enough") are not markedly different from the Victorian formulations ("I have no appetite" or "I feel bad when I eat"), there are significant new behavioral symptoms that mirror contemporary culture—namely, pervasive hyperactivity and competitiveness. Among affluent young Victorians food and eating were at the center of a web of associations that had a great deal to do with gender and class identity. The same is true today, but broad social and cultural forces, particularly the intensification of messages about the female body, have promoted the urgency of appetite control and generated a new experience of the disease in the twentieth century. Anorexia nervosa used to be an isolated and idiosyncratic disorder; over the past few decades it has become both more familiar and more formulaic, and its physical symptoms are now more acute.[9]

The historical study of anorexia nervosa also demonstrates that different explanations of a disease can exist simultaneously. This was true in the distant past and it is true today. In the 1980s we are still debating the determinants of human behavior. Much that is said in the familiar go-round over nature versus culture (now recast as biological versus social determinism) has relevance to anorexia nervosa.[10] Because the etiology of the disease remains unsettled, everyone asks which is the culprit, biology or culture. This unresolved state of affairs means that I could not write a "posthumous biography" of the sort written about cholera, chlorosis, pellagra, syphilis, and neurasthenia.[11] Because of the current high visibility of anorexia nervosa, as well as the prospect that new biomedical research may, at any time, revolutionize thinking about it, I forged my interpretation in an intellectual climate where there is no definitive answer to what the disease really is. The consistent pressure from the medical establishment for a biochemical explanation means that I had to think long and hard about what culture could or could not do to shape the lives of individuals.

In Chapter 1, I discuss the relative merits of the three major theoretical models (biological, psychological, and cultural) but I argue against any one model of causation. Anorexia nervosa is not a simple disorder; it does not reduce easily to a single etiological agent. But the fact that social and cultural factors play a role does not mean that it is a "phony" disease, a "mere social construction."[12] Anorexia nervosa has real physical consequences and involves a level of self-destructive behavior that makes it qualitatively different from chronic dieting. Rather than subscribe to any one theory of causation, I argue that there is a complex web of interactions of the sort described by Charles E. Rosenberg in a pioneering study of cholera in the nineteenth century: "A disease is no absolute physical entity but a complex intellectual construction, an amalgam of biological state and social definition."[13] In the case of anorexia nervosa, it is clearly time to drop the either/or approach and begin to think about the reciprocity of biology and culture.

In practice, rather than in principle, this book is biased in favor of an interactive cultural model. My bias seems to me appropriate, given our subject and the history I have uncovered. No explanation except a historical and cultural one begins to unravel the problem of the disease's increasing *incidence*. (Incidence, to be sure, is a different issue than etiology, and the two are not conflated here.) Culture is the critical variable that explains why and how anorexia nervosa became the characteristic psychopathology of the female adolescent of our day.

In the 1980s anorexia nervosa constitutes a modern credo of self-denial that has much to tell us about the situation of young women and about contemporary values. The disease starkly illustrates the predicament of the privileged but vulnerable adolescent female in a rapidly changing society that elevates thinness to the highest moral plane. From the vantage point of the historian, anorexia nervosa appears to be a secular addiction to a new kind of perfectionism, one that links personal salvation to the achievement of an external body configuration rather than an internal spiritual state.

1 · Anorexia Nervosa in the 1980s

The American public discovered anorexia nervosa only recently. Although the disease was known to physicians as early as the 1870s, the general public knew virtually nothing about it until the 1970s, when the popular press began to feature stories about young women who refused to eat despite available and plentiful food. In 1974, the "starving disease" made its first appearance as an independent subject heading in the *Readers' Guide to Periodical Literature*, a standard library reference tool that also provides a useful index to contemporary social issues. By 1984, the disease had become so commonplace that "Saturday Night Live" featured jokes about the "anorexic cookbook," and a comedian in the Borscht Belt drew laughs with a reference to a new disease, "anorexia ponderosa." In *Down and Out in Beverly Hills*, 1986 film audiences tittered at the predictable presence of an anorexic daughter in a lush suburban setting. Today nearly everyone understands flip remarks such as "You look anorexic." Anorexia nervosa has become common parlance, used as hyperbole by those outside the medical profession (particularly women) to comment on one another's bodies.

Our national education on the subject of anorexia nervosa can be traced to a variety of published popular sources in the decade of the 1970s. An early article in *Science Digest* reported on a "strange disease" in adolescent girls characterized by a "morbid aversion" to eating. Despite a new permissiveness in many areas of social behavior, parents in the 1960s were counseled against taking adolescent food refusal lightly or allowing it to continue.

In 1970, at the outset of a decade of national education about anorexia nervosa, the press warned American parents to seek professional medical intervention as soon as possible, because there was "no safe leeway for home-style cure attempts."[1]

Newspapers as diverse as the *New York Times* and the *Weekly World News* pursued the subject in their own inimitable ways. The *Times*'s first discussion of the disease was a synthetic overview of state-of-the-art medical treatment, defined as New York City and Philadelphia clinical practice. The *World News*, a tabloid equivalent of the *National Enquirer* and the *Star*, ran a provocative banner headline—"The Bizarre Starving Disease"—and featured a horrifying picture of a 55-pound woman in shorts and a halter. While the *Times* reported a fatality rate of 5 to 15 percent, the *World News* claimed 30 to 50 percent.[2] From whatever newspaper one draws information, anorexia nervosa has been taught to a variety of people from different class and educational backgrounds since the 1970s.

The disease has always had particular salience for women and girls. Not surprisingly, the three magazines that generated the largest volume of national coverage on anorexia nervosa—*People*, *Mademoiselle*, and *Seventeen*—all cater to the primary constituency for the disease: adolescent and young adult women. Another important source of information about anorexia nervosa suggests that the disease has a specific class constituency. Alumnae magazines from the elite eastern women's colleges took up the cause of the disease by alerting former students to the problem of anorexia nervosa on campus. Alumnae coverage provided information on what the typical anorectic was like: intelligent, attractive, polite, demanding of herself. In effect, she was the mirror image of much of their own student body.[3]

All of the women's magazines wrote about the disease with a common sense of urgency. Without being entirely certain of the data, they spoke of "epidemics," proclaiming that there were somewhere between one hundred thousand and one million Americans with anorexia nervosa. In addition, they reported that between 5 percent and 15 percent of anorectics in psychiatric treatment died, giving it one of the highest fatality rates of any psychiatric diagnosis. Although the notion of adolescent death through compulsive starvation seemed silly to some, anorexia nervosa was becoming a growing subject of concern among mothers in private discussions and among psychiatrists in clinical practice.

In 1978, after nearly three decades of clinical experience treating eating disorders, psychiatrist Hilde Bruch (1904–1984) published a book on anorexia nervosa for lay audiences. *The Golden Cage*, based on seventy case histories, was a popular success. Bruch began by saying: "New diseases are rare, and a disease that selectively befalls the young, rich, and beautiful is practically unheard of. But such a disease is affecting the daughters of well-to-do, educated, and successful families." She explained that "for the last fifteen or twenty years anorexia nervosa [has been] occurring at a rapidly increasing rate. Formerly it was exceedingly rare." As a practicing psychiatrist in Houston, Bruch observed that most of her colleagues "recognized the name as something they had heard about in medical school, but they never saw a case in real life." By the time her book was published, Bruch claimed that anorexia nervosa was "so common" that it was a "real problem in high schools and colleges."[4] Bruch's extensive knowledge of the condition, combined with her sense of urgency about the disease, contributed to the growing cultural perception of an epidemic. In effect, anorexia nervosa was the disease of the 1970s, to be obscured only by AIDS and the accompanying specter of contagion and pollution that absorbs public attention at this moment.

The Question of Epidemiology

Is an epidemic of anorexia nervosa in progress? When did the numbers of anorectics really begin to accelerate?

An increase in the number of cases of anorexia nervosa appears to have started about twenty years ago. During the Great Depression and World War II, in times of scarcity, voluntary food refusal had little efficacy as an emotional strategy and anorexic girls were a relative rarity in American clinical practice. A comment by Mara Selvini-Palazzoli, an Italian pioneer in the psychiatric study of anorexia nervosa, confirmed the relationship between anorexia nervosa and post–World War II affluence: "During the whole period of World War II in Italy (1939–1945) there were dire food restrictions and no patients at all were hospitalized at the Clinic for anorexia [nervosa]." After the war, however, "concurrent with the explosion of the Italian economic miracle and the advent of the affluent society," Selvini-Palazzoli did see hospitalizations for anorexia nervosa.[5]

By the 1960s wartime experiences of rationing, famine, and concentration camps were fading from memory. In the postwar culture of affluence many aspects of personal behavior were transformed: sexuality, relations between the generations, forms of family life, gender roles, clothing, even styles of food and eating. A discussion of these changes and how they affected the incidence of anorexia nervosa follows in later chapters. From a psychiatrist's perspective, the postwar years brought an increasing number of adolescent female patients who used appetite and eating as emotional instruments much as they had in early childhood. In the 1960s Bruch published extensively on the subject of anorexia nervosa, and her work was a bellwether that marked the beginning of a rise in the number of diagnosed cases, a rise that became even more precipitous in the next two decades.[6]

The dimensions of the recent increase are hard to ascertain, however, because of problems in collecting and interpreting data as well as lack of standardization in diagnostic criteria. Not all patients with anorexia nervosa have exactly the same symptoms in the same degree or intensity. Not all cases present exactly the same symptoms as those elaborated in the American Psychiatric Association's *Diagnostic and Statistical Manual*, the standard reference guide to modern psychiatric disorders. The DSM-III criteria are the following: refusal to maintain normal body weight; loss of more than 25 percent of original body weight; disturbance of body image; intense fear of becoming fat; and no known medical illness leading to weight loss.[7] Yet some clinicians differentiate between primary and secondary anorexia, some favor a less stringent weight criterion, and some include hyperactivity and amenorrhea as symptom criteria.[8] There is also the matter of how anorexia nervosa is related to bulimia, the binge-purge syndrome. Until 1980, when it was listed in DSM-III as a separate diagnostic entity, bulimia (from the Greek meaning ox hunger) was only a symptom, not an independent disease. But in 1985, in DSM-III-R, bulimia obtained independent disease status; according to the newest categorization, anorexia nervosa and bulimia are separate but related disorders. In the diagnosis of anorexia nervosa, there is increasing support for subtyping anorexic patients into those who are pure dieters ("restrictive anorectics") and those who incorporate binging and purging ("bulimic anorectics" and/or "bulimarexics").[9] Who gets counted (and who does not) is never entirely clear or consistent, so that diagnostic imprecision makes the numbers difficult to assess.

Despite these problems, the evidence does suggest that we have experienced an absolute increase in the amount of anorexia nervosa over the past two decades. For example, twenty years ago the University of Wisconsin Hospital typically admitted one anorectic a year; in 1982 over seventy cases were admitted to the same institution. A retrospective review of incidence rates in Monroe County, New York, revealed that the number of cases of anorexia nervosa doubled between 1960 and 1976.[10]

In terms of the general population, however, anorexia nervosa is still a relatively infrequent disease: the annual incidence of the disorder has never been estimated at more than 1.6 per 100,000 population.[11] Still, among adolescent girls and young women there is an increasing and disturbing amount of anorexia nervosa and bulimia; by a number of different estimates, as many as 5 to 10 percent are affected. On some college campuses estimates run as high as 20 percent.[12]

Two critical demographic facts about the contemporary population of anorectics are relevant to the question of an "epidemic." Ninety to 95 percent of anorectics are young and female, and they are disproportionately white and from middle-class and upper-class families. Anorexia nervosa can exist in males but with a quite different clinical picture. The rare anorexic male exhibits a greater degree of psychopathology, tends to be massively obese before becoming emaciated, and has a poorer treatment prognosis. Moreover, the male anorexic is less likely to be affluent.[13] Anorexia nervosa is not a problem among contemporary American blacks or Chicanos; neither was it a conspicuous problem among first-generation and second-generation ethnic immigrants such as Eastern European Jews.[14] As these groups move up the social ladder, however, their vulnerability to the disorder increases. In fact, the so-called epidemic seems to be consistently restrained by age and gender but promoted by social mobility.

In a similar vein, the "contagion" is also confined to the United States and Western Europe, Japan, and other areas experiencing rapid Westernization. A description of anorexia nervosa compiled by a Russian psychiatrist in 1971 was basically a report of clinical cases drawn from outside his country. Physicians looking for anorexia nervosa in developing nations or countries of the Third World have been unsuccessful in finding it, a fact which has led to its classification as a "culture-bound syndrome."[15] In other words, the anorexic population has a highly specific social address.

In the United States, as well as in Western Europe, the growth of anorexia nervosa is due in part to heightened awareness and reporting on the part of families and doctors. Rising numbers of anorectics do reflect "diagnostic drift"—that is, the greater likelihood that a clinician who sees a very thin adolescent female with erratic eating habits and a preoccupation with weight will describe and label that patient as a case of anorexia nervosa, rather than citing some other mental disorder where lack of appetite is a secondary feature (such as depression or schizophrenia).[16] Simple anorexia—meaning lack of appetite—is a secondary symptom in many medical and psychiatric disorders ranging from the serious to the inconsequential. For some girls an episode of anorexia is mild and transitory; others, perhaps as many as 19 percent of the diagnosed cases, die from it.[17] In the 1980s there may well be a medical tendency to place temporary and chronic anorexias under one diagnostic rubric precisely because of our familiarity with the disease. Most thoughtful clinicians agree that anorectics are not necessarily a homogeneous group and that more attention should be paid to defining and specifying their psychological and physiological characteristics.

This situation reflects a basic medical reality—that there are fashions in diagnosis. In 1984 Dr. Irving Farber, a practitioner in Jamaica, New York, wrote to his state medical journal about the overdiagnosis of anorexia nervosa: "In my experience, a significant number of girls and young women who have been diagnosed by professionals, and [girls] themselves, are not suffering from this disorder." A group of physicians from the Department of Pediatrics, Long Island Jewish–Hillside Medical Center, responded that Farber's point was "well-taken," although they disagreed with his analysis of a specific case.[18]

The statistical increase in the number of anorexics over the past two decades can be explained also by the amount of media attention paid to the disorder. Anorexia nervosa has become *au courant*, an "in" disease among affluent adolescent and young adult women, a phenomenon that confirms long-standing beliefs about the susceptibility of girls to peer influence. One prominent psychologist specializing in treatment of the disorder estimates that 30 percent of all current cases are what Bruch once called "me too" anorectics. Bruch herself wrote: "The illness used to be the accomplishment of an isolated girl who felt she had found her own way to salvation. Now it is more a group reaction."[19] This mimetic or copycat phenomenon is hard to assess statistically and only adds confusion to an already complex problem in psychiatric epidemiology. In sum: although the total number of actual anorectics is hard to assess and probably not enormous, incidence of the disorder is higher today than at any other time since the discovery of the disease over a century ago. In addition, among the constituency most vulnerable to the disease, bourgeois adolescent and young adult women, there is the perception of an epidemic—a perception fueled in part by messages coming from American popular culture.

The Influence of Popular Culture

In a society committed to hearing nearly everyone's story, the anorectic has come "out of the closet" like so many others—homosexuals, adopted people, substance abusers, molested children, born-again Christians and Jews. To be sure, the genre of disclosure has different ideological sources and purposes. Yet the current interest in experience and our self-confessional tendencies have generated a plethora of writing about anorexia nervosa, ranging from self-help books to autobiographical accounts to adolescent fiction. This concern for personal testimony and authenticity is revealed in the fact that the American Anorexia and Bulimia Association (AA/BA), founded in 1978, maintains a daily hot line across the country that provides telephone access to a recovered anorectic.

The disclosure in January 1983 that thirty-two-year-old popular singer Karen Carpenter had died of heart failure associated with low serum potassium—a consequence of prolonged starvation—fueled interest in the disease. Carpenter's tragic death confirmed the fact that anorexia nervosa could be fatal rather than just annoying. The news media emphasized that the best and most expensive medical treatment on both coasts had been ineffective against the disease. Although Carpenter's anorexia was described as a psychiatric disorder generated by her own insecurities and personality, she was also called a "victim" of anorexia nervosa, as if the disease were totally involuntary, or even contagious.[20] Carpenter's death focused national attention on the life-and-death drama of anorexia nervosa.

In the 1980s one can experience anorexia nervosa vicariously through films as well as books. Two made-for-television movies about anorexia nervosa have been shown in prime time on the major networks. The first, *The Best Little Girl in the World* (1981), had a screenplay by New York psychologist Steven Levenkron and was promoted with an advertisement that said simply, "A Drama of Anorexia Nervosa." The advertiser assumed that the disease was familiar and that its characteristic tensions and struggles generated audience involvement. At least one episode of "Fame," a program that portrays life at a select New York City high school for the performing arts, revolved around anorexia nervosa in a young student and its impact on her teachers and peers. In Marge Piercy's 1984 novel, *Fly Away Home*, the central character is a middle-aged, middle-class divorcée who is both a successful Boston cookbook author and the mother of an anorexic daughter.

Two other popular sources of information about anorexia nervosa are important for understanding the process of learning about the disease: fiction designed specifically for the adolescent market, and autobiographical accounts by sufferers. As a genre, anorexia stories are intended to provide adolescent girls with both a dramatic warning and a source of real information. The books are notable for their graphic descriptions of the anorectic's food preoccupations (for instance, never allowing oneself to eat more than three curds of cottage cheese at one sitting) and for their endorsement of medical and psychiatric intervention. In fact, the novel is used primarily as a device for getting adolescents to understand that professional intervention is imperative.[21]

In the typical anorexia story, psychiatrists and psychologists are portrayed as benign and compassionate figures whose only offense is that they ask a lot of questions. There is no real presentation of the classic battle for control that absorbs so much time and energy in psychotherapeutic treatment of the disorder. Nor is there any mention that patients with anorexia nervosa generate great anger, stress, and helplessness in the medical personnel who treat them. Clinicians report that anorectics have resorted to all of the following kinds of deceptions: drinking enormous amounts of water before being weighed; using terrycloth towels as napkins to absorb foods and food supplements; recalibrating scales; and inserting weights in the rectum and vagina. Consequently, anorectics are not popular patients, a fact confirmed by the comment of a New York physician: "Referral of an eating disorders patient to a colleague is not usually considered a friendly act."[22]

These stories are nearly formulaic: they emphasize family tensions and the adolescent girl's confused desire for autonomy and control, but they do not advance any particular interpretation of the cause or etiology of the disease. The plot almost always involves an attractive (usually 5 feet 5 inches), intelligent high school girl from a successful dual-career family. The mother is apt to be a fashion designer, artist, actress, or writer; the father is a professional or self-made man. In two of the novels the central characters say that they want to go to Radcliffe.

Naturally enough, the protagonist becomes interested in reducing her weight. Like virtually all American girls, she wishes to be slim because in American society slim is definitely a good thing for a female to be. Francesca, the principal character of *The Best Little Girl in the World*, cuts out pictures of models and orders them by thinness. Her goal is to be thinner than her thinnest picture. In each of the anorexia stories, for a number of different reasons all of which have to do with the difficulties of adolescence, ordinary dieting becomes transformed into a pattern of bizarre food and eating behavior that dominates the life of the central character. Some girls eat only one food, such as celery, yogurt, or dry crackers; others steal from the refrigerator at night and refuse to be seen eating. In one novel the parents are persuaded by their daughter to allow her to take supper alone in her room so that she can do homework at the same time. The mother acquiesces only to discover that for over a year her daughter has been throwing her dinner out the window of their Central Park West apartment.

In all of the fiction, girlhood anorexia curtails friendships and makes both parents extraordinarily tense, unhappy, and solicitous. Because the main characters are depicted as still in high school and living at home, mothers are central to the story. The fictive anorectic both dislikes and loves her mother and feels perpetually guilty about hurting and deceiving her. Mothers, not fathers, are the usual source of referral to professional help, a fact that is reflected in the real world composition of many anorexia nervosa support groups. Mothers of anorectics commonly join such groups to share their experiences; the AA/BA was founded by a mother for precisely that purpose.

Even though all of the novels move the story to the critical point of therapeutic intervention, few provide any valid information about the physical and emotional discomfort that lies ahead. In *Second Star to the Right* Leslie, age fifteen, is hospitalized in a behavior-modification program on a ward of anorectics where she is required to consume five glasses of liquid food per day or else she will be fed involuntarily. Her visits with parents and friends, as well as her television watching, are controlled and allocated on the basis of her weight. Yet the story stops short of describing the realities of forced feeding. By the end of the book Leslie wants to get well but has made little physical progress.

Most of the fiction for teenagers finesses the difficult, lengthy, and often unpleasant recovery period. With only one exception, none of the fictional anorectics die.

Personal testimonials provide another compelling perspective on anorexia nervosa. Between 1980 and 1985 a number of autobiographical accounts achieved wide readership: in particular, novelist Shelia MacLeod's detailed account of her anorexic girlhood in Britain and Cherry Boone O'Neill's intimate story of her anorexia, marriage, and dedication to the evangelical Christian faith.[23] Unlike the fiction, which protects its youthful readers from the harsh realities of the recovery process, these are testimonies to extraordinary and protracted personal suffering. Few details are spared. Boone, for example, describes an incident in which her eating behavior became so bizarre that she stole slimy scraps from a dog's dish.

In the effort to educate and raise public awareness about particular diseases, some contemporary celebrities have been forthcoming about their personal health histories. Rock Hudson's 1985 deathbed revelation that he had AIDS was a powerful and poignant example; Mary Tyler Moore, a lifelong diabetic, openly identifies herself with that disease. For the purposes of our story, Jane Fonda's 1983 disclosure that she suffered from bulimia was a critical public event. Fonda's revelation that she binged and purged throughout her years at Vassar College and during her early film career had the effect of imprinting bulimia and anorexia nervosa on the national consciousness.[24] Since then, many autobiographical narratives from contemporary bulimic women have surfaced. These are among the most disturbing and unhappy documents generated by women in our time. They describe obsessive thinking about food and its acquisition; stealing food; secret, ritualistic eating; and compulsive vomiting, often with orgiastic overtones.[25] Compared to the restrictive anorectic who typically limits herself to between 200 and 400 calories a day, the bulimic may ingest as much as 8,000 calories at one sitting. The public discovery of bulimia in the early 1980s meant that anorexia nervosa no longer stood alone as the solitary example of aberrant female appetite. Rather, it was the jagged, most visible tip of the iceberg of eating disorders.

The World of Eating Disorders

At a very basic level Americans are competitive even about disease. In the absence of a tightly conceived national health policy, the idea of promoting a disease is not unheard of, since medical researchers must routinely compete for funding. The availability of public and private money is often influenced by subjective social factors such as what type of person gets the disease and how much publicity it receives. Consequently, in contemporary American society many diseases have their own individual advocacy groups composed, typically, of people who have had direct experience with the disease either as sufferers or as family members. These individuals and organizations are understandably anxious to publicize their disease in order to garner more financial support. Because anorexia nervosa and bulimia were marginal (if not unknown) diseases until very recently, and because of their restricted age, gender, and class clientele, those who serve the cause of eating disorders must work aggressively to convince the public of their seriousness, especially when the competitors are AIDS, cancer, and Alzheimer's.

The most active advocacy group for eating disorders is the American Anorexia and Bulimia Association, founded in suburban Teaneck, New Jersey. The AA/BA sponsors an ever-expanding program of support groups and other activities designed to assist anorectics, bulimics, and their families. In 1985 the AA/BA had almost twenty different chapter affiliates in diverse locations across New York, New Jersey, Pennsylvania, District of Columbia, Virginia, North Carolina, Georgia, Florida, Louisiana, Texas, Colorado, and California. The organization publishes a newsletter that notes conferences on eating disorders, publishes excerpts from speeches given at professional meetings, reviews new books on the subject of anorexia and bulimia, reports on research done on the "doctoral level or higher," and lists successful publicity efforts by name and date of publication. "The world is learning about anorexia and bulimia," the newsletter states, and "our organization has been offered as a resource."[26]

The association's materials routinely state that anorexia nervosa and bulimia strike a million Americans every year and that one hundred fifty thousand die annually. AA/BA has lobbied the United States Food and Drug Administration against over-the-counter sales of Ipecac. Because of the wide availability of the drug and its speedy emetic action, Ipecac was abused, according to AA/BA sources, by an estimated thirty thousand young women last year.[27] In a world where adolescent eating disorders have often been trivialized, AA/BA has chosen to act aggressively, using powerful statistics to underscore the urgency of both its own mission and this emerging public health problem. The organization works energetically to keep anorexia nervosa and bulimia in the public eye and, in so doing, serves as a clearinghouse for the frenetic professional activity that characterizes the world of eating disorders.

There is a veritable army of health professionals involved in the treatment of eating disorders: internists, endocrinologists, psychiatrists, neurobiologists, clinical psychologists, social workers, family therapists, nurses, nutritionists, and student personnel specialists. As a result, the past two decades have seen an explosion of clinically focused research on anorexia nervosa and bulimia. Keeping up with the literature is a Herculean task even though an attempt has been made to centralize information in one publication. In 1981 the *International Journal of Eating Disorders* was founded to foster and publish research on anorexia nervosa, bulimia, obesity, and other atypical patterns of eating behavior and body-weight reduction. In its first four years the journal received over 270 submissions and experienced a 50 percent rise in the number of subscriptions.

Professional interest in empirical and clinical research on eating disorders cannot be confined, however, to a single journal or professional group. In 1984 alone, close to fifty different professional journals published articles and clinical research findings on anorexia nervosa.[28] The multiplicity of professionals interested in eating disorders reflects the currency of the issue and the increasing specialization of health-related knowledge and services. A deluge of publications and conferences since the late 1970s reveals a remarkable level of professional and intraprofessional competition in which each specialty has pushed for intellectual ascendancy.

Today, in the mid-1980s, various kinds of therapeutic services are offered by different kinds of professionals. What each conceives as the cause of anorexia nervosa has a critical impact on the treatment offered. In general, the three broad categories are medical, behavioral, and pharmacological therapy. Families can also choose among outpatient and inpatient facilities in a variety of institutions, both public and private. Costs may range from $25 per week for an outpatient counseling session in a community social service agency to $30,000 a month for residential treatment in a special eating disorders facility.

Before the late 1970s, most medical facilities placed individual patients with anorexia nervosa in a general medical setting or in a pediatric or adolescent unit. In the present decade, however, the concept of eating disorders provides a functional way of organizing comprehensive treatment. Special residential facilities, either within hospitals or free-standing, are devoted strictly to patients with eating disorders. These facilities allow for development of a coordinated approach to treatment that integrates different medical and psychotherapeutic approaches. Some of the nation's most prestigious university-affiliated teaching hospitals operate eating disorders units, as do important interests in the private-for-profit medical world. In 1985 the Renfrew Center, the country's first residential facility exclusively for the treatment of eating disorders, opened in an old Philadelphia estate refurbished and redesigned by architects. At the center patients who do not require acute medical or psychiatric hospitalization are counseled by a staff of forty professionals over a six-week to eight-week period. In Delray Beach, Florida, the dedicated parents of a young woman who died of anorexia nervosa are planning to open Villa Abrigo, a halfway house where girls with eating disorders can find a supportive environment away from home for as long as necessary. According to Charlotte Shatz, one of the founders, patients at Villa Abrigo will be charged according to their ability to pay.[29]

In a society where dieting constitutes a lucrative $5 billion a year industry, the private-for-profit interest in eating disorders should come as no surprise.[30] Corporations providing medical services on a fee-for-service basis, with the intention of extracting profits, understand on which side their bread is buttered. Patients with eating disorders will probably constitute an expansive market in the years ahead, particularly in newly affluent geographic areas. In the city of Miami at least two different private-for-profit organizations have ventured into the eating disorders trade: the Humana Corporation and the Counseling Centers of America, Inc. For a $25 registration fee the latter group offers an introductory daylong "Eating Disorders" seminar, publicized through a full-page newspaper advertisement that asks the question qua suggestion: "Does someone you love have anorexia nervosa or bulimia?" The ad explains that eating disorders can "destroy their victims" and "tear a family apart." In this seminar the Counseling Centers hope to provide introductory information on treatment approaches and "strategies for family survival" that will lead, ultimately, to a regularized outpatient treatment program in their offices.

Private-for-profit marketing of medical services is increasingly sophisticated and plays directly to the pain and pocketbook of affluent families. To publicize the services of the inpatient Anorexia-Bulimia Center at Humana-Biscayne Hospital, parents are given a well-designed promotional brochure entitled "She Has a Side No One Knows." The pamphlet outlines the basic symptoms of anorexia and bulimia, presents a rudimentary psychological interpretation, and offers tidbits of advice to the concerned parent, such as "Allow mental independence" and "Be patient." Little is said about what happens to the patient when she begins treatment, but the center claims that it can provide "stability and normalization of abusive eating patterns in a secure and caring environment." The last sentence is a warning: "Without the proper treatment, the side you know could be destroyed."

The Anorexia-Bulimia Center sells hope as well as fear. The last photographic image in the brochure holds out the promise of full recovery: a lovely, blonde adolescent—a version of Ralph Lauren's "American Girl"—is seated on a blanket outdoors, in the sunshine, in casual cotton pants and a loose sweater. The young woman is accompanied by a smiling and affectionate young man (who caresses her hand), a bottle of Perrier mineral water, and a picnic basket. Each element in the carefully constructed photograph portrays an ideal of recovery: normal social eating (the picnic basket); polite heterosexuality (the boyfriend); and a socially acceptable level of attention to the care and maintenance of an attractive body (the mineral water). The intent of the advertising is obvious: inpatient therapy at the Anorexia-Bulimia Center can make this idyll possible again for parents who have the sensitivity to devote attention and economic resources to recovery.

Because there is no single psychological therapy or drug that is uniformly effective with anorexia nervosa or bulimia, the health consumer is in a difficult predicament. Cures are not imminent, the cost is high, and many different treatment modalities are offered depending on the doctor, the therapist, the institution, the family's preferences and resources, and the severity of emaciation. Some treatments focus solely on weight gain as the absolute first step in recovery; others make weight secondary and emphasize psychological growth and awareness. The list of therapeutic options for the hospitalized anorectic goes on and on: drug therapy, psychoanalysis, dynamic psychotherapy, family therapy, behavior modification, peer counseling and support groups, social skills training, assertiveness training, projective art therapy, psychodrama, hypnosis, relaxation techniques, movement therapy, nutritional education, and even sex education.

Forced feeding is the most dramatic treatment in the medical armamentarium. In severe cases, where body weight falls to a dangerous level, parents and physicians may decide to remove the anorectic from home or school to a hospital where she will be forcibly fed. Forced feeding is accomplished with invasive tubes in the nose or by a new process called total parenteral nutrition. (In TPN an intravenous catheter is inserted so that its tip lies in a large vein near the heart, where the blood flow is relatively rapid. Then a concentrated fluid containing a balance of nutrients is infused at a steady rate. Not only glucose, but fat, protein, vitamins, and minerals may be infused in this way. It is thus possible to maintain, for relatively long periods of time, someone who will take nothing by mouth.) Forced feeding is justified by parents and doctors on the grounds that it will prevent death and restore the patient to a mental state that makes meaningful therapeutic interaction possible. In critical cases many physicians will recommend "renourishment" or "refeeding" because they believe that the biological effects of starvation create a psychological prison from which the patient cannot escape. In this view, the anorectic must gain a certain amount of weight before she can progress in psychotherapy or make rational decisions about treatment.[31]

The profusion of therapeutic treatments and the multiplicity of services available to anorexic women ultimately suggests confusion rather than confidence in the struggle with eating disorders. According to Harvard Medical School's David B. Herzog and Paul M. Copeland, treatments for anorexia nervosa and bulimia are among the "most unsatisfactory in clinical medicine." Thoughtful clinicians are as uncertain about the differential effects of various therapies as they are about the anorectic's ability to get well. Although two-thirds of the anorexic population will return to a normal weight, studies suggest that 50 percent of those hospitalized continue to have eating problems and show some level of "social and psychiatric impairment."[32] And if prognosis remains an issue, so does basic cause. There is much that is still unsettled in our thinking about this refractory disorder. Again, how one conceives the cause of anorexia nervosa has a critical impact on treatment.

Theoretical Models

There is little consensus on what causes anorexia nervosa. Current explanations generally fit within one of three models: the biomedical, the psychological, or the cultural. Much time and energy is expended by different professional groups in the attempt to establish a single paradigm of the "real" origin of the disease. No one model, however, explains the current rash of eating disorders and the place of anorexia nervosa in the long history of female food refusal. Anorexia nervosa is clearly a multidetermined disorder that depends on the individual's biologic vulnerability, psychological predisposition, family, and the social climate.[33]

Proponents of the biomedical model are drawn from the ranks of research-oriented physicians rather than from members of the mental health professions (that is, psychiatric social workers, clinical psychologists, family therapists). Advocates of the biomedical view assume that aberrations of human behavior can be explained by deviance or disorder in biological processes. They maintain that anorexia nervosa is generated by an organic cause, what some call somatogenesis.

Since the 1970s a number of different endocrinological and neurological abnormalities have been postulated as causes of anorexia nervosa: hormonal imbalance, dysfunction in the satiety center of the hypothalamus, lesions in the limbic system of the brain, and irregular output of vasopressin and gonadotropin. Most recently, research conducted at the National Institutes of Health reports that depressed patients and those with anorexia nervosa both oversecrete CRH, a corticotropin-releasing hormone produced in the hypothalamus that travels first to the pituitary and then to the adrenals to make cortisol. Normally, excess cortisol production occurs in response to fear and as a sign of stress.[34]

Although there is as yet no definitive answer to the puzzle of anorexia nervosa, the thrust of biomedical investigations leads to this conclusion: if anorexia nervosa is associated with an organic abnormality, the hypothalamus is the most plausible site for the origin of the dysfunction. The hypothalamus controls or modifies a variety of homeostatic processes including respiration, circulation, food and water intake, digestion, metabolism, and body temperature. It is sensitive to cultural patterning, and even the most zealous advocates of biomedicine acknowledge that environmental stress can result in emotional arousal and neuroendocrine changes that eventually may lead to pathologic changes in the organism.[35] The etiology or cause of anorexia nervosa, however, is still unclear: "At least three possibilities exist. It may be that starvation damages the hypothalamus, that psychic stress somehow interferes with hypothalamic function, or that the manifestations of anorexia nervosa, including the psychological aberrations, are relatively independent expressions of a primary hypothalamic defect of unknown etiology."[36]

If the case for somatogenesis were conclusive, our view of the patient would have to change: anorexia nervosa would then be an involuntary disease, perhaps even inheritable, and best treated by purely medical rather than psychotherapeutic techniques.[37]

Although the organic cause of anorexia nervosa has not been definitely established, proponents of a biomedical view have resorted to a wide variety of somatic remedies and drugs. At various points in the twentieth century anorectics have been given thyroid extract, implants of calf pituitary, vitamins, insulin, corticosteroids, testosterone, lithium carbonate, and L-dopa. The psychiatric literature also includes reports of shock therapy and prefrontal lobotomy.[38] Today, a sizable segment of the medical community sees the prospect of a cure in antidepressants combined with psychotherapy.[39] Yet a November 1986 summary of the literature concluded that "no drug treatment for anorexia nervosa has ever been found to produce better results than placebo in controlled double-blind trials."[40]

Physicians are justified in their close attention to the anorectic's body, because the disease is typically accompanied by characteristic physiological abnormalities. Anorexic patients experience hypothermia, edema, hypotension, bradycardia (slow heartbeat), and lanugo (excessive body hair). Because of the cessation of the menses, infertility is hypothesized. Patients who binge and purge may experience serious dehydration and electrolyte imbalance, the latter leading to abnormal heart rhythm and sometimes death. Furthermore, anorexia combined with bulimia can produce hiatal hernia, deterioration of tooth enamel, abrasions on the esophagus, swollen salivary glands, kidney failure, and osteoporosis.[41]

The question that biomedicine must address, however, is not whether the disease has somatic components (it obviously does) but whether these symptoms are primary or secondary in the etiology of anorexia nervosa. Research has yet to establish a common biological characteristic of the anorexic population that is unambiguously a *cause* and not a consequence of extreme weight loss and nutritional deprivation. This is the old chicken-and-egg problem: which came first, hormonal imbalance or starvation?

A second problem is that the biomedical model fails to explain why young women (and not young men) are affected by the particular biochemical disturbances that are implicated in anorexia nervosa. (In the context of the recent NIH study, we might ask why young women, but not young men, are producing excess

CRH.) Although the issue of women's supposed biologic vulnerability to anorexia nervosa remains largely a mystery, there are a few very simple physiological (as opposed to biochemical) facts that are relevant to the issue of gender skew. In puberty and adolescence a major portion of a young woman's weight gain derives from fat rather than muscle. While boys are developing muscles as a consequence of biological development, girls experience an increase in adiposity, particularly in the breasts and hips. This increased fat is a necessity for the menstrual cycle.[42] In our fat-phobic society, where female self-worth is so intimately tied to a slim figure, these biological differences have critical and distinctive emotional consequences.

For adolescent boys, growing larger is frequently a source of pleasure and power; for girls, an increase in size is often confusing, awkward, and stressful. In her influential treatise *The Second Sex* (1949), Simone de Beauvoir noted the normal adolescent girl's fear of "becom[ing] flesh . . . and show[ing] her flesh . . ." This distaste is expressed by many young girls through the wish to be thin; they no longer want to eat, . . . they constantly watch their weight. Others become pathologically timid . . . From such beginnings psychoses may now and then develop."[43] In this sense, normal maturation in our society "sets up" young women for anorexia nervosa.

A third limitation of the biomedical model is that it does not address important social characteristics of the anorexic population. To repeat: with only rare exceptions, anorectics are found among the middle and upper social classes in "developed" countries of the West and in Japan. Anorexia nervosa is certainly not a universal disease. A medical interpretation that isolates the etiological agent within the hypothalamus simply does not square with these social facts, nor does it acknowledge the interactive nature of the hypothalamus and the environment.

The final critical limitation of the biomedical model is that it does not deal with the question of incidence: why are there so many anorectics now, at this particular moment in time?

Psychological models of anorexia nervosa fall into three basic groups born of psychoanalysis, family systems theory, and social psychology. In the first two in particular, anorexia nervosa is seen as a pathological response to the developmental crisis of adolescence. Refusal of food is understood as an expression of the adolescent's struggle over autonomy, individuation, and sexual development. "Anorexia [nervosa] is a pathology of the ordinary issues of adolescent passage," writes a contemporary clinician.[44] Much of current psychotherapeutic thinking about anorexia nervosa takes its direction from Sigmund Freud and, more recently, from Hilde Bruch. Freud regarded the anorectic as a girl who feared adult womanhood and heterosexuality. In 1895 he wrote: "The famous anorexia nervosa of young girls seems to me (on careful observation) to be a melancholia *where sexuality is undeveloped*" (italics added). In Freudian terms, eating, like all appetites, is an expression of libido or sexual drive. Clinicians confirm the direction of the Freudian interpretation: anorectics generally are not sexually active adolescents.[45]

Hilde Bruch, in the spirit of Freud and his early followers, considered the contemporary anorectic unprepared to cope with the psychological and social consequences of adulthood as well as sexuality. Because of the anorectic's paralyzing sense of ineffectiveness and anxiety about her identity, she opts, furiously, for control of her body. Bruch argued that the anorectic makes her body a stand-in for the life that she cannot control. She experiences a disturbance of "delusional proportions" with respect to her body image, and she eats in a peculiar and disorganized fashion. By refusing food, the anorectic slows the processes of sexual maturation: her menses stop and her body remains childlike. The preoccupation with controlling her appetite directs the young woman inward so that she becomes increasingly estranged from the outside world. She lives a bizarre life, obsessed with thoughts of food, while struggling with her parents over her right not to eat.[46]

We have seen that there have been numerous efforts to place anorexia nervosa within other established psychiatric categories such as schizophrenia, depression, and obsessional neurosis. Recent psychoanalytic literature suggests that anorexia nervosa is a popular form of classic obsessive-compulsive disorder. Unlike depression, where there is a true reduction of appetite, in anorexia nervosa the patient is constantly aware of her hunger. Simultaneously, she ruminates about calories and exercises frantically, all the while dwelling on images of the very food that she fears. These preoccupations can become excessive and involuntary. Patients usually are stubborn, rigid, and strongly defensive about their behavior, and they espouse elaborate and highly intellectual theories about food and exercise. Many display other behavior patterns associated with obsessive-compulsive disorders: perfectionism, excessive orderliness and cleanliness, meticulous attention to detail, and self-righteousness.[47] The anorectic is, then, a "good girl" who alternates between compliance and rebellion. In the beginning, at least, her refusal to eat is a form of overcontrol that is subtly hostile and rebellious in its nature.

In the 1980s a great deal of attention is being paid also to values and patterns of interaction within anorexic families. Indeed, family systems therapy provides one of today's most important theoretical perspectives on anorexia nervosa. According to family systems theorist Salvador Minuchin, certain kinds of family environments encourage passive methods of defiance (for example, not eating) and make it difficult for members to assert their individuality. Minuchin describes this "psychosomatic family" as controlling, perfectionistic, and nonconfrontational, adjectives that apply equally well to their anorexic daughter. On the basis of clinical work with these families, mental health professionals have come to describe the anorectic as "enmeshed," meaning that the normal process of individuation is blocked by the complex psychological needs of the girl, her parents, even her siblings. In family systems theory not just the patient has anorexia nervosa: the family too has the disease.[48]

When a parent *is* implicated in anorexia nervosa, it is almost always the mother. Kim Chernin, a psychoanalytically inspired feminist writer, argues that eating disorders are rooted in the problems of mother-daughter separation and identity. Mothers and daughters, she writes, express emotions around issues of food and eating rather than sexuality. The "hunger knot" experienced by so many modern daughters represents issues of failed female development, fear, and the daughter's guilt over her desire to surpass her mother. Chernin asserts that women who have disordered relationships to food are unconsciously guilty of symbolic matricide and their obsessive dieting is an expression of their desire to reunite or bond with the mother.

Other recent discussions of anorexia nervosa by psychiatrists suggest that anorectics may have mothers of a certain kind. It has been suggested that the mother of the anorectic is all of the following: frustrated, depressed, perfectionistic, passive and dependent, and unable to "mirror" her child.[49] (The inability to mirror means that the mother is unable to see and reflect her daughter as an independent being. Consequently, a specific conflict emerges within the child, between her invisible sense of self and her visible body. Refusing to eat and losing weight is a desperate appeal to her mother to make emotional contact with the unseen person.)

Research in social psychology and in the field of personality also proposes interesting approaches to anorexia nervosa. At least two different predictive tests for eating disorders have been developed since the late 1970s: the Eating Attitudes Test (EAT) and the Eating Disorders Inventory (EDI). The EDI evaluates an individual on a number of different subscales including drive for thinness, body dissatisfaction, sense of ineffectiveness, perfectionism, interpersonal distrust, and maturity fears.[50] A 1984 study by University of Toronto psychiatrist David Garner used the EDI to compare eating habits, weight-related symptoms, and psychological characteristics of anorectics with two other groups: women who were highly weight preoccupied and those who were not. The study concluded that while weight-preoccupied women and anorectics were indistinguishable on many of the test subscales, the anorexia nervosa group had significantly higher scores on measures of ineffectiveness.[51] Some theorists propose an actual cognitive problem with body imaging.[52] Others, following Carol Gilligan's theory of female moral development, regard the anorectic as a young woman in conflict with the dominant male values of her society, while yet another group posits that anorectics are overly socialized to the feminine role, as indicated by their scores on the Bem Sex Role Inventory.[53]

Another fascinating and potentially promising line of research utilizes models drawn from the study of addiction and substance abuse. Anorexia nervosa does involve a habitual behavior (starvation) which, like intoxication or drug addiction, alters the individual's psychological and physical state. Although each of the behaviors may be unpleasant initially, they can, with prolonged indulgence, come to feel "right." Even when the behavior is patently self-destructive, the anorectic and the alcoholic will characteristically deny the problem—a response that stands in marked contrast to neurotic disorders, in which patients apparently exaggerate the abnormality of their symptoms. According to George I. Szmukler and Digby Tantam, British psychiatrists, anorexia nervosa is most usefully conceived as a dependence disorder, specifically as "an addiction to starvation." In effect, individuals with anorexia nervosa may be dependent on both the psychological and the physiological effects of starvation.[54]

In the end, no single psychological model provides a full explanation of anorexia nervosa. The psychological paradigm is incomplete, just as the biomedical model is, in that it fails to provide an adequate answer to the same thorny problems of social address, changing incidence, and gender. After reading the psychological literature, one still asks: Why is the anorexia nervosa "epidemic" restricted by class and confined to societies like our own? Why are we experiencing more anorexia nervosa today than we did fifty or one hundred years ago? Why is it that adolescent girls and not adolescent boys engage in this form of developmental struggle? These particular questions suggest that we look closely at what the cultural model has to offer.

The cultural explanation of anorexia nervosa is popular and widely promoted. It postulates that anorexia nervosa is generated by a powerful cultural imperative that makes slimness the chief attribute of female beauty. In casual conversation we hear this idea expressed all the time: anorexia is caused by the incessant drumbeat of modern dieting, by the erotic veneration of sylphlike women such as Twiggy, and by the demands of a fashion ethic that stresses youth and androgyny rather than the contours of an adult female body. The common wisdom reflects the realities of women's lives in the twentieth century. In this respect the cultural model, more than any other, acknowledges and begins to explain why eating disorders are essentially a female problem.

Important psychological studies by Susan and Orlando Wooley, Judith Rodin, and others confirm that weight is woman's "normative obsession."[55] In response to the question, "How old were you when you first weighed more than you wanted?" American women report a preoccupation with overweight that begins before puberty and intensifies in adolescence and young adulthood. Eighty percent of girls in the fourth grade in San Francisco are dieting, according to researchers at the University of California. At three private girls' schools in Washington, D.C., 53 percent of the students said they were unhappy with their bodies by age thirteen; among those eighteen or older, 78 percent were dissatisfied. In the same vein, a 1984 *Glamour* magazine survey of thirty-three thousand women between the ages of eighteen and thirty-five demonstrated that 75 percent believed they were fat, although only 25 percent were actually overweight. Of those judged underweight by standardized measures, 45 percent still thought they were too fat. Clinicians often refer to people with weight preoccupations of this sort as "obesophobic."[56]

The women in the *Glamour* survey confirm that female self-esteem and happiness are tied to weight, particularly in the adolescent and young adult years. When asked to choose among potential sources of happiness, the *Glamour* respondents chose weight loss over success at work or in interpersonal relations. The extent to which "feeling fat" negatively influences female psychological adjustment and behavior is only beginning to be explored. A 1984 study, for example, demonstrates that many college-age women make weight a central feature of their cognitive schema. These women consistently evaluate other women, themselves, and their own achievements in terms of weight. A 1986 study revealed that "feeling fat" was significantly related to emotional stress and other external stimuli. Obviously, being and feeling thin is an extremely desirable condition in this culture, whereas feeling fat is not: "I became afraid of getting fat, of gaining weight. [There is] something dangerous about becoming a fat American."[57]

All indications are that being thin is particularly important to women in the upper classes. (This social fact is reflected in the widely quoted dictum, attributed to the Duchess of Windsor, "A woman can never be too rich or too thin.") A study by Stanford University psychologist Sanford M. Dornbusch revealed a positive correlation between gender, social class, and desire to be thin. Controlling for the actual level of fatness, Dornbusch's data, based on a nationwide sample of more than seventy-five hundred male and female high school students, showed that adolescent females in higher social classes wanted to be thinner more often than those in the lower classes. (Not surprisingly, most obese women come from the working class and the poor.) By contrast, the relationship between social class and the desire to be thin was minimal in males. Because body preference differs among girls according to social class, those from middle-class and upper-class families are the most likely to be dissatisfied and troubled by the normal development associated with sexual maturation.[58]

According to the cultural model, these class-specific ideas about body preference pervade the larger society and do enormous harm. The modern visual media (television, films, video, magazines, and particularly advertising) fuel the preoccupation with female thinness and serve as the primary stimulus for anorexia nervosa. Female socialization, in the hands of the modern media, emphasizes external qualities ("good looks") above all else. As a consequence, we see few women of real girth on television or in the movies who also have vigor, intelligence, or sex appeal. Young girls, fed on this ideological pablum, learn to be decorative, passive, powerless, and ambivalent about being female. Herein lies the cause of anorexia nervosa, according to the cultural model.

The most outspoken and influential proponents of this model of the etiology of anorexia nervosa are feminists, often therapists, concerned with the spectrum of eating disorders that ranges from overeating to noneating. In the work of Kim Chernin, Marcia Millman, Susie Orbach, and Marlene Boskin-White and William C. White, the obese, the anorectic, and the bulimic all receive sympathetic treatment.[59] The tendency of these authors is to avoid casting the behavior as pathological. Instead, they seek to demonstrate that these disorders are an inevitable consequence of a misogynistic society that demeans women by devaluing female experience and women's values; by objectifying their bodies; and by discrediting vast areas of women's past and present achievements. Both overeating and noneating are a "protest against the way in which women are regarded in our society as objects of adornment and pleasure."[60] A strain of Socialist feminism, popular in women's studies scholarship, also marks these and related critiques. To wit, our society's exaltation of thin, weak women expresses the inner logic of capitalism and patriarchy, both characterized by the sexual division of labor and female subordination. In response to these brutal economic and cultural imperatives, women turn to an excessive concern with food as a way of filling their emptiness and dealing with their fear and self-hate.

Following the organizational models of the contemporary feminist movement (that is, collective consciousness raising and networking), advocates of the cultural model suggest that above and beyond psychotherapy women with eating disorders should (1) talk with other women who are similarly afflicted and (2) organize to educate the public about their problem. The AA/BA, for example, sponsors such groups in a number of different metropolitan areas. Many former anorectics and bulimics attribute their recovery to the experience of listening and sharing with others. Group therapy and peer support groups for anorectics and bulimics are common. In May 1986 in New York City, Susie Orbach, a leader in the feminist therapy community, organized a Speak-Out against eating disorders, an event that sought to bring the experience and pain of eating disorders to a larger audience through the presentation of personal statements and testimonials. In its most simplistic form, the cultural model suggests that merely by speaking up about sexism and subordination, women with eating disorders can cure themselves and society.

The popular feminist reading of anorexia nervosa has much to commend it. First and foremost, this interpretation underscores the fact that a total reliance on medical models is inadequate. Because of feminist sensitivity to the interrelationship of culture, gender, and food, the impact and meaning of weight obsession in women's lives is now a serious area of theory and research in the academic disciplines and in the mental health professions. Before Chernin, Orbach, and Millman, women's dieting and weight concerns were trivialized or interpreted as masking a strictly individual psychological problem without consideration of the ways in which culture stimulated, exacerbated, and gave shape to a pattern of problematic behaviors.[61]

This contemporary feminist analysis has a literary analogue in the writing of academic feminist critics on nineteenth-century women, medicine, and madness. Their interpretation is rooted in the study of nineteenth-century medical texts and the male physician's view, in that era, of the female body. The analysis is confined to examination of the discourses and representations that evolved in the discussion of women and their diseases in nineteenth century Britain and the United States.[62] In this mode of analysis the primary focus is on epistemology, or how we conceptualize mental disorder. Following Michel Foucault, these scholars argue that women's bodies are a locus of social control; that in the nineteenth century male-dominated medicine created nosologies that marked women as deviant; and that "female diseases" are socially constructed states that symbolize both the hegemony of scientific medicine and Victorian social constraints on women.[63] In conditions such as anorexia nervosa, where there are no discernible lumps, lesions, or germs, there are those who question whether there is a disease at all. The problematic behavior, in this case refusal of food, is interpreted strictly as a form of symbolic interaction. Thus, anorexia nervosa is painted as a young woman's protest against the patriarchy—that is, as a form of feminist politics.

The strength of this analysis is that it identifies a troubling, if not misogynistic, set of ideas about women's bodies and minds that was part of the intellectual world of Victorian medical men and, inevitably, shaped some part of their clinical practice. While I respect the contribution of feminist literary critics to our understanding of the discourse that surrounded medical treatment in the nineteenth century, I am disquieted by the tendency to equate all female mental disorders with political protest. Certainly we need to acknowledge the relationship between sex-role constraints and problematic behavior in women, but the madhouse is a somewhat troubling site for establishing a female pantheon. To put it another way: as a feminist, I believe that the anorectic deserves our sympathy but not necessarily our veneration.

Feminist insistence on thinking about anorexia nervosa as cultural protest leads to an interpretation of the disorder that over-emphasizes the level of conscious control at the same time that it presents women and girls as hapless victims of an all-powerful medical profession. Anyone who has worked with anorectics or read the clinical literature understands that food refusal becomes increasingly involuntary as the physiological process of emaciation unfolds. In full-blown cases of anorexia nervosa, the patient cannot eat even when she wants to. The cultural model denies the biomedical component of this destructive illness by obscuring the helplessness and desperation of those who suffer from it. After years of treatment a disheartened anorexic student wrote to me: "I too hope more than one could ever express that one day I will be well and my future will be bright and fulfilling. The frustration and fear I feel now is tremendous, as each day is a struggle for survival." This is hardly the voice of social protest.[64]

The romanticization of anorexia nervosa (and female mental disorders in general) can lead to some unwise and counterproductive therapeutic strategies. For example, in 1978 when Susie Orbach declared fat a "feminist issue," some took her to mean that feminists should allow themselves to get fat, thereby repudiating both patriarchal and capitalist imperatives. More recently, as the number of anorectics and bulimics has grown, some writers, in a well-intentioned but desperate attempt to dignify these all-too-frequent disorders, have tried to transform anorexia nervosa into the contemporary moral equivalent of the hunger strikes associated with early-twentieth-century English suffragists such as Emmeline and Sylvia Pankhurst.[65]

In the *Wisconsin Law Review* (1984) Roberta Dresser, an attorney and professor of law, argued that all medical and parental orders for renourishment of anorectics should be opposed on civil libertarian grounds. Dresser's intention, to make the case for minimizing state intrusion in personal medical decisions, was altogether admirable, but her understanding of anorexia nervosa was naive (in terms of both the psychology and the physiology of the disorder) and insensitive (in terms of historical precedents). Dresser based her argument on the idea, drawn from literary analysis, that "socio-cultural explanations of anorexia nervosa challenge the notion that the condition is a mental illness attributable to sources within the individual."[66] She posited that anorectics and early-twentieth-century hunger strikers were essentially the same and that anorexia nervosa is a freely chosen method of communicating and asserting power—in essence, an exercise of free will. (Dresser did not consider that anorectics may become physically unable to eat and that at some point the behavior may become involuntary.)

Although some earnestly believe that anorexia nervosa is a conscious and/or symbolic act against sexism that follows in a direct line from early-twentieth-century feminism, it is difficult from a historical perspective to see the analogy between the articulate and life-affirming political strategies of the Pankhursts and the silent, formulaic behavior of the modern Karen Carpenters.[67] The suffragists had a specific political goal to achieve, at which point food refusal ended. In contrast, the anorectic pursues thinness unrelentingly (in the same way that a paranoid schizophrenic attempts to elude imagined enemies), but she has no plan for resumption of eating. If the anorectic's food refusal is political in any way, it is a severely limited and infantile form of politics, directed primarily at parents (and self) and without any sense of allegiance to a larger collectivity. Anorectics, not known for their sisterhood, are notoriously preoccupied with the self. The effort to transform them into heroic freedom fighters is a sad commentary on how desperate people are to find in the cultural model some kind of explanatory framework, or comfort, that dignifies this confusing and complex disorder.

Finally, there is a strain of cultural analysis that implicates recent social change in the etiology of anorexia nervosa, particularly increased educational, occupational, and sexual options for women. In *The Golden Cage* Hilde Bruch suggested such a connection. In 1978 she wrote: "Growing girls can experience . . . liberation as a demand and feel that they have to do something outstanding. Many of my patients have expressed the feeling that they are overwhelmed by the vast number of potential opportunities available to them . . . and [that] they had been afraid of not choosing correctly."[68] Yet, as a sophisticated clinician, Bruch did not blame social change or feminism for anorexia nervosa.

She understood that confusion about choices was only a partial explanation, for most young women handled the same array of new options with enthusiasm and optimism and did not develop the disease. Some antifeminists will still insist, however, that feminism is to blame for the upsurge in eating disorders. This interpretation usually asserts, incorrectly, that anorexia emerged for the first time in the late 1960s and 1970s, at the same time as the modern women's movement. To the conservative mind, anorexia nervosa might go away if feminism went away, allowing a return to traditional gender roles and expectations. The mistaken assumption is that anorexia nervosa did not exist in past time, when women's options were more limited.

In sum, the explanatory power of the existing cultural models is limited because of two naive suppositions: (1) that anorexia nervosa is a new phenomenon created by the pressures and circumstances of contemporary life and (2) that the disease is either imposed on young women (as victims) or freely chosen (as social protest) without involving any biological or psychological contribution. Ultimately, the current cultural models fail to explain why so many individuals *do not* develop the disease even though they have been exposed to the same cultural environment. This is where individual psychology as well as familial factors must come into play. Certainly, culture alone does not cause anorexia nervosa.

In order to understand anorexia nervosa, we must think about disease as an interactive and evolving process. I find the model of "addiction to starvation" particularly compelling because when we think about anorexia nervosa in this way, there is room for incorporating biological, psychological, and cultural components. Let me demonstrate. An individual may begin to restrict her food because of aesthetic and social reasons related to gender, class, age, and sense of style. This constitutes the initial "recruitment" stage. Many of her friends may also be doing the same thing, because in the environment in which they live being a fat female is a social and emotional liability. Being thin is of critical importance to the young woman's sense of herself. Contemporary culture clearly makes a contribution to the genesis of anorexia nervosa.

An individual's dieting moves across the spectrum from the

normal to the obsessional because of other factors, namely emotional and personality issues, and personal physiology and body chemistry. If refusing food serves a young woman's emotional needs (for instance, as a symbolic statement about herself, as a bid for attention, as a way of forestalling adult sexuality, as a means of hurting her parents or separating from them, as a form of defiance), she may continue to do so because it seems like an efficacious strategy. It becomes more and more difficult to back off and change direction if the denial and control involved bring her emotional satisfaction. In some families the symptom (not eating) and the girl's emaciated appearance are overlooked or denied longer than in other families, thereby creating a situation that may actually contribute to the making of the disorder.

After weeks or months of starvation the young woman's mind and body become acclimated to both the feeling of hunger and nutritional deprivation. This constitutes a second stage of the disorder. There is evidence to suggest that hunger pangs eventually decrease rather than intensify and that the body actually gets used to a state of semistarvation, that is, to a negative energy balance. At some unidentified point in time, in certain girls, starvation may actually become satisfying or tension relieving—a state analogous perhaps to the well-known "runner's high."[69] Certain individuals, then, may make the move from chronic dieting to dependence on starvation because of a physiological substrate as well as emotional and family stresses. This is where biochemical explanations (such as elevated cortisol levels in the blood or some other neuroendocrine abnormality) come into play. The fact that many anorectics seem unable to eat (or develop withdrawal symptoms when they begin to eat regularly) suggests that something biological as well as psychological is going on.

Obviously, only a small proportion of those who diet strenuously become addicted to it, presumably because the majority of young women have neither a psychic nor a biological need for starvation. For most, even normal dieting, for short periods, is an unpleasant necessity that brings more frustration than it does satisfaction (hence the current rash of popular women's cartoons about eating as a form of forbidden pleasure and self-expression, and dieting as a futile endeavor).[70] Yet in alcohol and drug dependence and in anorexia nervosa, there appears to be a correlation between the level of exposure and the prevalence of a dependence. Simply put, when and where people become obesophobic and dieting becomes pervasive, we can expect to see an escalating number of individuals with anorexia nervosa and other eating disorders.[71] Thus, we have returned full circle to the cultural context and its power to shape human behavior.

For this study the critical implication of the dependency-addiction model is that anorexia nervosa can be conceptually divided into two stages. The first involves sociocultural context, or "recruitment" to fasting behavior; the second incorporates the subsequent "career" as an anorexic and includes physiological and psychological changes that condition the individual to exist in a starvation state.[72] The second stage is obviously the concern of medicine and mental health professionals because it is relatively formulaic and historically invariant. Stage one involves the historian, whose task it is to trace the forces and events that have led young women to this relatively stereotypical behavior pattern.

History is obviously important in understanding how and why we are where we are today vis-à-vis the increasing incidence of the disorder. A historical perspective also contributes to the debate over the etiology of anorexia nervosa by supplying an interpretation that actually reconciles different theoretical models. Despite the emphasis here on culture, my interpretation does not disallow the possibility of a biomedical component in anorexia nervosa. In fact, when we take the long history of female fasters into account, it becomes apparent that there are certain historical moments and cultural settings when a biological substratum could be activated by potent social and cultural forces. In other words, patterns of culture constitute the kind of environmental pressure that interacts with physiological and psychological variables. What history provides is a new perspective on critical questions of changing incidence, social address, and cultural origins. To that end, Chapter 2 turns to another time and place where refusal of food was also a notable aspect of female experience.

2 · From Sainthood to Patienthood

In medieval Europe, particularly in the years between 1200 and 1500, many women refused their food and prolonged fasting was considered a female miracle. The chronicles and hagiographies of this period tell numerous stories of women saints who ate almost nothing or claimed to be incapable of eating normal earthly fare. The best-known of these saints, Catherine of Siena (1347–1380), ate only a handful of herbs each day and occasionally shoved twigs down her throat to bring up any other food that she was forced to eat. Thirteenth-century figures such as Mary of Oignes and Beatrice of Nazareth vomited from the mere smell of meat, and their throats swelled shut in the presence of food. Other women saints covered their faces at the sight of food, refused to partake of family meals, and some—such as Columba of Rieti (fifteenth century)—actually died of self-starvation. Somewhat later, in the seventeenth century, Saint Veronica ate nothing at all for three days at a time but on Fridays permitted herself to chew on five orange seeds, in memory of the five wounds of Jesus. Although fasting and restrictive eating was a widely noted characteristic of medieval spirituality, it did not engage both genders in the same manner or to the same degree. There are few cases of male saints who claimed or were claimed by others to be incapable of eating.[1]

In the medieval period fasting was fundamental to the model of female holiness. The medieval woman's capacity for survival without eating meant that she found other forms of food: prayer provided sustenance, as did the Christian eucharist—the body and blood of Christ—ingested as wafer and wine. Women who were reputed to live without eating—that is, without eating anything except the eucharist—were particularly numerous in the thirteenth through fifteenth centuries, a time when food practices were central to Christian identity.[2] By the seventeenth and eighteenth centuries, however, scientifically minded physicians began to pay close attention to food abstinence, so common among women of the High Middle Ages. They called it both inedia prodigiosa (a great starvation) and anorexia mirabilis (miraculously inspired loss of appetite).[3]

Some medical writers and historians claim that anorexia mirabilis and anorexia nervosa are really one and the same. In other words, they would have us believe that Karen Carpenter and Catherine of Siena suffered from the same disease. Advocates of this view naively adopt and apply the biomedical and psychological models of anorexia nervosa as if there was absolute certainty about the etiology of the disease and as if there were complete, verifiable case histories available on historic subjects. In actuality, the documentary evidence for the congruence of anorexia mirabilis and anorexia nervosa is exceedingly weak and usually rests either on interpretative acts of faith or on inconclusive medical "evidence" such as the fact that the individual lost her appetite, did not eat, or stopped menstruating. (This sequelae of symptoms need not necessarily mean anorexia nervosa.) In effect, most of those who argue literally for anorexia nervosa in the far distant past have ignored the two-stage process noted in Chapter 1, recruitment and career. It may well be that in stage 2, particularly after chronic starvation has set in, the medieval ascetic and the modern anorectic have the same biomedical experience—that is, they are actually *unable* to eat. But it is abundantly clear that on the issue of recruitment the routes to anorexia mirabilis and anorexia nervosa are quite different.

There are some who would disagree. In *Holy Anorexia* medievalist Rudolph Bell uses modern psychological theory to explain medieval fasting. The argument is predictable. According to Bell, Catherine of Siena, Margaret of Cortuna, and other holy women were engaged in "anorexic behavior patterns" that closely resemble the modern disorder anorexia nervosa. Bell claims that there is a psychological (rather than a biomedical) continuity across the centuries: anorexia mirabilis and anorexia nervosa, he writes, are "psychologically analogous" states in medieval and modern women.[4] (The underlying assumption here is that the psychology of women is fixed in time and that past and present are the same.) The critical fact that anorexia mirabilis was *not* restricted to adolescent or young adult women does not deter Bell from arguing that there is a consistent pattern across time. In his view, both anorexia mirabilis and anorexia nervosa are part of a larger quest for female liberation from a patriarchal society.

Others with less sophistication than Bell argue on the basis of biomedical evidence that they have found anorexia nervosa in unlikely places and that the disease explains historical personalities and/or events. A British psychiatrist, for example, claims that Wilgefortis, the bearded medieval female saint, had anorexia nervosa. Her hirsutism, he says, was actually the lanugo found in chronic cases of the disease. And a recent article in *World Medicine* asked earnestly, "Was Byron anorexic?" The author argues that the nineteenth-century poet did indeed have anorexia nervosa and that the disease was the source of his Romantic spirit. In addition to fasting, feasting, and purging, Byron was hyperactive, a symptom demonstrated in his famous swim of the Hellespont.[5]

In order to understand fully the long tradition of female food refusal, one must do more than merely "lay on" psychological constructs drawn from modern life or search out look-alike symptoms. First and foremost, lack of appetite is a common secondary symptom in many emotional and organic illnesses. When anorexia, lack of appetite, or refusal of food presents as a symptom, it need not always imply anorexia nervosa.

Much of what is taken to be the true or hidden history of anorexia nervosa does not discriminate between primary and secondary loss of appetite. Nor does this kind of writing recognize that in anorexia nervosa the appetite is not really lost; rather, in the initial stages, it is under extreme control. Nowadays, whenever a young woman will not eat, we seem to think that the diagnosis is unequivocal. This tendency leads to some unsatisfying and debatable medical history. For example, Hilde Bruch, Eugene Bliss, C. H. Hardin Branch, Joseph Silverman, and other doctors claim that anorexia nervosa was first identified in 1694 by Richard Morton in *Phthisologia; or, a Treatise on Consumptions*. Morton, physician to James II, did indeed describe the existence of a form of nervous consumption (phthisis nervosa) caused by "sadness and anxious cares" and presented two case histories of adolescents: an eighteen-year-old girl, "Mr. Duke's daughter of St. Mary Axe," and a sixteen-year-old boy, the son of a Presbyterian minister.

In making the case for Morton's "discovery" of anorexia nervosa, a recent article by Silverman concentrates on the case of the girl.[6] Mr. Duke's daughter was so severely emaciated that she looked "like a skeleton only clad in skin." Still, she did not appear to suffer from the fever, cough, or respiratory problems so common in consumption. She did experience "total suppression of her Monthly courses" and she complained of "coldness of the body," both natural consequences of chronic starvation and symptoms of anorexia nervosa. Silverman concludes on the basis of the report that Richard Morton deserves credit for the discovery of anorexia nervosa. What he does not consider is the discordant information: first, that Mr. Duke's daughter also suffered from periodic "fainting fits" and apparently died from one and, second, that Morton himself said that he saw a great deal of this condition in "those who have lived in Virginia." This peculiar connection indicates that Morton did not conceive of phthisis nervosa as an adolescent female condition or as a rare disorder. What he described included some of the symptoms of anorexia nervosa; but he saw other symptoms that are not part of the modern diagnosis. In effect, our modern sensitivity to anorexia nervosa makes for a situation in which it is altogether too easy to lead the historical evidence.

This is definitely what has happened in the reinterpretation of anorexia mirabilis offered by Rudolph Bell. The alternative treatment of medieval women provided by medievalist Caroline Walker Bynum suggests that Bell's approach focuses attention on only one small aspect of medieval women's behavior and, in so doing, obscures the totality of their experience. Catherine of Siena, for example, did more than just fast: her life was filled with a program of austerities that included self-flagellation, scalding, and sleeping on a bed of thorny substances. "It is only modern historians," Bynum writes, "who have given food-rejection its startling and privileged place in medieval women's piety."[7]

As Bynum demonstrates in *Holy Feast and Holy Fast: Food Motifs in the Piety of Medieval Women*, fasting and the cults of eucharistic devotion were only one part of a larger complex of food practices central to female piety and Christian identity in the medieval world. Because medieval culture associated women and the female body with food, female spirituality was expressed in food language and imagery and in eating and feeding practices, as well as in fasting. Some pious women did deny themselves ordinary food in order to become receptacles for the food that was God, but power and service to others, through "holy eating," was the ultimate goal.

Many medieval women spoke of their "hunger" for God and their "inebriation" with the holy wine. Many fasted in order to feast at the "delicious banquet of God." Many of the voices that we hear from the women of this distant world seem to be conscious of the interconnection of food practices and religious symbols. Through extraordinary eating and extraordinary feeding, medieval women offered help and assistance to their fellow human beings. Angela of Fogligno, for example, who drank pus from sores and ate scabs and lice from the bodies of the sick, spoke of the pus as being as "sweet as the eucharist." Other women saints were reported to miraculously multiply food for the devout, filling empty casks with drink and turning a few crumbs into food enough to feed a hungry multitude. The bodies of women were also a source of food: mystical women exuded oil from their fingertips, lactated even though they were virgins, and cured disease with the touch of their saliva.

In sum, medieval women's legendary asceticism—the pattern of renunciation and austerity—is not the whole story. In the medieval world, as Bynum has astutely and sensitively demonstrated, women were preoccupied with eating and with noneating because food practices provided a basic way to express religious ideals of suffering and service to their fellow creatures. Thus, medieval culture promoted a specific form of appetite control in women, anorexia mirabilis, which symbolized the collective values of that age. Anorexia nervosa expresses the individualism of *our* time, a point to which I shall return later in this book.

Nevertheless, the existence of a female tradition of anorexia mirabilis does have implications for how we understand anorexia nervosa. From a historical perspective, it becomes evident that certain social and cultural systems, at different points in time, encourage or promote control of appetite in women, but for different reasons and purposes. (This is the recruitment theme I have suggested before.) In the history of Western civilization there have been at least two periods in which noneating and control of appetite have been notable aspects of female experience: in Catholicism in the thirteenth to sixteenth centuries, and now in the postindustrial age. In the earlier era, control of appetite was linked to piety and belief; through fasting, the medieval ascetic strove for perfection in the eyes of her God. In the modern period, female control of appetite is embedded in patterns of class, gender, and family relations established in the nineteenth century; the modern anorectic strives for perfection in terms of society's ideal of physical, rather than spiritual, beauty.

Although Catherine of Siena and Karen Carpenter do have something in common—the use of food as a symbolic language—it is as inappropriate to call the former an anorectic as it is to cast the latter as a saint. To describe premodern women such as Catherine as anorexic is to flatten differences in female experience across time and discredit the special quality of eucharistic fervor and penitential asceticism as it was lived and perceived. To insist that medieval holy women had anorexia nervosa is, ultimately, a reductionist argument because it converts a complex human behavior into a simple biomedical mechanism. (It certainly does not respect important differences in the route to anorexia.) To conflate the two is to ignore the cultural context and the distinction between sainthood and patienthood.

Once we understand the special meaning and significance of anorexia mirabilis, we can assert the following: the modern anorectic is one of a long line of women and girls who have used food and the body as a focus of their symbolic language. Although there are some important biomedical continuities in female fasting behavior, anorexia mirabilis and anorexia nervosa are not literally the same.

Miraculous Maids

By the seventeenth and eighteenth centuries fasting was on the decline as the result of the breakup of medieval culture, the Protestant Reformation, and the scrupulous efforts of religious reformers to disavow traditional practices such as the worship of saints. During the Reformation, prolonged abstinence was taken as the work of Satan (rather than God) and female fasters were frequently regarded as victims of evil delusion or possession. In the postmedieval world, harsh ascetic practices were discouraged and acts of autonomous female piety—such as prolonged fasting or extraordinary food miracles—came under special scrutiny from male clerics.[8] The renunciation of food, once experienced and explained as a form of female holiness, was increasingly cast as demoniacal, heretical, and even insane.

Still, medieval superstition and belief did not disappear overnight. Faith in the idea of miraculous fasting actually coexisted with Protestant iconoclasm and the behavior continued, remarkably, into the modern world. The historical record reveals that a considerable number of women from the sixteenth through the nineteenth centuries continued to behave in a way that supported the belief that they did not need to eat. This cultural fiction surely served to empower some women by drawing public attention to them, and in some cases it brought them material rewards.[9]

In the early modern period, formulaic stories of miraculous fasting maids came primarily from continental Europe, where the Catholic tradition remained strong. Typically, these women were young and humble, characteristics that made their rejection of food still more astonishing.[10] All of them claimed to avoid normal earthly fare, and if they ate, they ate only delicate things. One fasting girl allegedly "din'd on a rose and supt on a tulip"; another took only aqua vita as a mouthwash; and still another was said to live by her olfactory sense, inhaling only the "smell of a rose." The symbolic diet of the maiden underscored her purity.[11]

The claim of prolonged or total abstinence in that era was remarkable enough to generate questions. When a young woman asserted that she did not eat, the claim had to be verified because, first, it raised the possibility of miracles (or satanic influence) and, second, it implied autonomy or "radical holiness" on the part of the faster, a dangerous concept in the highly structured and deferential society of the early modern period. Consequently, miraculous maidens stimulated around-the-clock investigations conducted not only by clergymen but by civil magistrates, physicians, dukes, bishops, even kings.

During these watches the maiden's body and character were given careful scrutiny. Typically, "miraculous maids" were presented with elaborate enticements that involved the presentation of delectable foods. In 1599, for example, Eva Fleigen, the "Fasting Woman of Meurs," was brought to the luxuriant garden of the local nobility, where she was seduced into tasting exquisite fruits from nearby trees. But no sooner had Fleigen plucked a cherry, tasted, and ingested it, than she became ill and nearly died.[12] Authenticity was an emerging concern in seventeenth-century stories, and apparently in real life as well. In Germany in the sixteenth century, a fasting maiden was executed when it was discovered that she did actually eat on the sly.[13]

In the sixteenth and seventeenth centuries, as printing became widespread in Europe, continental stories of inedia prodigiosa and anorexia mirabilis were translated and published in England, where they became the subject of heated discussion among clergymen, doctors, and civil authorities. As a result, even iconoclastic Protestants became intrigued with the subject of prolonged abstinence and its meaning. For example, in 1635, Protestant George Hakewill, anxious to demonstrate the authority of his own church, called attention to the existence of Protestant women who performed fasting miracles. In his *Apologia*, Hakewill asserted that such "wonderful works of God as these [maids] should not pass us without consideration especially considering that the greatest and most notable part of the examples alleged have been of the Protestant religion."[14] Hakewill, it seems, simply could not allow anorexia mirabilis to remain an exclusively Catholic claim.

Stories of miraculous fasting women constituted a popular folk tradition in both Protestant and Catholic countries well into the eighteenth century. By and large, these stories were religious, in that they always testified to the divine providence of God, but they were not theological; they made little distinction between Protestant and Catholic doctrine. All of the stories rested on a common narrative principle: the faster did not die despite inanition and refusal of food over periods of time ranging from weeks to decades. Life without food was the miracle at the heart of the story. Chroniclers of both Protestant and Catholic perspectives concluded their tales with statements such as the maid "liveth through the singular, pure, and incomprehensible grace of Almighty GOD" or "what beyond compasse of all man's reason God inwardly nourisheth all."[15]

By the seventeenth century cases of prolonged abstinence aroused as much skepticism as wonder. In 1600 Jacob Viverius, a French physician, observed the case of Jane Balan, the fourteen-year-old daughter of a locksmith who claimed to take "neither eate or drinke" for close to three years. The case must have been well-known because the king (probably Henri IV) sent his "best and chiefest" physician to evaluate the girl's fast in order to see if the abstinence be "by deceit or not." By this time physicians as well as clergy were regarded as appropriate persons to judge the circumstances of the case. This evolution in the nature of who was expert in interpreting fasting cases marked the beginning of the long historic process of the medicalization of human behavior.

Jane Balan's emaciation was graphically described by observers: "The inferior part of her belly is in such manner grown lean, and dried up in her, as down from her sides, and so along her navel, there remaineth nothing of the belly she had before . . . [Here is] a Cartilage or gristle, hanging pointed down from the thorax, or sternum, after the manner of an eaves of a penthouse." Viverius paid attention to the girl's anatomy, but he was particularly interested in seeing if he could find feces or urine, the hard medical evidence of food intake. On the basis of the absence of excrement ("her privy parts were cleaned thence nothing fell to ground") Viverius concluded that Balan must be a "miraculous maid," whose continued life was an act of God.[16]

If Viverius accepted a supernatural explanation of anorexia

mirabilis, there were many others in the seventeenth century who did not. In 1668 Thomas Hobbes, best known as author of *The Leviathan*, reported seeing a young woman at Over Haddon so thin that her "belly touches her backbone." The girl's emaciation, explained her mother, was due to loss of appetite dating from six months earlier. Unwilling to take sustenance other than water brushed on her lips with a feather, the obvious question was, how did the girl sustain life? In evaluating the claim to total abstinence, Hobbes looked, as did many other emerging rationalists of his day, for a phenomenon that he could see—passage of food wastes. The case was clouded, however, by the conventions of modesty and decorum. Hobbes wrote: "To know the certainty there may be many things necessary which cannot honestly be pryed into by a man. Whether any excrement pass, or none at all."[17] Unlike Viverius, Hobbes called the girl "manifestly sick" even though her talk was "most heavenly" and some local people regarded her as a kind of saint.

In the seventeenth century prolonged abstinence more and more was linked to organic causes and regarded as illness. In this way loss of appetite became a general symptom of disease rather than a sign of preternatural intervention. The burden of proof was on the skeptics, who had to demonstrate one of two things: either that there was a medical explanation of the faster's long survival without normal food or that the claim to noneating was fraudulent.

An examination of the arguments involved in the case of Martha Taylor, the famed "Derbyshire Damsel," reveals a growing level of skepticism and sophistication in the evaluation of abstinence cases. In 1668–1669 nineteen-year-old Martha, a young woman of "mean" or poor parentage, attracted the attention of local clergy and physicians because she allegedly took no food "except now and then a few drops of the syrup of stewed prunes, water and sugar, or the juice of a roasted raisin." Although she slept little, it was said that her "countenance [was] fresh and lively." Her body, however, was in a sorry state: she was emaciated "into the ghastliness of a skeleton"; her lower body was immobile ("languid, and unapt for motion"); and her skin was dry with a "prurignous scurf." Almost totally confined to her bed, Martha Taylor's body was washed with milk by her mother.

Many people came to Taylor's humble home in the village of Bakewell simply to see the young woman who was said to live without eating. In 1668 and 1669 two religious pamphlets were published that told the story of Martha's abstinence from food and proclaimed her a "wonder of the world" and a miracle which God intended as an exhortation to sinners.[18] The popularity of this view prompted John Reynolds, a Protestant with connections to London's Royal Society of Physicians, to offer a rebuttal that now stands as perfect testimony to the style and logic of seventeenth-century medical rationalism. Reynolds' *Discourse on Prodigious Abstinence* demonstrates the tensions between magical, religious, and scientific interpretations of fasting behavior.[19]

John Reynolds used Martha Taylor's own mentality, what he called her "non-pretensions to revelation," as a starting point in his argument. He was quick to point out that Taylor had only recently learned to read the Bible and that she made no explicit preternatural claims despite the fact that many religious persons who came to her bedside tried to influence her with tales of "sacred mysteries." Reynolds praised the girl because she was not taken in by these visitors: she pretended "nothing of enthusiasm" and did not think of herself as a miraculous maid or saint. Convinced that Taylor's affliction originated in her body, Reynolds spoke of the girl's inability to eat as an illness and argued aggressively that virtuoso fasting should be exorcised forever from its "supernatural asylum."

Reynolds' first assault was against the "miracle mongers," those who believed that Martha Taylor was fed by angels, fairies, or benign spirits.[20] Reynolds made quick work of this interpretation by indicating his incredulity that "such a favor should be shown to persons of no known sanctity." In fact, the anonymity of the miraculous maids and their lack of articulate spirituality led Reynolds to suggest that they were inappropriate recipients of the supernatural gifts of God. Moreover, there was the issue of whether fairy food was visible or invisible. If the food was visible, it should have been seen as either "ingress at the fore door" or "excrementitious egress at the back door." If fairy food was invisible, then it was "altogether incongruous to our bodies," nonnutritional and hence miraculous. This returned the argument full circle to Reynolds' central question of the "miracle mongers": why favor with miracles young women of undistinguished parentage or accomplishment?

Reynolds' second attack was leveled at those who found an explanation in feeding by demons rather than by fairies, a position associated with the American Puritan divine and scientist Cotton Mather (1663–1728). To Reynolds' mind, a demonological view implied that Martha Taylor was bad although she was not. There are "no footsteps of such a possession" in the Taylor story, Reynolds wrote. Reynolds argued that Satan looked for "wider markets" than simple, rural young women. "It would be strange," he said, "if the devil should grow so modest as to content himself with a single trophy [such as Martha Taylor]."

Cotton Mather, on the other hand, always maintained that Satan cast his net as widely as possible. From his provincial outpost in the Massachusetts Bay Colony, Mather kept abreast of scientific developments in Europe; thus, he knew about the Darbyshire Damsel. On the basis of his own experience in Massachusetts with the witchcraft cases of Mercy Short and Margaret Rule, Mather concluded that "long fasting is not only tolerable, but strangely agreeable to such as have something more than ordinary to do with the Invisible World." Mather contended that Rule was assaulted as she fasted by eight "cruel specters," pinched by "vassals" of the devil, and encouraged to touch a "red book" as a symbol of fealty to Satan. In passing, Mather observed that "one sex may suffer more trouble . . . from the invisible world than the other."[21]

John Reynolds dismissed both demonology and Christian miracle as an explanation of the Taylor case. Still, he was careful not to discredit all scriptural accounts of fasting behavior, pointing instead to the need for discrimination: "True it is, the fast of Moses, Elijah and the Incarnate word was miraculous, and possibly some others; yet why we should make all miracles, I understand not." There were two important distinctions between scriptural fasting and the Taylor case. First, fasting in the Bible had a point, whereas Martha Taylor's behavior seemed to have no purpose at all. "Certainly the infinitely wise Operator labors not for nought," Reynolds wrote, "abstinents [such as Taylor] if miraculous, should confirm some doctrine rejected, or refuse some error received." Second, Reynolds argued that "our blessed Savior and his prodromi [followers] procured not the least detriment to their health," whereas Martha Taylor grew emaciated and ill.

The scientific explanation of Taylor's prolonged abstinence, and the one favored by Reynolds, was to be found in the theory of fermentation, a relatively new explanation of health and disease introduced only a decade before by Thomas Willis (1621–1675), a follower of Sir William Harvey (1578–1657).[22] Reynolds' explanation focused on the role of physiological changes caused by "ferment in the seminals," a recognition of the ovarian activity that was part of the young woman's reproductive development. According to Willis in *Of Fermentation of the Inorganical Motion of Natural Bodies* (1659), the seminal vessels and the genital parts were filled, as were other major organs, with fermentative particles made up of salt, spirit, sulfur, earth, and water. These bodily elements could ferment, much as grains do in the process of becoming beer, within the organs and then move throughout the body in the blood, making the blood volatile and hot. Those women whose ferment was in good order displayed a rosy skin color; where ferment was lacking, or where there was disequilibrium, women were pallid, short of breath, and lethargic. Blood that became too rank from fermentation, as in "turned" beer, was sloughed off every month during menstruation. In men, ferment in the seminals generated heat, strength, voice changes, and facial hair—all characteristics of sexual maturation.

Fermentation theory, combined with a Harveian conception of blood as a reusable fluid, led Reynolds to conclude that Martha Taylor probably could survive without eating. Ferments within the body independently enriched her supply of recirculating blood without the addition of new chyle produced by eating and digestion. Moreover, when her excretion was reduced, as it was in the case of marathon fasters, the body actually conserved elements already in the blood. Thus Martha could continue to live without eating and yet not be a miraculous maid.

Interestingly, Reynolds linked the ability to live without eating normal food to the process of adolescent female development. "It will strengthen our hypothesis to observe," he said, "that most of these damsels fall to this abstinence between the ages of fourteen and twenty years, when the seed hath so fermented the blood, that various distempers will probably ensue without due evacuations." By the eighteenth century the female proclivity for fasting was part of the established medical canon. Erasmus Darwin (1731–1802) concurred that food abstinence was associated with "young ladies," and Albrecht Von Haller (1708–1777) wrote in his influential text: "All medical history from the earliest time is filled with men, but especially women, who for whole entire months, in fact even years, lived without food."[23] Without subscribing to Reynolds' specific fermentation theories, scientific rationalists agreed that women seemed to be the primary constituency of inedia prodigiosa and anorexia mirabilis.

Ann Moore's Anorexy

In order to assess the authenticity of fasting claims, doctors had to have some sense of how long a person could actually live without eating. Consequently, there was a great deal of attention to the issue of abstinence in the scientific literature of the seventeenth, eighteenth, and nineteenth centuries. Abstinence was also an important clinical question. How long a person could survive in a seriously malnourished state had implications for routine practice. In effect, scientific rationalism required that physicians collect and describe medical cases of all kinds. These cases would become, particularly in the nineteenth century, the basis for elaborate nosologies and classifications of diseases.

Physicians and those interested in science culled the historical record for cases of long abstinence and for medical judgments on how long humans could go without food. Although Hippocrates admitted the possibility of total abstinence for about six days and Pliny allowed a slightly longer time, Democritus was said to have lived for forty days simply by smelling honey and warm bread.[24] Because they found so little consensus in classical sources, physicians developed an eclectic, anecdotal chronicle of human abstinence that borrowed from many different sources.

Cases of shipwrecked sailors who lived without eating and drinking for many days, stories of individuals trapped without food by natural disasters, crude ethnological reports of the trances and burials of the fakirs of India, and accounts of fasting women and girls from the medieval and early modern periods were all part of the medical and scientific literature on abstinence.[25] The question of what constituted the real limit of human abstinence apparently had answers so various, and often so extraordinary, that it was hard to codify findings. Some argued that seventy-two hours was the outer limit; some figured a month, as long as water was provided; and a few still clung to stories of fasters who survived for years without eating. At the beginning of the seventeenth century Licetus of Padua wrote a treatise "On Those Who Can Live a Long Time without Food." It contained various chapters on "those who lived eight days," "those who lived a month," "those who lived three months," "those who lived from one year to eight years," and "those who lived more than twelve years."[26]

The most cautious medical men reasoned that the ability to sustain life without food was idiosyncratic and depended on the constitution of the individual as well as his or her natural environment. Nonetheless, many spent time trying to calculate the actual number of ounces of solid nutriment required to sustain life in different situations. Cornaro, for example, lived fifty-eight years on twelve ounces of food and fourteen ounces of light wine every day; three women caught in a stable by an avalanche survived thirty-seven days on only a few ounces of goat's milk; and a young man lived twenty-six days in a canoe on Long Island Sound eating only a pint of barnacles and some snow.[27] Obviously, mathematical calculations of food intake were becoming a basic part of the literature on human abstinence.

By the eighteenth century, abstinence was a medical problem to be resolved by a set of predictable empirical validation techniques: around-the-clock watches, calculations of food intake, observation and measurement of excrement, and weighing of the body. The case of Ann Moore, the "Fasting Woman of Tutbury," exemplifies how scientific and medical rationalism transformed the nature of abstinence cases. Ann's fame was actually transatlantic; after 1813, American and English editions of her story circulated on the east coast of the United States and a "likeness in wax" was exhibited at the Columbian Museum in Boston.[28]

In the winter of 1807, Ann Moore's "anorexy" first became public. The daughter of a laborer, Ann married James Taylor at the age of twenty-seven but she soon separated from him. Within a few years she had two illegitimate children by her employer, with whom she lived "at service." When she was not working as a domestic servant, she supported herself and one daughter, Mary, by "beating cotton"—probably in a cottage industry or in one of the textile mills that had already begun to change the landscape of her Midlands home. By 1807 she was poverty-stricken and receiving a small allowance from the parish.

Many in the village of Tutbury were convinced that Moore was a good woman despite her sexual nonconformity. According to sympathetic reports, her loathing of food was a direct result of unpleasant domestic work, particularly her duties as a servant washing the bedclothes of Samuel Orange, a young man afflicted with a "scrophulous complaint" (probably open ulcers). "The offensiveness of the smell was so disgusting," wrote one of Moore's supporters, "that no other person but Ann would undertake it." She remained with Orange, doing the foul work, for nearly a year. Subsequently, whenever she took any food it smelled to her of his body. Her "disgust" had the "effect of causing her to vomit up a kind of slimy matter, resembling that proceeding from [Orange's] wounds."[29] An 1809 account by physician Benjamin Granger reported that Moore's refusal of food resulted from difficulty in swallowing and the fact that she experienced debilitating stomach pains after eating, sometimes severe enough to send her into convulsions. According to Dr. Granger, Moore's last food before her abstinence began was either gruel or coarse bread but, according to Moore, who sought to identify herself with the tradition of miraculous maids, her final food was a few delicate black currants.[30]

Local sympathy for Ann Moore was compounded by her ability to convince others that the fast was a symbol of her moral reclamation. This she did by making a "religious profession," by ad-mitting the sinfulness of her past ways, by espousing Christian principles in an articulate manner, and by beseeching God and the local clergy for salvation. As she was watched by local clerics and doctors, Ann Moore said and did just the right things—that is, she demonstrated "intelligent piety . . . and more than ordinary share of religious knowledge." Despite the fact that she did not read, a sympathetic account presents her as reading "Burkitt, on the New Testament, and other valuable books . . . [for] her study, pleasure, and amusement."[31] Ann was obviously an autodidact, a person able to draw, appropriately and often, on things she heard from others. The ability to say the correct thing, or at least to utter the right responses, "disposed many respectable and amiable individuals to conclude that she was upright in what she asserted, both as to her mental and bodily state. The one seemed to be a test of the other."[32] Supporters found in Moore's modest and pious deportment both reason to believe her claims and material to construct a new persona as religious doyenne rather than as town pariah.

The initial investigation of the case, supervised by physician Robert Taylor, a member of the Royal College of Physicians, had all the makings of a community celebration. Surrounded by "her enemies," Ann Moore was literally watched from every side, day and night, by one hundred seventeen different persons—all of whom validated her claim. After the first forty hours placards were posted throughout the town, announcing that she had as yet taken no nourishment and inviting the incredulous to "disprove the fact" and "watch for themselves."[33] The invitation to come to Tutbury and see Ann Moore in person apparently brought "immense numbers" and redounded to her economic benefit. By one estimate Moore collected £400; by another, she managed to save £200.[34] At first, her capital accumulation was viewed in a benign light, probably because she could be taken off the rolls of the town's poor.

There were at least four different interpretations of Moore's behavior: that her condition was a manifestation of God's super-natural power, that she "lived on air," that she suffered from a disease of the esophagus that made it impossible for her to eat, and that her fast was a fraud. Her celebrity status and her steadily improving financial condition attested to the fact that many people in the region still credited the first explanation.

The second and third interpretations deserve attention because they were emblematic of the state of contemporary science and medicine. An 1811 account of the case advanced the idea that Moore lived on elements in the atmosphere—specifically hydrogen, which she drew from air and water. "The atmosphere is not a simple substance," the unnamed author explained. "Chemists have ascertained that hydrogen [in the air] is the basis of animal fat." With this in mind, the author asserted that fermentation theory, as advanced by John Reynolds in the Taylor case, was an unlikely explanation:

> From the extremely emaciated state of [Ann Moore's] body, and the length of time she has been without any kind of aliment, it is impossible that she can have any internal source from whence a supply of the necessary juices can be obtained. Air seems to be the means by which life is still maintained, as she cannot endure without a fresh current of it continually admitted into her room, for which purpose the chamber window is always open, even in the coldest weather.

Moore's life was sustained by something outside her body: "she collects from the decomposition of both [air and water], a sufficient quantity of animal oil to preserve the body in existence."[35]

An alternative medical view held that an impairment inside Ann Moore's body was causing her anorexy. One common but largely unelaborated version of this interpretation said simply that there was something wrong with her throat or stomach. Some doctors, however, were more precise about the relationship between anorexia and disease. Recall that Richard Morton in the seventeenth century described lack of appetite as a symptom of consumption. An even more elaborate typology was developed by Erasmus Darwin, who placed women without appetite in three general categories: anorexia epileptica (loss of appetite with fits), anorexia manicalis (loss of appetite with insanity), and cacositis (a general aversion to food). Benjamin Granger regarded Ann Moore as a case of inedia prodigiosa, but he was uncertain about the somatic cause of the starvation even though it had been seen many times before.[36]

By 1813, after five years of visitors and notoriety, some important local authorities, both religious and secular, called for
"stricter scrutiny." Despite her religious mien, Ann Moore was
not necessarily an asset to the local scene. From the perspective
of her critics, Moore's presence kept alive a popular (but ignorant)
belief in the miraculous and made a mockery of scientific learning
and authority. The woman put Tutbury on the map, so to speak,
but for the wrong reasons. The second investigation was spear-
headed by Legh Richmond (1772–1827), the well-known evangelical rector at Turvey, an Oxford graduate, and a disciple of
William Wilberforce.[37] Assisted by the Vicar of Ashbourne and a
gentleman friend from London, Richmond approached Ann
Moore to see if she would accede to the proposition of a second
watch.

After some negotiation over terms, Moore agreed to a carefully
conceived watch of one month. It was her undoing. By the end
of the first week she lay gravely ill and was expected to die within
hours. Her daughter requested that the watch be stopped, but the
determined mother insisted on issuing an affidavit attesting to her
sincerity: "I declare that I have used no deception, and that for
six years I have taken nothing but once, the inside of a few black
currants; for the last four years and a half nothing at all."

Despite the fact that death seemed imminent, the watchers
persisted; after ten days they got their first hard evidence of
Moore's insincerity. An investigator discovered Ann Moore sitting
on a blanket, wet with urine, "through to the bed." Then she was
seen taking sustenance from a handkerchief moistened with vinegar and water. (Mary Moore had sustained her mother's life by
providing the handkerchiefs and transmitting small morsels of
food through kisses.) Finally, the watchers saw red stains on the
bodice of an undergarment, indicating that Ann Moore had been
drinking medicine applied to relieve soreness of the throat. When
she attempted to substitute one garment for another, she was
caught.[38]

Moore was forced by local authorities to testify to her imposture. On May 4, 1814, she put her mark to this statement: "I,
Ann Moore, of Tutbury, humbly asking pardon of all persons
whom I have attempted to deceive and impose upon, and above

all with the most unfeigned sorrow and contribution imploring the Divine Mercy and Forgiveness of that God whom I have so greatly offended, do most solemnly declare, that I have occasionally taken sustenance for the last six years." Once the fiction of total abstinence was deflated, few were interested in how she managed to exist on so little food. Moore survived her confession and the cancellation of the watch. Of her later life we know only that she was in "gaols" at some point for "robbing her lodgings."[39]

Throughout the nineteenth century Ann Moore stood as a symbol of female cunning and deceit. She was decried by everyone as a fraud and cited in medical books as evidence of the scurrilous nature of religious fasting claims. Here was a woman who made a mockery of Christian piety and scientific learning, employed her own daughter in the service of her deceit, and drew substantial material gain from the earnest gifts of the pious. These were odious and reprehensible acts that were not easily forgotten.

For Legh Richmond, the rector, victory over Ann Moore had wide implications. Both "science and morality," he said, were served by this important investigation and its resolution.[40] Had he been asked, Richmond would probably have concluded that the fraudulence of Ann Moore meant the death knell of anorexia mirabilis. What he could not foresee, however, was the manner in which a set of ambiguous cases of prolonged abstinence was to become a central arena for the intellectual and professional "boundary wars" that characterized popular religion and medicine in the middle to late nineteenth century. In effect, the long transition from sainthood to patienthood was yet incomplete. A battle still had to be waged.

3 · The Debate over Fasting Girls

In the last three decades of the nineteenth century, the tradition of anorexia mirabilis was again called into question by a series of public cases involving women who did not eat. "Fasting girls" were widely discussed in Anglo-American medicine and in the popular press. In 1869 in the popular magazine *All the Year Round*, Charles Dickens observed that "it seems to be little known how frequent the[se] instances . . . have been, in past years." Moreover, Dickens confirmed that "fasting women and girls have made more noise in the world than fasting men."[1] Similarly, in the 1880s, while the city of New York was caught up in the case of a local fasting girl, the *Times* observed: "It is a singular fact that in all the ages of the world it is not the strong and healthy men who have been reported to fast for long periods, but in most cases, [fasters] are weak and emaciated girls . . . In modern times, one or more [of the fasting girls] . . . is before the public at nearly all times."[2]

The term "fasting girl" was used by Victorians on both sides of the Atlantic to describe cases of prolonged abstinence where there was uncertainty about the etiology of the fast and ambiguity about the intention of the faster. Regardless of whether the faster was a mature woman or an adolescent, if she or her family allowed any form of public attention to her behavior, or if especially long abstinence was claimed, medical men responded by calling her a fasting girl (a term used facetiously by some and as an epithet by others). The generic use of the term "girl" also conveyed the notion of hysteria, for girlhood was a time of life that Victorian physicians regarded as particularly susceptible to nervous disorders.

Of course, the designation also evoked the history of female asceticism and anorexia mirabilis, but it mocked rather than honored that tradition. While nineteenth-century medical dictionaries continued to include the term "anorexia mirabilis," this anachronistic diagnostic category was not used in clinical situations or in popular discourse.[3] By the 1870s doctors rejected both the designation and the concept; still, they were not entirely certain how to differentiate among other possible sources of lack of appetite. As a result, the years between 1870 and 1900 constituted a transitional moment when the long, historical tradition of anorexia mirabilis still had some popular relevance and anorexia nervosa was largely an inchoate formulation. In this period, at least in public discussions, "fasting girl" was the term of choice.

Although doctors generally spoke of fasting girls with skepticism, many lay people took the claims of these girls in earnest (although total abstinence was obviously hyperbolic).[4] Not eating could mean eating irregularly, eating small amounts, or eating outside the normative food categories. In a number of cases there was a curious pattern of exempting fruit. In the same breath that she said her daughter had eaten nothing at all for six months, the mother of a fasting girl noted that her daughter took pieces of watermelon, pears, or strawberries. Physicians, suspicious of exaggerated abstinence claims, noted this deception: "You are often deceived by the patient's friends, who will sometimes state that no food has been eaten for days, and who do not consider that beef-tea, milk, or any other liquid should be called food."[5]

Others, continuing to believe in the veracity of fasting girls, would take "all such accounts as they would Gospel truth and herald [these individuals] as a return to the miraculous periods."[6] Sometimes the girls themselves facilitated the celebration of their special powers and enjoyed the status and material gifts that came with their notoriety. Among certain segments of the Victorian religious community, fasting girls and the fiction of total food abstinence became a way of sustaining belief itself. Many who were pietists or pious Catholics embraced the cause of a particular fasting girl, either because her story reinvigorated the tradition of anorexia mirabilis and Christian miracles or because her existence demonstrated the independence of the spirit from the flesh, a central tenet of Victorian Spiritualism.

In the United States in the late nineteenth century, Spiritualism was a significant and influential religious movement that held the promise of ultimate moral perfection through demonstration of the healing powers of the spirit world. "It was not just the half-baked, the uneducated and the credulous who appeared at séances or spirit circles," writes a historian of the movement. Spiritualists, who believed in direct communication with the dead or with disembodied spirits were often scientific and reform minded; moreover, both Spiritualist assemblies and mediums were disproportionately female.[7] In the United States in the 1880s and 1890s, fasting girls were often interpreted and understood as exemplars of the Spiritualist quest for transcendence over the material body. To live without eating was, of course, to deny one's need for material support or earthly connection. In late-nineteenth-century America the continuing fascination with fasting girls must be understood in terms of both a sophisticated urban Spiritualism and a lingering strain of rural or provincial pietism.

Claims to prolonged food abstinence provoked a natural curiosity among most persons, regardless of whether they were skeptics or believers. After all, the ability to live without eating constituted a provocative challenge to a fundamental premise of human existence—that life required food. The controversy over fasting girls exacerbated a set of preexisting ideological tensions about the relationship between mind and body that were central to the Victorian debate between religion and science.[8] By entertaining the possibility that any individual could live months or years without eating, the Victorian public was considering a fundamental and radical revision of the material facts of life as they knew them. Women and girls who claimed not to eat provided both a symbolic denial of the laws of science and a point of connection to the past and to the tradition of religion as a miracle-working process. For these reasons reputable medical men on both sides of the Atlantic became actively involved in public brouhahas over fasting girls.

The Welsh Fasting Girl

Sarah Jacob, the "Welsh Fasting Girl," was the best-known English example to catch public attention in the 1870s. The Jacob case provided a point of reference for public discussion of other food-refusal cases throughout the century, and that discussion was consistently informed by the legacy of Ann Moore. As a result, fraud and tricksterism became a basic concern in the medical evaluation of women who came to public attention because of prolonged abstinence.

Sarah Jacob was one of seven children of Evan and Hannah Jacob, crofters who farmed one hundred twenty acres near Pencander, Wales, at the rent of £61 per year.[9] As a premenstrual girl of twelve, Sarah began to fast in October 1867, when she reduced her food intake to "nothing but a little apple, about the size of a pill, in a teaspoon." Soon, according to parental report, she ceased to take any food at all. At the mention of food she became "excited" and often "when it was offered . . . would have a fit." Sarah's father claimed she passed neither stool nor urine after December 1867, except on one occasion when she became agitated over the simultaneous death of her grandfather and a family cow. The girl was intermittently watched by the local Anglican vicar, the Reverend Evan Jones, and by medical examiners who inspected the bedclothes for the signs and smells of excretion. The Reverend Mr. Jones attested to her good character in that she attended Sunday school and was "never particularly seeking the society or play of the other sex."

Although Jacob lived in rural Wales, her fast was widely known throughout Britain and the United States. In 1869 a letter from the Reverend Mr. Jones to the *Welshman* brought to the attention of a larger public the "wonderful little girl" who lived without eating. The vicar's letter stated that Sarah Jacob had not "partaken of a single grain of any kind of food whatever for over sixteen months." After noting that "medical men persist in saying that the thing is impossible," the earnest vicar went on to declare his confidence in the truth of the girl's claim. The celebratory letter constituted the vicar's personal declaration of faith and, at the same time, subtly laid down the gauntlet, challenging medical authority on the interpretation of Sarah's behavior. Between March 22 and April 5, 1869, the girl was subjected to a watch by two local men who worked shifts from 8 A.M. to 8 P.M. Both men, described as initially skeptical, left the girl's home, a thatched farmhouse in Carmarthenshire, declaring that the Welsh Fasting Girl was authentic, that Sarah Jacob did not eat.

Throughout 1869 and 1870 the emaciated girl was visited in her bed by hundreds of strangers, who brought her gifts and money. According to some reports, the visitors created something of a boom on the local railway. One visitor described village men and boys, waiting on the railroad platform to receive the pilgrims, wearing large caps bearing strips of paper that said "To the Fasting Girl." Another described the wasted Sarah in bed: "She had a victorine about her neck, and a wreath about her hair." Her bed, strewn with ribbons, flowers, and religious books, was also adorned with a small crucifix—despite the fact that the family worshipped as Protestants in the nearby Congregational chapel. Ritualism with overtones of Catholic practice was combined with a degree of commercial showmanship. Hannah Jacob began to dress her daughter in "fantastical" attire and multicolored ribbons. Some visitors came only to touch the girl, to feel her hands and face, or to rub her palms with oil. The *Cambria Daily Leader* sent a photographic artist to the house to take a likeness of the girl, but the parents asked twenty pence for the privilege and so the artist declined.

The presence of visitors on the farm changed the nature of the case from a private family agony to a public event that generated intimate, graphic descriptions of the starvation process, Sarah's excretory history, and her clothes. Little attention was paid to the family, except to substantiate their reputation as honest people. Among all the family members, the mother was most involved in the daily care of the girl. She told the Reverend Mr. Jones that medical men were probably impressed with mortification of the flesh in a child so young, suggesting an essentially religious conception of her daughter's behavior. The fact that pilgrims came to see her bolstered the widespread notion that Sarah had anorexia mirabilis.

Despite, or perhaps because of, the circuslike aspects of the case, Sarah Jacob's condition provoked serious discussion by reputable medical men. Most physicians recognized that the phenomenon was not something new. The author of a book on the Welsh fasting girl told his readers, "Instances of asserted fasting have been by no means rare in the history of the world." In fact, doctors made easy reference to the long tradition of religious austerities and its cast of female characters. Despite the continuity of female fasting in human experience, doctors were basically skeptical. "So much superstition and chicanery surround many of the examples of alleged wonderful fasting, that no possible reliance can be placed on the assertions which have been made concerning them."[10]

Distaste for the hoopla surrounding Jacob was only one component of professional hostility to the fasting issue. More crucial than either crass commercialism or the lingering patina of Catholicism was medical skepticism about any claim to live without food, which to most Victorian physicians suggested the primitive and the miraculous. These doctors failed to consider that the total abstinence claim might be hyperbolic; to them hyperbole was tantamount to deceit. Citing metabolic studies, they refused to admit that any human being could survive for more than a few weeks without food and water. Marathon fasting was denied outright since neither "the temperature [nor] the development of tissue could [be] maintained without any waste or change of substance."[11] From their understanding of nutrition and metabolic processes, doctors discredited the entire notion of anorexia mirabilis and painted Sarah Jacob as a fraud, calling up references to the case of Ann Moore whenever possible. "Some fifty years ago the fasting girl at Tutbury was exciting just such a stir," the *Lancet* reminded its readers. On another occasion a letter to the editor said Ann Moore's case was "perfectly parallel" to the one in Carmarthenshire.[12]

In the summer of 1869, after a faith healer had tried to cure Sarah Jacob by laying on hands, Robert Fowler, a graduate of the medical college at Edinburgh and a member of the Royal College of Surgeons, journeyed to Wales from London for a summer holiday. As part of his journey he paid a call on Sarah Jacob.

(Fowler's experiences became the basis of his 1871 account of the case, *A Complete History of the Welsh Fasting Girl*, published in London.) In the presence of the girl's family, Fowler attempted to examine the girl, whom he found "pretty" but with the restless eye movements that, he said, characterized hysteria. The mother apparently intervened at a number of points, restricting Fowler's access to Sarah. Unaccustomed to sophisticated medical examination, she was openly disturbed by Fowler's tapping of her daughter's body with instruments and his application of the stethoscope. The physician, by contrast, felt a professional responsibility to give as complete an anatomical examination as possible. Fowler determined that Sarah Jacob was not in poor health; he found some subcutaneous fat and heard a gurgling sound in the stomach, evidence of digestive activity. He concluded that Sarah Jacob was a hysteric and advised that "no sensible medical man, unless guaranteed perfect control and means, would undertake the treatment of such a case in the cottage in which the girl lives."[13] Fowler regarded those adults who believed Sarah's claim as either superstitious or disingenuous. "Being made an object of curiosity, sympathy, and profit is not only totally antagonistic to the girl's recovery," Fowler wrote, "but also renders it extremely difficult for a medical man to determine how much of the symptoms is the result of a morbid perversion of the will, and how much is the product of intentional deceit."[14] In order to restore the girl to normalcy, the patient needed to be removed to a more scientific setting, such as a hospital or county infirmary, where those who believed in her were stripped of their power.

The tension between the growing authority of professional medicine and lingering folk belief in the miraculous was demonstrated in the Jacob case where the patient literally was killed by empirical design. In November 1869, at the request of a committee of concerned locals, the London medical establishment arranged to send to Wales four reliable nurses from Guy's Hospital in order to determine the authenticity of Sarah Jacob's claim. The conditions of the medical watch were negotiated by the committee with a willing family and the farmstead's floors, ceilings, and windowsills were checked for hidden foods. Sarah's youngest sister,

Margaret, was no longer able to sleep with her and her parents' bed was removed from the sleeping room in the effort to control access to her.

When the Guy's nurses arrived at the farmhouse in early December, they found their patient cheerful and communicative. Reportedly she called them "nice ladies." One of the nurses, Anne Jones, was Welsh speaking. On the head of the famous girl was a garland of flowers, with a yellow streamer flowing down the side of her face. On top of an embroidered nightdress with a black cloth jacket, Sarah wore a white woolen scarf fastened at the neck with a brooch. The room where she lay had been carefully prepared; no food had been found except for an old turnip beneath the parents' bed. In accordance with the wishes of the parents, who maintained that Sarah was additionally debilitated by being urged to eat, the nurses were instructed not to offer food—no matter how the situation developed.

Because it was a cold, damp time of year, the nurses sat by a small fire, with hot bricks and flannels at their feet, watching the girl day and night as candles flickered near her head. Within the first thirty-six hours, the nurses reported seeing urine and a feces-stained nightdress, but whenever a doctor appeared to see the girl, the father objected to any examination of either her tongue or her body parts beneath the bedclothes. After the sixth day, as the patient grew observably weak, the nurses appealed to the doctors and to the family to cancel the endeavor so that Sarah might have the chance of getting nourishment the way she did before, however that was. The doctors agreed that the girl needed to be fed and recommended brandy and water, but no one could convince the parents either to force-feed the girl or to call off the watch. In response to Dr. Fowler's advice on the matter, the father queried: "How can you London doctors make my child eat, without making a hole in her?"[15]

To the end, the parents maintained that they would not violate their promise to Sarah: because unsolicited food provoked "fits," they would not offer her food until she asked for it. When the family doctor, Henry Harries Davies, a surgeon, counseled the father to stop the watch so that whatever method had been used to sustain life could now be resumed, Evan Jacob was angered by the imputation of dishonesty. On the ninth day, when Sarah's cold body began to experience the ultimate effects of sustained starvation, her naked six-year-old sister, Margaret, was put to bed with her in order to provide warmth. Approximately ten days after the watching began, on December 17, 1869, Sarah Jacob died of starvation.

An editorial deplored this atavistic event: "It appears to us monstrous that such an occurrence should have taken place in the nineteenth century."[16] All along, medical men had urged the parents to consider hospitalization, but they steadfastly maintained that God would take care of their daughter. Evan Jacob was later found guilty of criminal negligence for his failure to compel his daughter to eat.[17] "Had the girl been in Guy's Hospital," a senior physician wrote in the London *Times*, "she would have been fed had she desired it or not, and no veto on the part of a parent could have prevented our taking measures to preserve her life."[18] The *Lancet* editors, who maintained that a cure could have been "induced by moral means, easily accomplished in the wards of a hospital," reminded their readers that informed medical opinion had been rejected as an "arrogant expression of professional prejudice."[19]

Medical Opinion

In the Jacob case the medical consensus was that Sarah died as the result of starvation associated with girlhood hysteria, hysteria provoked by undue publicity and by religious enthusiasm generated by an "addiction" to religious reading.[20] The *Lancet*'s explanation of her demise was characteristic of informed opinion on the case:

> A girl in a weakly state of health, with a highly impressionable, emotional nervous organization, that has been unduly stimulated as well as disordered by religious reading and the sympathy of visitors, and having her vanity gratified by fuss, flowers, and ribands, will simulate anything almost well enough to deceive herself into believing it. And this case leads us to say that Perversions of Volition, similar to those observed in Hysteria, are by no means uncommon among children.[21]

Others were more explicit about the connection between hysteria and female adolescence. The attorney at a postmortem inquiry told the court that in 1867 Sarah Jacob was "affected by what is not uncommon in girls of her age, that is, fits of Hysteria." "I use [the] popular phrase," Gifford went on, "because I believe there is in some of the Depositions a quantity of scientific words which mean the same thing, but which you would not so well understand."[22]

Medical men unequivocally supported the notion that the adolescent girl was at risk for mental as well as medical disease. In women, puberty and the onset of the menses were believed to mark the beginning of a period of profound psychological as well as physiological crisis that would continue until menstruation was regularized or "firmly established." Anglo-American medical advice urged both girls and their parents to consider the need for special care and protection in puberty. Because of the "large demands upon the resource of the female adolescent system," doctors generally advised close parental supervision of the diet, clothing, exercise, sleep, and mental and moral training of girls. In this context many physicians (as well as clerics) regarded reading as a potentially dangerous activity. To be sure, romantic and sentimental novels were widely regarded as too stimulating for delicate young women, but pietistic religious tracts were also considered inflammatory.[23]

Fowler explained that girlhood hysteria frequently manifested itself as a localized nervous affection—that is, as a physical disorder centered in the stomach or throat. Only a year before, at the annual meeting of the British Medical Association, Sir William Withey Gull, a prominent London physician whom we shall see emerge as a major figure in Chapter 4, spoke of a nervous stomach condition in young women that included lack of appetite and emaciation "to the last degree." In 1868 Gull called that condition "hysteric apepsia."[24] Fowler told of his clinical experience with another variant of localized nervous disease: he called it globus hystericus, or a ball in the throat, attributable to a "spasmodic action of the gullet." For nervous girls such as Jacob, who complained that they could not eat because they could not swallow, Fowler recommended a specialist in diseases of the throat.[25]

The inability to swallow was certainly not an organic condition, but rather a function of the girl's frame of mind: "I expect that with an hysterical girl with that habit of fasting and simulation, the attempt to swallow food would bring on that sensation [of a ball in the throat], which might be followed up by the rejection of food and might produce an indisposition and determination not to take food in public." Fowler had seen the symptom many times before and had his own explanation; he told the London *Times*, "The cunning stratagems and deceptions sometimes practiced by young girls afflicted with this form of hysteria are well known to medical men." And when asked by the court, "Have you in your experience noticed that there is a secretive tendency in these people [hysterics], especially girls?" Dr. Fowler answered, "I have."[26]

Fowler drew evidence for the deceptive nature of hysterical fasting from the Jacob autopsy. The postmortem examination revealed the existence of fecal matter that predated the period of medical surveillance. Furthermore, a curious indentation under the girl's right arm, supposedly the same shape and size as a half-pint bottle, suggested that Sarah had a regular nutritional supplement, however small. While her heartbroken parents continued to assert that she took no food or drink for over twenty-six months, the doctors now had proof to the contrary: Sarah Jacob did not live without eating because when she was systematically denied all food for less than two weeks, she died. Clearly, medical materialism could undermine the total abstinence claim; could it provide an explanation of Sarah Jacob's motivation?

Robert Fowler regarded the deceit of the hysterical girl as an instrumental technique for gaining special attention within the family. In addition to the "morbid perversion of the will" involved in hysteria, Fowler believed that most adolescent fasters were also "night feeders." Fowler supplied an infrequently used term: "Children that don't take food in the presence of their parents are generally called 'night feeders,' and the disease of want of hunger is called 'Asitia.' My opinion of [Sarah Jacob] was—that she was a 'night feeder.'"[27] In Fowler's rendering, Sarah Jacob was forced to eat on the sly in order to maintain the powerful fiction that she did not eat at all.

How and why food refusal became so potent a preoccupation within the Jacob family is not something Fowler ever attempted to explain. He assumed that noneating generated a pattern of parental coaxing and indulgence that reinforced the behavior. In certain kinds of family and community settings, particularly among the uneducated, a hysterical girl's ability to live on small amounts of food could become exaggerated and subsequently transform her into a "miraculous child." This attention and sympathy, Fowler wrote,

> soon engendered in Sarah Jacob's wrongly-balanced mind, notions of merely ideal creation. The oft expressed wonderment and surprise of the ignorant household around her, as to the very little food she had lately lived upon, tended to give a morbid direction, form, and shape, to these visions of the mind. The occasional refusal of some temptingly-offered article of sick-diet, was followed by more parental coaxings, endearments, indulgences and pettings. The resultant self-gratification, the feelings of childish pride at treatment so different to that of the other children, conduced, for the same ends, to a more frequent declining of food when offered. Gradually thus became acquired the power of fasting, without distress, for unusual periods.[28]

The doctor concluded that the "cultivation of this habit" brought rewards which led to acts of "simulation and deception." By the time of the second watch, Sarah Jacob was on the "border land of insanity": "she had got herself into that state of mind in which she believed she could last out the fortnight without food, . . . but she got on too far to hark back."[29]

Sophisticated British physicians did not regard Sarah Jacob as anomalous. A decade after her death Samuel Fenwick wrote: "Cases of this description have been recognized for centuries, and have afforded material for wonder or superstition. They have been frequently described as 'fasting girls' and have been sometimes regarded as persons especially gifted with the power of dispensing with the necessity for food, whilst in other cases they have been looked upon as imposters trading upon the credulity of the public." As a spokesman for the scientific point of view, Fenwick concluded, "A careful perusal of many of their histories will, I believe, convince any unprejudiced person that, in the first instance at least, these individuals have been the victims of disease, and that it was only when the wonder excited by their abstinence stimulated their avarice, or aroused their vanity, that they added deception to support their popularity."[30]

Despite medical skepticism, other fasting girls attracted the attention of the British reading public in the last decades of the century. In addition to Lancashire's Ellen Sudworth, a shoemaker's daughter who claimed to have eaten no solid food for over four years, there was a second "Welsh Fasting Girl" (a fifteen-year-old with the family name of Morgan); Maggie Sutherland, fourteen, of the Orkney Islands; Martha White, seventeen, the "Market Harborough Fasting Girl"; and Christinia Marshall, thirteen, of Glasgow—all of whom received attention in the London and regional newspapers as well as in the medical journals of the day. In 1871, approximately one year after the close of the Jacob case, the mayor of Preston, a northern industrial town, asked the home secretary for power to remove a local fasting girl, Ann Riding, to "some public institution, where she [would] receive all the attention and assistance that the peculiarities of her case required."[31] Because public fascination with these cases seemed not to ebb, British medicine was aggressive in its efforts to instruct the public in the proper medical interpretation of the behavior: "No one can be considered sane who, without cause, starves so as to endanger health and life. Should cases of 'fasting girls' continue to crop up, I think it would be well if the subject were brought under the notice of the Commissioners in Lunacy."[32]

Somatic Neurology and Religious Women

The most vocal American medical critics of the fasting girls came from the emerging specialty of neurology. The somatic neurologists, so named because of their insistence on the centrality of the physical operations of the spinal cord and nerve systems, paved the way toward modern psychiatry. In the United States they were located in large urban centers on the east coast, where they built lucrative private practices that catered to the nervous disorders of middle-class and upper-class women.[33]

Anglo-American neurologists regarded lack of appetite and food refusal as a common symptom in functional nervous disorders such as hysteria. They had little tolerance for anorexia when it was linked, either by the faster or by observers, to personal piety, to claims of extraordinary abstinence, or to public notoriety. The neurologists openly attacked the fasting girls as hysterics, as symbols of popular superstition, and as perpetrators of outright deceit. The distinguished American neurologist George Beard (1839–1889) reflected medicine's characteristic skepticism and familiarity with fasting girls: "The stories that periodically arise of young girls who live without food, may probably be explained partly by fraud, and partly by ignorance."[34] Throughout the colorful controversy over the fasting girls the neurologists clung to the hope of persuading the public that, on the basis of the scientific laws of metabolism, prolonged abstinence from food was fraudulence at worst or sickness at best.

The neurologists insisted on a clinical and comparative perspective. The male body, they said, operated rationally, according to the laws of scientific metabolism.[35] Those who failed to eat, died. Among women, however, the outcome seemed less predictable. A New York neurologist wrote:

> I am not aware that this power has been claimed to its fullest development for the male of the human species. When he is deprived of food he dies in a few days, more or less, according to his physical condition as regards adipose tissue and strength of constitution: but if a weak emaciated girl asserts that she is able to exist for years without eating, there are at least certificates and letters from clergymen, professors, and even physicians, in support of the story. The element of impossibility goes for not [sic] against the bare word of such a woman.[36]

Consequently, when the claim to "live without eating" was raised, it sounded to the ears of most male physicians like a cry for irrationality and for a peculiar and archaic form of female empowerment. In this way, fasting girls posed a basic challenge to the ideological and professional structure of modern science.

Confronted by a ground swell of interest in fasting girls, the neurologists boldly asserted the primacy of medicine as the best interpreter of human behavior. They took to the popular press, explaining their position in New York dailies and even in book form. In so doing, they always recapitulated the history of female asceticism and the phenomenon of anorexia mirabilis, but they recast that history in terms of superstition, chicanery, and mental illness.

To the Victorian physician, anorexia mirabilis constituted a distinctive form of female religious empowerment that was incongruent with the material facts of the contemporary world. Religious behaviors, especially acts of intense personal piety, were suspect. "The outpouring of the Spirit of God," wrote one doctor, is too often "only another name for epilepsy, chorea, catalepsy, ecstasy, hysteria, or insanity."[37] Sophisticated neurologists displayed an intolerance for Christian miracles, for intense religious experience of almost any kind, and for the irrational. Significantly, women were central in all these domains, a fact that the neurologists did not fail to underscore and incorporate into their biomedical view of the female sex. In fact, the history of medieval religious women was used by the emerging psychiatric specialties as evidence for demonstrating women's propensity to mental disorders. In doing so, Victorian medicine used religious history to cast female piety as pathology.

By the 1870s, when fasting girls became a public issue, both old and new forms of female religious activity were irksome to medical professionals striving to promote a scientific view of human behavior. Whatever expansion the Protestant religious establishment experienced in post–Civil War America, it was an expansion fueled by women rather than by men. In the decades after the war three major American religious movements—Spiritualism, Seventh-Day Adventism, and Christian Science—involved large numbers of women and gave them leadership roles, nationally as well as locally. In each of these traditions, as well as in the contemporaneous Methodist Holiness movement, the women emerged as important interpreters of doctrine and experience.

Significantly, each of these major religious movements incorporated some basic challenge to medical authority.[38] Spiritualism raised questions about what constituted being "medically dead" and proposed the existence of the soul apart from the flesh; Seventh-Day Adventism, which was outwardly hostile to medical professionalism, spread the gospel of whole grains, exercise, fresh air, and pure water—all things that were readily accessible and demanded no special knowledge to employ; and Christian Science, by asserting the spiritual rather than the physical dimensions of healing, eliminated doctors altogether. Because of the feminized nature of the Victorian religious establishment and its close connection to issues of health and disease, the neurologists' analysis of fasting girls must be seen as part and parcel of the politics of science, professionalization, and gender.

One man wrote more on the subject than any other nineteenth-century physician: William Hammond (1828–1900), a former surgeon general of the United States and founder of the New York Neurological Society.[39] Impatient with the lingering vocabulary of faith, superstition, and spiritual transcendence, Hammond used the public discussion of fasting girls to promulgate the new discourse of medicine. In *Fasting Girls: Their Physiology and Their Pathology* he wrote: "Strange to say the ability to live on the eucharist and to resist starvation by diabolical power, died out in the middle ages, and was replaced by 'fasting girls' who still continue to amuse us with their vagaries."[40] In his view, neither the saints nor the fasting girls were miraculous. They were merely hysterical, and they required medical intervention.

This is not to suggest that Hammond was either irreligious or a convinced atheist. Like most physicians of his class, he was a liberal Protestant whose taste in religious observance was bland; he shied away from excess in any form. Always careful to assert his respect for the underlying morality of Christianity and disclaiming any basic hostility to religion, Hammond stated authoritatively: "There can be no conflict between pure science and pure religion; for the one is truth and the other is faith in truth." False religion, he said, "distorted facts and misinterpreted phenomena," creating "gross and senseless delusion" in women and in weak-minded men.[41]

Religious excitement was dangerous because it had the power to induce emotional and physical changes of an extraordinary nature. In Hammond's view "intense mental concentration on some one particular subject—generally, one connected with religion"—contributed to hysteria. He described hysteria as the predominance of the emotional "subforce" over the intellect or will.

Furthermore, according to the precepts of somatic neurology, religious exaltation could become "so intense as to interfere with sensibility of various parts of the body, or to derange the contractility of muscles." Religion that emphasized emotionality at the expense of the other subforces could generate in its adherents different types of hysterical disorders such as catalepsy, hystero-epilepsy, and ecstasy. Ecstasy, which he found more common in women than men, was a "cerebral and spinal preoccupation—a kind of setting of the current in one direction, whereby all other occupation is for the time prevented."[42] Fasting girls were ecstatics, according to Hammond's morphology.

"[I have] no great respect [for] religion based upon emotion," Hammond wrote at the same time that he carefully reconstructed the annals of Catholic miracle makers and Protestant enthusiasts.[43] Rather than hide or ignore the historical record of feminine spirituality, Hammond brought this history into the light of day and then used it to fashion what he believed to be an empirical critique of Christian miracles, as well as an explanation of gender differences. By depicting women as the primary actors in the pageant of the miraculous, Hammond associated them with outmoded systems of belief and with a spirit of mental delusion unfit for the progressive life of the nineteenth century.

Newspaper coverage of cases of fasting girls provided physicians with the opportunity to demonstrate their virtuosity as diagnosticians and their rhetorical power as spokespersons for the scientific perspective. In his medical diagnosis of the spiritual state of female religious figures, Hammond implied that religion itself was an epiphenomenon. In short, somatic neurology suggested that piety was not piety at all. Rather, spirituality in women would be understood, in the modern world, as a form of irrationality rooted in the peculiar organization of the female synapses. For this reason the claims of Brooklyn's Mollie Fancher were particularly vexing to Dr. Hammond.

The Brooklyn Enigma

The public debate over female fasting behavior reached new intensity in Victorian New York in the case of Mollie Fancher, known in her youth as the "Brooklyn Enigma" and in maturity as "America's Most Famous Invalid." Although the Fancher case shares many characteristics with that of Sarah Jacob, it was distinguished by its own cast of characters, a cast that reflected both the contours and the texture of American intellectual and professional life. That cast included a middle-class Brooklyn schoolgirl (Mollie) whose alleged abstinence from food became part of an extensive repertoire of supernatural skills; the feisty New York neurologists (men such as William Hammond and George Beard) who were willing to speak publicly, through interviews in popular metropolitan dailies, about Fancher and other fasting girls; eccentric believers (such as Spiritualists), pious clergy, and physicians of secondary status who all rejected the neurological canon on prolonged fasting; and a receptive reading audience that was fascinated with the enigmatic relationship of body and mind posed by Fancher's case.[44]

Born Mary Fancher in Attleboro, Massachusetts, in 1848, Mollie (as she was known from childhood) was the eldest of five children in the family of James and Elizabeth (Crosby) Fancher. At some point in her childhood the family moved to Brooklyn, New York, where her father became a prominent merchant. After her mother's premature death Mollie was raised by her maiden aunt, Susan Crosby, and attended the reputable Brooklyn Heights Seminary. By all reports, she was a fine student blessed with good looks and the modicum of poise and style befitting a respectable bourgeois family. A local newspaper declared her a "fine looking [girl], capable . . . [and] of great apparent promise."[45] But at age sixteen, in a manner typical of Victorian adolescents, her health began to fail: "Her trouble was pronounced nervous indigestion, her stomach rejecting most kinds of food: She had wasted away and become weak, and was the subject of frequent fainting spells."[46] Her dyspepsia was apparently so extreme that the girl left the seminary and became a semi-invalid. Eventually her doctor found a cure: "Her physician pronounced her trouble indigestion; and horseback riding was advised as just that kind of exercise which would likely produce beneficial results."[47] Until she reached the age of nineteen, her medical problems were essentially a private family matter.

Fancher's story first appeared in the "public prints" on June 7, 1866. In a lengthy article describing "A Remarkable Case," the *Brooklyn Daily Eagle* reported the existence of a young woman in that city who had gone "seven weeks without food" as a result of extreme "nervous prostration." (The *Eagle* was quick to point out that the girl was not likely to be an entrepreneurial type. Rather, she was the daughter of a "moderately circumstanced, respectable, intelligent and well connected family.") The *Eagle* described her as looking "more like parchment than flesh and blood."

What accounted for the unidentified sufferer's nervous prostration and her rejection of food? According to the *Eagle*, the local case merely illustrated a national trend: most Americans "abuse their nerves from the cradle to the grave" as a result of overwork and overstimulation.[48] But, the risk of nervous exhaustion was particularly great among young people, that is, adolescents, in the process of coming to maturity. "Those to whom are confined the education of our youth of both sexes" were warned about the "unhealthy action" that resulted from too much stimulation of mental faculties.

The girl in Brooklyn was definitely such a case. The *Eagle* said of the young Mollie Fancher: "Her books were her delight . . . she neglected all for them, and would arise late in the morning in consequence of weakness, hasten away to school without breakfast, fearful of being tardy, and then at evening, in her anxiety to learn her lessons, again neglect a meal for which she felt no inclination." In this way Fancher's "vitality gradually ebbed."

The girl's fragility did not stop her from attempting a normal round of activities. Her "mistaken enthusiasm" for education took her out of the house, and as a result she suffered two accidents.[49] She had her first accident in May 1864 when, challenged by an unruly horse, she fell from the animal. Although she experienced some double vision, she recovered adequately. Later she became engaged to a young man by the name of John H. Taylor, whom she met through attendance at the Washington Avenue Baptist Sunday School. In June of 1865 she was seriously injured in another accident, this time involving a streetcar. Her petticoats became affixed to a trolley, which dragged and banged her against the pavement and the streetcar. She was immediately removed from the street to a nearby residence and then to her home, where began a long recuperative period marked by a constellation of symptoms that defied medical men of different therapeutic traditions. In response to Fancher's reported loss of all the senses— sight, sound, touch, taste, and smell—her father and aunt brought in a range of nineteenth-century practitioners, from homeopaths (who tried to administer pills and tonics to an "almost hermetically closed throat") to hydropaths (who showered the girl with cold water and froze her spine with ice) to an allopath (who forced food and nourishment under her cuticles).[50]

Fancher's gradual assumption of the invalid role was accompanied by extraordinary claims to specific "powers." In fact, by her early twenties she was transformed from a nervous, dyspeptic schoolgirl to a fully empowered female mystic and clairvoyant. A chart of her postaccident biography constitutes a roster of bizarre medical symptoms coupled with impressive supernatural skills. For example, Fancher's supporters said that even though the girl was periodically blind, she could "see without use of eyes" and hear although she was deaf; reportedly, she also endured periodic contortions of the limbs. It was said that she could tell the exact time simply by passing her hand over the crystal of a watch, and she could read by rubbing the cover of a book. Mollie claimed to anticipate events, such as the chime of fire bells or the ringing of her own front doorbell. Sealed letters placed under her pillow were allegedly read verbatim by the invalid. Scenes and conversations that occurred miles away were said to be reported with astonishing accuracy. In addition to her mind-reading skills and her general prescience, Fancher endured long trances and told of visits with her mother and other deceased spirits in heaven. The *Eagle* article stated that Mollie Fancher was "what would be termed *spirituelle*."

Although her behavior catered to a large constituency of Spiritualists who maintained a belief in communication with spirits of the dead through human mediums, Fancher always disassociated herself from the Spiritualists. She identified instead with evangelical Presbyterians and Methodists. In 1878 it was noted that Mollie Fancher dreaded "being classed in any manner with clairvoyants or second sight seers or spiritualists." Rather, she described herself as an "earnest Christian."[51] Despite her efforts to separate herself from female mediums who were paid for their services, her critics consistently tried to cast her as one of the flotsam and jetsam of Victorian Spiritualism.

Because late-nineteenth-century Spiritualism attempted to "sell itself by language and deed as a scientific endeavor," many of its followers regarded Fancher as empirical proof that the "laws of science" were not laws at all. Of course, this interpretation annoyed the somatic neurologists, who had an entirely different version of the meaning of Spiritualist practices such as somnambulism and trance.[52] Somatic neurology regarded these states as nervous disorders rooted in malfunction of the spinal cord. Consequently, William Hammond was absolutely opposed to the Spiritualist credo, to its spirit-gathering practices, and to its functional use of women's alleged "greater sensitivity" for the role of medium. The fact that thousands saw Spiritualism as a legitimate form of scientific religion galled him for decades. In 1876 he wrote a book on the connection between Spiritualism and nervous derangement. From Hammond's perspective, Spiritualism was the worst religious bugaboo of the post–Civil War era.[53]

By the late 1870s Fancher's food abstinence was allegedly as awesome as her clairvoyance. She apparently ate very little or nothing at all. In one six-month period, her recorded intake was four teaspoons of milk punch, two teaspoons of wine, one small banana, and a piece of a cracker. Although two Brooklyn doctors treated her as though she were a classic case of female hysteria and used a stomach pump to force-feed her, Mollie Fancher would not resume a normal eating pattern. "She refused food when offered to her saying it made her sick," was the *New York Sun*'s description of her behavior.[54]

Fancher quickly became a Victorian celebrity. According to an 1893 deposition, an agent from P. T. Barnum came to Brooklyn because he "wanted to exhibit Mollie" but was unsuccessful in recruiting her. Fancher's refusal to join a traveling show as a hunger artist or as a clairvoyant did not herald rejection of *all* commercial applications of her fame, however.[55] Her name was formally associated with George F. Sargent Company, a manufacturing concern that specialized in prosthetic products geared to the needs of invalids. A supporter explained that while Mollie Fancher "does not pretend to despise money," her chief object in endorsing Sargent's products was "the development of devices for the relief of suffering humanity."[56] Still, in her second-floor bedroom Fancher did other things to bring material gain and recognition. Confined to her bed, on her back, with one arm immobile and her hand held rigidly above her head, Mollie Fancher practiced the popular Victorian art of waxflower making. By all reports, she fashioned beautiful if lachrymose designs—"windows filled with flowers and vines and butterflies, bouquets, crosses and anchors." She formed from memory the leaves and flowers that she could not see; and she tinted the waxes in subtle colors. A Harvard professor allegedly invented "a peculiar knife, with a rounded blade for cutting the leaves . . . specifically fitted to [her] closed left hand."[57] Fancher's handiwork attracted much attention and brought visitors and buyers to her house at Myrtle Avenue and Downing Street. There she sold her mournful waxflower arrangements, as well as her embroidery and crochet work, to those who desired "some memento of their visit."

Fancher achieved enormous notoriety, and her claim to abstinence from food extended to fourteen years. All of the major New York City newspapers gave some attention to her alleged ability to live without eating. Eventually, Fancher's flamboyant claims that she did not need food in order to sustain life posed a problem that was critical to the Victorians' understanding of the world: what is the relationship between the mind and the body? This question dominated late-nineteenth-century intellectual life and was a major preoccupation of the Victorians. Fancher was provocative because, like many female fasters before her, she believed she could transcend the flesh.

For the somatic neurologists of New York City, the claims of the Brooklyn fasting girl were a special irritation. This kind of theatrical behavior demanded an appropriate response. So Hammond proposed, in the pages of the *New York Sun*, that he place a certified check for a sum of money exceeding $1,000 inside a single paper envelope and place it on a table in Fancher's bedroom. Hammond was willing to allow the envelope to be taken in hand by Mollie or to be placed in contact with her body. The arrangement specified that within one half-hour Fancher would be expected to produce an accurate description of the check—its number, the date, the bank on which it was drawn, the amount, and the signature. If the description was complete and accurate, the physician agreed to give the amount of the check to a charitable institution of Fancher's choosing or to "otherwise dispose of it in accordance with her wishes." The conditions of the experiment were relatively simple: the envelope could not of course be opened, nor could it pass out of the sight of a team of three validators—Hammond and two other members of the New York Neurological Society.[58]

In his public challenge Hammond said he would rethink the nature of modern science if he were proved wrong. If Mollie Fancher "succeeds in this test," he wrote, "I will admit that heretofore in my denunciations of such performances as hers I have been in error, and that there is a force in nature which ought to be investigated." Always the empiricist, Hammond explained that if Fancher read the check correctly he would pay the money without chagrin and with complete satisfaction. Fancher did not, in fact, respond to Hammond's provocative challenge. The reason cited in the *Times*, based on interviews with her friends, was that Mollie doubted the efficacy of her own powers in the presence of someone as "gross and materialistic" as Dr. Hammond.[59]

The issue of how to test Mollie Fancher's abstinence from food was particularly difficult, given popular knowledge about the outcome of the Sarah Jacob case. Two years earlier, in 1876, Hammond had predicted that "it would be perfectly possible to reenact in the City of New York the whole tragedy of Sarah Jacob should ever a hysterical girl take it into her head to do so."[60] But Hammond was not deterred from the validation technique that had proved fatal in Wales. He proposed another watch: relays of members from the New York Neurological Society were to monitor Fancher day and night for thirty days. At the end of the month the doctor promised to give Fancher $1,000 if she had not taken food "voluntarily" or "as a forced measure to save her from dying of starvation."

Hammond's familiarity with the contemporary medical litera-

ture convinced him that he could not lose. Throughout the brou-
haha over Fancher he remained a consummate materialist. Repeatedly he told the public that Mollie Fancher had to be eating
something, that the claim to fourteen years of abstinence was
preposterous. Fancher was neither miraculous nor specially empowered; she was simply hysterical.[61]

As a somatic neurologist, Hammond was more interested in the
medicine of the Fancher case than in its psychology. Because he
never met or examined her, Hammond reasoned that Fancher's
physiological condition was probably the result of a severe injury
to the spinal cord, which had caused paralysis in the lower
extremities.[62] Secondary injuries to the sympathetic nerve and the
brain were implicated in her mental condition. Mollie's refusal of
food except for minute bits of milk punch, crackers, and fruit was
congruent with Hammond's general notion that "hysterical
women are able to go for comparatively long periods without
food."[63] Confined to her bed, often in a state of insensibility,
Fancher had limited food needs, but nevertheless they existed.
According to Hammond's reading of the literature on inanition
and metabolism, absolute deprivation of food and drink could
not be endured by a healthy adult for longer than ten days. Even
a person as inactive as Fancher required food in order to sustain
her vital functions. Rejecting the notion that life and food could
be separated, Hammond declared that "all the teachings of science
and experience are against her claim."[64]

The Testimony of Nonexperts

The neurological explanation for fasting girls was not accepted
without suspicion. In fact, it generated strong hostility among
those who, for one reason or another, found the neurologists'
pronouncements discordant with their own beliefs, overly confident, or too materialistic. An amorphous community of supporters—drawn from the evangelical Protestant churches, Spiritualism, and Catholicism—continued to pay attention to Mollie
Fancher and respect her claims to abstinence. These claims, coupled with reports of clairvoyance, made her a public personality
whose activities received attention in the press for over three

decades. She died in February 1916, only eight days after the celebration of what was billed as her "Golden Jubilee in Bed," an occasion marked by a letter of greeting from President Woodrow Wilson.[65]

Fancher's personal character was consistently under attack from medical men who stated that she had to be either fraudulent or hysterical. William Hammond explicitly charged her with deceit: "Miss Fancher undoubtedly lives because she eats" and "at night . . . when she thinks she is unobserved, she rises from her bed and with the agility of a cat moves around her chamber."[66]

Deceit was at the core of Hammond's conception of female hysteria because it was the rational way to explain long abstinence. "Many ecstatics pretend that they do not eat," he reported in his medical textbook. "There are hysterical patients who apparently live for months without food or drink and would certainly die of inanition," he said, "were it not for food which they surreptitiously obtain."[67] In a series of interviews in the *New York Sun* Hammond again and again reiterated the same point. He proclaimed that Mollie Fancher (by this time thirty years old) was not "the first girl that has deceived learned and good men: . . . I can read you case after case where they [hysterical girls] have deceived thousands." Less virulent medical skeptics echoed the association between female hysteria and deception, rooting their comments in clinical experience. For example, Dr. Meredith Clymer told the *Sun* that "an entire perversion of the moral faculties" accompanied hysteria. "I have known young girls, good, pure, and charming [become] just the opposite—coarse, vulgar, obscene. There is no keeping pace with the cunning of such [hysterical] girls." Dr. E. C. Seguin reiterated the same theme in reference to Fancher and the fasting girls: "I know that these patients are sometimes very tricky. I had one in the hospital who did not eat; food was nauseating to her. She pretended not to eat anything. But one day I gave her an emetic, and up came a nice lot of nuts that she had been eating."[68]

Local supporters who knew the Fancher family in Brooklyn felt compelled to express a rather different view of Mollie Fancher, the woman. Professor Charles E. West, her former teacher and principal of her alma mater, unequivocally rejected the notion of deception in the Fancher case. West, who described himself as a "common sense man," a "physicist and a chemist . . . dealing with facts" all his life, actively promoted the idea that Fancher was a medical anomaly. In answer to the question "Are you quite sure that you are not deceived by Mollie Fancher?" he replied:

> I can't imagine how I could be deceived. I have known Miss F. for years . . . I have subjected her to severe tests and I have never seen a single deception, or an attempt to deceive. She has always been the same good, loving Christian girl. She is a member of the Church. She is honest, if anyone is honest . . . I can place my hand on her abdomen and feel her backbone. Is there any deception there?[69]

For West, who felt Fancher's backbone both literally and metaphorically, survival was extraordinary: "[Mollie Fancher] is simply a miracle. She says she is a miracle, and I know she is one. The entire scientific world should know about her."[70]

In 1878 the earnest Professor West proposed that a commission of scientific men come to Brooklyn to study Mollie Fancher. Specifically, he named British physicist John Tyndall, British anatomist Thomas Henry Huxley, and American zoologist Louis Agassiz.[71] The proposal was rejected. George Beard, a leader in the field of neurology, spoke for his colleagues when he suggested that the men named by West "knew nothing about the subject at hand" and that Agassiz (who by then was dead) "was filled with superstition."[72] Dr. Beard and Professor West obviously differed on what constituted a man of science. Beard wanted a proper three-month scientific investigation of the Fancher case, at a cost of $1,000; but neurologists, in his view, were the only scientists appropriate to conduct the empirical inquiry:

> The testimony of non-experts amounts to nothing . . . If we accept non-expert testimony there can be no science. The first step in any science is the rejection of all average non-expert human testimony relating to it.[73]

As an indication of the emerging professional *mentalité*, Beard's statement is a classic demonstration of where specialization could lead, and his repeated insistence on this formulation served to alienate as many as it convinced. Disclaiming any personal animosity, but refusing to qualify his evaluations of the generalist, Beard told the *Sun*:

These physicians in Brooklyn are my personal friends; they are able men in their line, but they are not experts, and their testimony goes for naught. The number who testified to Mollie Fancher's wonderful performances makes no difference. A naught has no value, two naughts has no value, 500 million of naughts has no value.[74]

The fact that neither Hammond nor Beard ever saw or spoke with Fancher galled many, such as West, who doubted their claims to empiricism-at-a-distance. Ultimately Beard drew the cord of specialization so tight that West gagged: "Do they [the physicians] know everything?" he asked. "Have they universal knowledge?"[75]

Neurological arrogance and somatic determinism left many unconvinced that regular medicine could explain the fasting girls or the relationship between the mind and the body.[76] The Reverend Joseph T. Duryea, pastor of Brooklyn's Classon Avenue Presbyterian Church, gave his sanction to the publicity that surrounded Fancher on these ideological grounds: "I like to see such peculiar manifestations of the mind and the body made public. They teach the difference of existence between the spirit and the flesh and the superiority of one over the other."[77] Fancher's 1878 public utterance, "There is nothing of me to die," and her friends' confirmation that her spirit was already "released from the bondage of the flesh" fueled the idea that food refusal and prolonged abstinence could be understood as a function of the duality of the mind and body, or as a result of a "disturbance in their usual relations."[78] The Spiritualist community, of course, basked in Fancher's pronouncements.

Yet another view of the case was proposed by J. R. Buchanan, who held a chair in Physiology and Anthropology at the Eclectic Medical College of New York. Eclectic physicians rejected, in general, the materialism of regular medicine and, in particular, the somatic determinism of the neurologists. Buchanan, for example, argued that "man is more than a physical machine." According to the eclectics, the body and soul were in "deeply interesting correlation." However, in the average person, they were so tightly united that the flesh "completely masked" the spirit. Nonetheless, changes in that relation could occur such that flesh and spirit were separated—"the body lying as if inanimate, while its vital principle, which is spiritual, acts independently."[79] For the eclectics, the soul was a legitimate arena for scientific investigation; moreover, food was not essential to the existence of the soul. Thus, fasting girls such as Mollie Fancher raised issues of medical interpretation between neurologists and eclectics as well as articulating differences between the religious and the secular communities.[80]

Ultimately, Dr. Buchanan explained the Fancher case much as had the Reverend Duryea. Unlike the Brooklyn pastor, however, the eclectic physician never regarded Fancher as new or anomalous. He took the position that "medical annals contain many authentic cases of abstinence from food, some even for longer periods than in the Fancher case." Additionally, he faulted the medical profession for its general ignorance on the subject of fasting, an ignorance born of medical parochialism and professional solidarity. Buchanan's language was strong:

> [Medical men and schools] know no more of the psychic universe than the mole does of astronomy. To ask one of these skeptics, who considers mind a secretion of the brain, as bile is a secretion of the liver, his opinion of Miss Fancher's case, would be as profitable as to ask a description of the climate of Cuba from one of the learned monks in the days of Columbus, who denied the existence of the Western Hemisphere.[81]

In addition to its wrongheadedness on the mind-body issue, Buchanan found regular medicine to be deliberately narrow-minded, manipulative, and meanspirited. His analysis actively discredited the neurologists' claim to authority by virtue of scientific objectivity. Instead, he reported a very different kind of professional behavior and activity. Medical authors and medical schools, he wrote, "have their infallible dogmas and everything contrary to these dogmas is fiercely assailed by the whole phalanx, discredited in every possible way, right or wrong, and scrupulously expurgated from the medical literature." And then, as if he had a particular example close at hand, he concluded, "The ease and energy with which a trained professor repels unlimited amounts of testimony, facts and even the most authentic statistics can be compared only to the energy that we find in the heels of a spirited mule—excuse the coarseness of the metaphor, for a coarse illustration is necessary for a coarse subject."[82]

Buchanan's mule in all probability was the New York neurological community headed by William Hammond and George
Beard. Only the week before, both had delivered major public
pronouncements on Fancher. Hammond's analysis, widely circulated in both the *Times* and the *Sun*, was distinguished for its
heavy emphasis on Mollie's deceit and its patronizing view of
her supporters. When asked by the *Times* how he might explain
enthusiastic testimony on Fancher's behalf by reputable clergymen
and physicians, Hammond responded: "Oh, that's nothing. Clergymen are the most gullible men in the world and physicians who
have not made a study of nervous diseases are apt to be imposed
upon by these girls."[83]

In the summer of 1881, when the Fancher fascination was at its
height, eclectics and neurologists brought the battle over food
abstinence to center stage. As the result of a public challenge from
Hammond an eclectic physician from Minneapolis, Henry S. Tanner, rented Clarendon Hall in New York City and proceeded to
fast for forty-two days, taking only alcohol vapor baths and
charging twenty-five cents admission to all persons outside the
medical community. Tanner's original intention was to invalidate
the time limits on human abstinence that were at the basis of the
neurological interpretation of Mollie Fancher. (Regular physicians
who were skeptical about fasting girls tended to set a numerical
limit, usually twelve to fifteen days, on the time a human being
could live without food.) Rejecting the idea that human life could
be reduced to this simple material calculation, Tanner undertook
his fast in order to demonstrate the power of the mind over the
body and to illustrate the independence of the soul from physical
functions. He took to public fasting in defense of Fancher because
he wanted to provide scientific proof that her claims were not the
impossibility that the neurologists asserted.[84]

If Dr. Tanner died or failed to reach his goal, Hammond and
others could claim that prolonged fasting was an impossibility,
that fraud lay at the core of the historical and religious record,
and that deception must be implicated in hysterical loss of appetite. During the monitored forty-day fast, Tanner took only an
occasional alcohol vapor bath which, his critics later claimed,
constituted food and acted as a stimulant. In the final days of his

ordeal the doctor from Minneapolis suffered greatly but refused to either eat or desist. Tanner's intimate behavior was carefully scrutinized, including measurement of urine and feces, and although Tanner expected progressive starvation to bring with it prophetic dreams, visions, or other "psychical phenomena," nothing of the sort occurred. When he finally broke his fast, Tanner was simply debilitated and hungry.

Because of the alcohol vapor baths and the "imperfect nature" of Tanner's supervision by a "parcel of doctors whom very few ever heard of," neither Hammond nor Beard ever acknowledged the fast as a success. The *New York Times* called the event Tanner's Folly, submitting that the eclectic doctor gained neither any sizable amount of money for himself nor legitimacy for his school of practitioners. "No physiological principle of any importance was deduced from the undertaking," reported the *Times*.[85]

Tanner felt differently about the implications of his "achievement." Using a faulty analogy drawn from the animal kingdom, he asserted that his Clarendon Hall fast revealed man's capacity to exist in a state of "suspended animation," much like the hibernation of a bear and requiring neither food nor water. To Tanner's mind, suspended animation meant that the only "sure and infallible sign of death was decomposition." Thus, he used the fast to argue against what he considered "hasty" burials of those pronounced medically dead. In fact, a number of late-nineteenth-century physicians were interested in fasting girls precisely because they were similar to a phenomenon classified as "hysterical lowered vitality," that is, a condition that mimicked death. In these cases physicians had to be careful about pronouncing a patient dead and risking premature interment.[86]

Throughout the 1880s different types of medical men offered interpretations of Fancher's fasting behavior—much to the chagrin of the New York neurologists who felt that only those who studied nervous disorders should comment on the case. Throughout the twenty-year controversy over fasting girls, regular medicine continued to be concerned with the technical problems of abstinence, deceit, and validation; in other words, the authenticity of the symptoms superseded serious questions of etiology. The doctors did not address the critical behavioral questions of why fasting girls chose to avoid food (or eat secretly) and of the resemblance of these girls to the emerging clinical reports of a newly named disease, anorexia nervosa. Because of their own ideological commitments and a host of intraprofessional rivalries, American physicians were sidetracked from the basic issues raised by these cases. Ultimately, the neurologists prevailed with their assertion that refusing food was less a miracle than a functional nervous disorder, a symptom of hysteria. But, as the next section demonstrates, the public controversy over Mollie Fancher constituted a crescendo, and not a coda, in the long cultural preoccupation with women who did not eat.

The Coda

As late as 1910, cases of fasting girls appeared in popular American news reports. In Fort Plain and Covert, New York; in La Crosse, Wisconsin; in Bremerville, New Jersey; and in San Francisco, fasting girls received the attention of the press.[87] Each of the fasting girls was designated with a place-name so that the cases could be differentiated and compared. Fasting girls became local celebrities and brought notoriety to their places of residence, which, more often than not, were rural settlements or small towns.

Wherever sustained food refusal was still regarded as a supernatural event rather than a medical disorder, fasting girls were a possibility. While no hard and fast rules governed their appearance, late-nineteenth-century fasting girls were generally not the daughters of the urban, educated, or secularly minded bourgeoisie. (The latter, by contrast, were apt to be treated for poor appetite by medical doctors seeking a physical explanation of their emaciation. This is the story of the next chapter.) Although an exact determination of the religious affiliations of the fasting girls is nearly impossible, it is accurate to describe them in this way: they fed on a lingering strain of piety in a world where mystery was still alive. Their existence did not depend so much on a particular church affiliation as it did on a familial and community *mentalité* that allowed the possibility of the miraculous.

Surprisingly, fasting girls spoke to the antimodernist impulses of a set of Protestant intellectuals, that is, men and women who were associated with Episcopalianism, with Anglo-Catholicism, and with the High Church movement. The antimodernists were uneasy and unhappy with the direction of late-nineteenth-century bourgeois society and its doctrines of material progress, scientific positivism (personified by the neurologists), and self-absorption. They actually were yearning for the kind of intense religious experience (anorexia mirabilis) that fasting girls recalled. Drawn to both medievalism and Catholicism because of their mystical, ecstatic, and ascetic tendencies, the antimodernists shared some of the fascinations of the more plebeian community of the devout.[88]

Consequently, fasting girls received attention from both the educated and the uneducated, the elite and the ordinary. In nearly all instances they generated a familiar discussion replicating the themes and cadences of the earlier, more famous cases. In 1881, for example, in Bremerville, New Jersey, twenty-one-year-old Lenora Eaton stopped eating and died after refusing food for forty-five days. The attending physician and the girl's friends were mystified by her refusal to eat. Eaton had given no explanation for her starvation and her physician could not provide any organic explanation of her inanition. The attending doctor did not mention hysteria or any other emotional or mental disorder. People in her town, individuals described as reputable citizens, promoted the notion that Lenora Eaton had actually "lived without eating," marking her as a special person and as a symbol of their faith in the miraculous.[89] The persistence of the total abstinence claim, in the face of scientific incredulity, reveals that acceptance of the medical explanation of food refusal was not universal. Clearly, belief was not yet dead nor medicine completely triumphant.

By the turn of the century, however, a scientific view of the fasting girl as hysteric had penetrated even into rural areas and into general practice. In 1886 the death of Adeline (Lina) Finch, twenty-one, stimulated much interest in the rural Finger Lakes community of Covert, New York.[90] A report entitled "Long Fasting" in the local *Homer Republican* observed that Lina Finch "had been for several years afflicted with a strange disease, which affected her body and mind." In late adolescence, the account went, "she became imbued with the idea that it would be better not to eat, and it is said [that] for 86 days before her death she had not tasted food." Finch's chronic refusal of food set the small community astir. When an autopsy disclosed that the organs of the body were absolutely healthy, the local physician concluded that the girl had died of voluntary starvation. As an explanation of her behavior, the Homer paper reprinted an analysis from the nearby Seneca Falls *Reville*: "It is probable that the condition in which she had been so long was the result of a mental or nervous affection." Just what the "mental or nervous affection" was and how it was generated was left unspecified by the anonymous Seneca Falls author. The newspaper report suggests, however, that even in a rural agricultural community there was popular acquaintance with the concept of hysteria and some rudimentary notion of functional nervous disorder, however imprecise the formulation.

In the 1880s the case of Kate Smulsey, the "Fort Plain Fasting Girl," recapitulated many of the medical and social dilemmas raised in the Jacob and Fancher cases. Smulsey, an obscure twenty-year-old seamstress, achieved regional notoriety for her refusal of food.[91] Known to be a "bright and industrious girl" with "an excellent reputation among the good people of [her] vicinity," she came from a family of "hardworking Germans" whose veracity was never explicitly questioned. Her father, George Smulsey, a laborer in his sixties, probably worked in one of the town's leading industrial and manufacturing establishments (the Fort Plain Spring and Axle Company or the Fort Plain Hosiery Mill). Her elder brother, Adam, a clerk in Dillenbeck's dry goods store, was quick to tell the local paper, "No, sir: we are not believers in Spiritualism."[92] The mother, portrayed sympathetically by the local press as a woman of good character and a member of the German Lutheran Church, signed an affidavit sworn before a notary that her daughter ate nothing for over six months except for a "small piece of watermelon not to exceed two inches square" and a "bit of beefsteak" described as the "size of a caramel." (Mrs. Smulsey claimed that Kate never ingested the meat. Allegedly she swallowed only the juice and abstained from the flesh.)

According to local and regional newspapers, Kate Smulsey fasted for nearly a full year. Stories of her abstemiousness drew over a thousand visitors to the Smulseys' "small but neat cottage" on the west side of the Fort Plain village. Visitors purportedly came from New York, Albany, Troy, Utica, Rochester, the Cherry Valley, and neighboring towns; the family and the attending physician, William Zoller, a graduate of Hahnemann Medical College in Philadelphia, were overcome by letters of inquiry and telegrams from places as far afield as Japan.[93]

According to the *New York Times*, which covered the story throughout 1884–1885, Kate Smulsey became sick in 1882 and took to her bed. Her illness appeared at that time to be some variant of hysteria, accompanied by strange, regular, rolling movements of the body. Then, in March 1884, she reputedly stopped eating altogether. "The parents and every member of the family . . . coaxed and implored the girl to swallow some food, but without avail."[94] Silently and recalcitrantly, Kate lay in her bed, pallid against the sheets, wearing blue glasses to protect her sensitive eyes, and turning away "the most tempting morsels," declaring that "she could eat nothing." Smulsey explained her lack of appetite in somatic terms, saying that food, water, and conversation all made her "turn purple and bloat." Some local residents regarded her behavior as "miraculous" and "remarkable"; others "expressed the opinion that the girl is possessed of the devil."[95]

Throughout 1884 the press maintained an ambivalent attitude about the fasting girl in Fort Plain. As if they were hedging all their bets, the local newspapers and the urban dailies vacillated between taking the case seriously (by issuing solemn reports on the faster's condition intermixed with reputable medical opinion) and painting the whole business as an absurdity. For example, the *New York Morning Journal* poked fun at Smulsey, facetiously recommended emaciation as a new strategy for romance, and implied that the girl was an actress.

If Miss Kate Smulsey, dressmaker of Fort Plain, N.Y. and her friends are to be believed, Miss Kate has not partaken of food or drink, not even of the cream that freezes or the soda that effervesceth, for 167 days. This beats Tanner's best fasting record by 118 days. If Miss Smulsey goes on as she has begun she will in time become a transparent woman. This is a class of person which has long been looked for and desired. Lovers who have found it difficult to understand their wayward flames might perhaps persuade them to undertake a little starvation. Such a course would have the further advantage of rendering them ethereal and beautiful. Sarah Bernhardt owes her wonderful popularity and fame to thinness of this character.[96]

Even in Smulsey's home region, there was an occasional ray of levity as a reporter or editor, in this case from the *Amsterdam Daily Democrat*, amused himself with a headline or quip about their local attraction:

Faster and Faster
Kate Smulsey is the champion faster. To-day is her 176th day. A poor specimen in Stranstown, Pennsylvania died of starvation after going without food for 48 days. Montgomery County leads the world.[97]

For physicians, however, the business of diagnosis was serious, whatever hoopla or amusement the girl generated. For William Zoller, the family doctor, the case was "puzzling" but it involved no deceit or attempt at commercial exploitation. Zoller maintained that while it was "contrary to the laws of nature for a human being to live without subsistence," Smulsey clearly did: "During the long period [I] attended the case, [I have] never seen her eat a morsel nor discovered any indications whatever that she did so."[98] Zoller thought that Smulsey might be suffering from dropsy. Another local doctor, Douglas Ayers, a graduate of Albany Medical College, cast her as the victim of a peculiar form of St. Vitus' dance, a neurological manifestation of acute rheumatic fever. As a consequence of widespread skepticism about the case and a lack of medical clarity on what was wrong, the Amsterdam newspaper suggested community subscription to support a watch by reliable nurses in order to ascertain the veracity of Kate Smulsey's bizarre behavior.

Although the watch never took place, physicians from outside the immediate area engaged in speculation about the case in response to reporters' eager questions. Some doctors actually traveled to the girl's bedside; others made their diagnosis from afar. One visiting medical man suggested that Smulsey's illness was related to venereal disease: the girl had "spinal disintegration, or a species of locomotor ataxia, [that is,] a wasting of the nervous system" that destroys all desire for food and the power of the stomach. (Locomotor ataxia was commonly used to describe the symptoms of tabes dorsalis—chronic syphilis of the central nervous system.)[99] Another doctor said Smulsey had chorea, a disease characterized by involuntary, uncontrolled, dancelike movements, but he did not explain her refusal to eat. A medical man from nearby Albany likened Kate Smulsey to Sarah Jacob and turned his attention to her bodily excretions. By measuring them, he determined that she was eating something and recommended a hospital where, under "kind but firm" care, she would begin to eat again. J. A. Smeallie, a physician from neighboring Canajoharie, visited Kate twice and then recapitulated the professional sentiments of Robert Fowler and William Hammond. Smeallie insisted that Smulsey was a hysteric who should be removed from her home. "No sensible or thinking person will give any credence to [this story]," he said. "Humbuggery seems to be the order of the day."[100]

Smulsey died in April 1885, to the end claiming abstinence and special powers. "News of the girl's death brought hundreds to the scene," was the word from the local paper. Many came to view the emaciated corpse, which weighed about 75 pounds. Some weeks later an autopsy report was issued. Heading the medical team was Theodore Deecke, a well-known pathologist from the state lunatic asylum at Utica, and at least six other doctors from Montgomery and adjoining counties. Two reporters were admitted to the room where the procedure was done.

The importance of the postmortem clearly demonstrated the new power of scientific explanations of behavior. In the organs of the dead girl, medicine expected (and promised) to find a definitive somatic explanation of the "Fort Plain Fasting Girl." Instead, the postmortem added to the confusion. Although Deecke's report stated authoritatively that the twenty-year-old girl had died of tuberculosis (suggesting that her lack of appetite and emaciation were the result of organic disease), the girl's stomach and intestines in actuality were empty. In the end, the examining doctors said ambiguously, "The girl could have lived a long time upon a small amount of food."[101] A headline from the local paper captured the confusion surrounding the Smulsey case and fasting girls in general: "Is She a Fraud? Who Shall Decide When the Doctors Disagree?"

Because they were regarded as both a curiosity and a medical mystery, fasting girls presented entrepreneurial opportunities for sharp promoters. An undisguised case of commercial intent involved Josephine Marie Bedard, seventeen, a poor French-Canadian girl from Lewiston, Maine. Described as a modern Cinderella, Bedard grew up unhappily in the home of her father, a stepmother, and numerous siblings. Apparently, she communicated directly with her deceased mother's spirit and consistently sought her advice and counsel. According to newspaper reports, the miserable girl had eaten nothing for a period of seven years: "She had no more desire to eat than other people would have to chew iron." Testimonies taken from community supporters affirmed that she ate no solid food but consistently drank tumblers full of water.[102]

In December 1888, when two different Boston promoters learned of the nearby fasting girl, each sent his own representative scurrying north to Lewiston, to offer money to exhibit the girl at their respective establishments—the Nickelodeon on Court Street and Stone and Shaw's Museum on Tremont Row. C. H. Webber, who eventually made himself Marie Bedard's "guardian," cast his employer, the proprietor of the Nickelodeon, as a man of science: he was "always upon the look out for curiosities and wonders of Nature, [and] he felt that there might be some grain of truth in the [Lewiston newspaper's] account." Bedard was undoubtedly a desirable property: the two establishments eventually went to court over who had first right to offer her as an attraction. Webber, in promoting his protégée's significance, did not fail to capture the impact of the litigation: "Without a doubt [Marie] will go down in the annals of science as the greatest marvel the world has ever known, and her introduction to the public by lawsuit will not make her case one whit the less interesting."[103]

Much as the neurologists had predicted, commercialism and chicanery were observable motifs in the Bedard case. Poor and uneducated fasting girls like Marie Bedard were vulnerable to exploitation so long as their behavior was accompanied by provocative claims or suggestions. (Because of her class background, Bedard was probably unlikely to receive regular medical attention or careful clinical analysis.) When an individual girl with the compulsion to starve—or hide her eating from public view—was supported by either earnest believers, clerical authority, or crass promoters, the situation became volatile. The complicit patient then moved out of the private realm into the public arena. This notoriety, of course, was something that reputable middle-class people sought to avoid and that most physicians disdained.

By the close of the nineteenth century fasting girls in any guise but that of medical patients violated prudence and propriety. Prolonged fasting for commercial gain had been discredited ever since the case of Ann Moore, but in Victorian society religious motives were equally suspect. Religiosity increasingly was cast as an exercise for consenting adults and their children, in the privacy of their homes, and not in the "public prints." Fasting girls and other displays of pietistic virtuosity were sharply disdained.

In the history of female fasting behavior, the nineteenth century was a crucial divide. During those hundred years food refusal was transformed from a legitimate act of personal piety into a symptom of disease. This was a matter of behavior as well as classification. Food refusal because of so-called divine empowerment became so infrequent that it was easily cast as a form of aberrant behavior by the emerging psychiatric specialties. In 1896 a physician confidently observed, "At the present day, religious fervor accounts for but few of our remarkable instances of abstinence, most of them being due to some form of nervous disorder, varying from hysteria and melancholia to absolute insanity."[104] By 1910 the religious delusionary had disappeared entirely from classifications of malnourished individuals.[105] This development suggests that the locus of appetite control and food-refusing behavior had moved from the religious realm to the secular: patients were simply not articulating reasons of faith when they did not eat.

Driven by imperatives for rationality and authority, Victorian medicine did not miss the opportunity to reclassify the ambiguous fasting girls and move them, in that process, from the realm of piety to disease, that is, from anorexia mirabilis to anorexia nervosa. This was a transformation that medicine self-consciously helped to engineer by its willingness to enter the imbroglio surrounding girls who refused their food.

What the physicians did not anticipate was the degree to which even the most blatant hucksters were incorporating an approximation of scientific discourse into their salesmanship. Marie Bedard, the Lewiston fasting girl, was sold to Boston audiences as a curiosity but also as a figure in the "annals of science." The commercial expropriation of science (rather than religion) as a backdrop for the fasting girls suggests a critical turn in popular modes of explanation and confirms a gradual transfer of cultural leadership from the clergy to men of science, particularly professional medical men.

The transformation of fasting behavior from piety to disease captures the parallel processes of secularization and medicalization. Doctors eventually prevailed over clergy, and biomedical "facts" superseded faith.[106] My account differs from much previous work in the history and sociology of religion in that it moves the secularization process beyond the confines of formal, organized church life into the realm of basic individual behavior. Rather than concentrate on the shrinking reach of churches, pastors, and declining membership rolls, I use food refusal and control of appetite as an indicator of *mentalities* in transition.

There is a final point to the story: there were, in fact, no "fasting boys." That women and girls, even as late as 1900, continued to claim prolonged abstinence through divine empowerment suggests that secularization may move at different rates depending on gender. It is not that there is anything about the cognitive abilities of women that makes them incapable of understanding or embracing modern scientific rationalism. Rather, the social and cultural experiences of women prepared them to "march to a different drummer," to mark out a somewhat different cadence in the change to a secular worldview. The existence of fasting girls well into the late nineteenth century suggests that some women clung to supernaturalism, belief, and ritualistic practices longer than men. They seemed to have needed, either as ideological sustenance or as opiate (depending on one's point of view), the supports that religion can provide. Deprived of many worldly sources of empowerment, some Victorian girls chose to draw instead on the lingering tradition of anorexia mirabilis. In this way the nineteenth-century fasting girl was a provocative relic, in a secularizing age, of an older female religious culture.

4 · Emergence of the Modern Disease

The nineteenth century was notable for the identification, classification, and description of many diseases. The clinical differentiation of scarlet fever from diphtheria, typhoid from typhus, and syphilis from gonorrhea constituted definitive medical advances. "New" diseases, bearing the names of the physicians who first described them, took their place in the medical armamentarium: Bright's, Addison's, Hodgkin's, and Parkinson's diseases were (among others) nineteenth-century creations.[1] In the 1870s anorexia nervosa emerged as a new disease, and its appearance reflected medicine's increasing empiricism and sophistication in the business of distinguishing one ailment from another. Both the intellectual push for new nosologies and the clinical process of differential diagnosis are central to an understanding of how anorexia nervosa emerged as an independent disease entity.

Dunglison's 1865 dictionary defined anorexia as "absence of appetite" and specified that this symptom need not be accompanied by any articulated distaste or pronounced "loathing" for food. Dunglison said simply: "Anorexia or want of appetite is symptomatic of most diseases."[2] In clinical practice most nineteenth-century doctors regarded anorexia as a simple and obvious sign of disease. Medical journals confirm that physicians saw lack of appetite in many different physical conditions: in tuberculosis and a related pulmonary condition known as phthisis, cancer, stomach diseases, anemias such as chlorosis, chronic diarrhea, and the nausea of pregnancy. Anorexia was a particular symptom of patients suffering from diseases that were marked by "wasting"—that is, either temporary or persistent loss of flesh.[3] In short, anorexia was a general medical symptom, a sign of disease, but not a disease in its own right.

The question then is, How was anorexia nervosa gradually distinguished from other symptoms involving loss of appetite? For an answer we must turn to the experience of three different groups of physicians: public asylum keepers in the United States; elite British medical consultants; and early French psychiatrists. It is important to remember that, at least in the Anglo-American world, nineteenth-century medicine was highly stratified by social class. Middle-class people (or those who aspired to that status) normally avoided public institutions such as asylums and hospitals because their inmates were apt to be the poor, the diseased, and the chronically insane. Physicians who worked among that clientele were accorded lower status than those who catered to bourgeois patients and their ailments.[4] Although anorexia nervosa was seen in both public and private settings, the disease ultimately fit within the clinical purview of high-status practitioners because of social considerations that shaped the experience of illness, the individual's access to the health care system, and the nature of treatment itself.

Anorexia in the Asylum

Among the depressed, the disoriented, and the disorderly who came to the nineteenth-century lunatic asylum were a substantial proportion who presented anorexia (lack of appetite) as a symptom. In fact, the public and private asylums that began to appear in the late eighteenth and early nineteenth centuries supplied physicians with their major experience with patients who refused to eat. Robert Fowler's public bout with Sarah Jacob and William Hammond's set-to with Mollie Fancher were more showmanship than medicine compared to the hands-on experience that asylum doctors acquired.[5]

For all physicians the symptom of anorexia posed a serious problem because it implied a sequence of events that could lead eventually to death by starvation.[6] For American asylum superintendents, who were accountable to the public, the specter of death by starvation was particularly frightening.[7] Mortality statistics from public asylums were published in professional medical journals and also abstracted in newspapers for the general reading audience. A high death rate within the asylum was a serious indication of failure. Among the British, asylum keepers (known as alienists because of their patients' strange or alien ideas) demonstrated a similar concern. As a consequence, superintendents in Anglo-American institutions had a pragmatic need to feed that was linked to the very legitimacy of the asylum undertaking. In both England and the United States alienists paid close attention to anorexia. As a result, the first crude classifications for what we now call eating disorders emerged at midcentury from among the American asylum superintendents and the British alienists.

Differentiating the physical from the mental causes of anorexia was often hard for asylum doctors. Luther Bell, chief medical officer of the private McLean Hospital near Boston, confessed that it was a "most embarrassing difficulty" in his mental asylum.[8] Asylum doctors described a number of different kinds of mental patients who displayed the symptom of anorexia, but the emphasis was almost always on outward behavior rather than etiology. Their classifications of food-refusing patients usually fell into three categories: patients with a "morbid appetite"; those who believed their food was poisoned; and those whose "religious monomania" or preoccupations precluded their eating.[9] Beyond these specific behaviors, the insane were thought to experience a breakdown of normal physical function with respect to appetite and digestion.

As the psychiatric specialities (such as asylum medicine and neurology) developed, physicians came to see the wide spectrum of situations in which patients presented anorexia as a symptom. Lack of appetite and refusing food cut across the formal diagnostic categories that informed early psychiatric medicine. Aspiring asylum doctors were told: "In studying mental diseases we must . . . take into account instincts and appetites, e.g., love of life, sexual functions and reproduction, social instincts, appetite for food and drink. Disturbances of all these instincts and appetites are found in mental diseases."[10] Moreover, as diagnostic techniques became more informative and as diseases were labeled more precisely, a general medical symptom like anorexia was understood to be part of a constellation of symptoms rather than an isolated problematic.

Among nineteenth-century doctors who were conversant with mental diseases, anorexia and food refusal were always loosely linked to melancholia, a generalized form of mental depression that often included "paralysis of food appetite." Severe melancholics were known to be suicidal and anorexia was part of their "suicidal intent." Acute melancholics were prone to combine anorexia with aphonia (lack of voice) and overt attempts at suicide using asylum bed sheets, cutlery from the dining room, or their own clothes. Melancholia, a popular diagnosis in the nosological grab bag, incorporated a variety of depressive disorders, mild and severe, which did in fact inhibit normal appetite.[11]

In short, the management of anorexia (no matter how it was classified) became a specialty of asylum medicine. "Unquestionably the medical officers of asylums see far more of, and [have] therefore more experience in overcoming attempting starvation than any other part of the profession."[12] In this context forced feeding, an invasive procedure in which pulverized food was spooned, dripped, pushed, or pumped into the orifice of a patient, was not uncommon. The reports of nineteenth-century asylum keepers reveal a personal reluctance to force-feed patients but a managerial commitment to the procedure as a practical technique to prevent unnecessary death. Forced feeding was a dramatic type of intervention that the asylum doctors justified on the basis of medical concerns. An editorial in the 1883 *American Journal of Insanity* forthrightly stated that forcible feeding of the insane was "sometimes an absolute necessity for the saving of life."[13]

Asylum doctors recognized forced feeding also as a psychological technique of intimidation that could break recalcitrant patterns of anorexia. They repeatedly told of cases where the mere presentation of the feeding apparatus so terrified the patient that he or she agreed to eat. One noted physician went so far as to claim that the intimidation strategy was successful 99 percent of the time. "In only one instance have I found it requisite to order use of the stomach pump," he wrote, "and if sufficient firmness is displayed by the attendants, such a measure will be scarcely ever necessary."[14]

For families and general practitioners who were stymied by the wasting of particular individuals, the asylum's reputation for forced feeding made it a magnet and a last resort.[15] A case from the records of the Hartford Retreat suggests how the asylum was used as a "forced feeder." Between 1891 and 1894 Liza, a young woman diagnosed as suffering from primary dementia, was admitted and discharged from the Hartford Retreat on three separate occasions; anorexia was a prominent symptom in the patient's condition. After an abortive attempt to restore her sanity and appetite at a friend's home in Vermont, the girl was sent to the asylum in Hartford where she began eating, albeit reluctantly, under the threat of tube feeding. When she returned home for a two-day visit, however, she resorted to her former behavior and refused to eat. After four months in the institution the girl seemed on the path to normalcy; she was discharged in the care of her family and remained on the outside for over a year and a half. Then she was returned to the asylum because she was acting strangely and again refusing food. This time tube-feeding was employed and Liza remained for another five months. She was discharged for the second time in March 1894 but was recommitted only a month later by her desperate father. Apparently her food refusal had begun anew: "[Liza] has remained at home since her discharge, and recently refused to eat; on account of which her father brings her back to the retreat."[16] However much the asylum was feared or despised, some families obviously did turn to it for assistance with chronically recalcitrant eaters.

Sitomania among High-Born Families

In 1859, in the *American Journal of Insanity*, William Stout Chipley (1810–1880) published the first American description of sitomania, a "phase of insanity" characterized by "intense dread of food." ("Sitomania" and "sitophobia," from *sitos*, Greek for grain, were interchangeable terms and they were included as diagnostic categories in American medical dictionaries.)[17] Chipley, who originally read his paper before colleagues at the Association of Medical Superintendents of American Institutions for the Insane, was chief medical officer of the Eastern Lunatic Asylum of Kentucky, then the oldest and largest public provision for the insane in the West.[18] His observations on sitomania were based on his clinical experience at that institution.

When Chipley took over as superintendent of the eastern Kentucky hospital, he found it grim and disorderly. His early administrative and medical efforts focused on establishing classifications of patients and arranging for their appropriate placement within the institution. Chipley's 1859 description of sitomania should be seen as part of a larger push by the early asylum superintendents for clarity in the classification and differentiation of mental diseases. It was also an expression of nineteenth-century asylum medicine's interest in enlarging the definition of insanity.

Chipley regarded sitomania as a phase of insanity "rather than a distinct form," and he cast the refusal to eat as a secondary symptom in various forms of insanity. Chipley said of food refusal: "It is remarkable that a feature of insanity of such frequent occurrence, and fraught with so much interest in the patient, and indescribable anxiety to the practitioner, should have received so little attention. Other phenomena of insanity, far less gráve and important, have received more attention, and become the subjects of elaborate research."[19] Chipley's clinical description of sitophobics made the usual distinctions between organic and moral causes, and in the latter category he elaborated the two most predictable types: those who feared poison in their food and those who sustained "belief in a divine command, or other supernatural direction, not to eat."

The significance of Chipley's commentary for the prehistory of anorexia nervosa is that he specified the existence of another type of food refuser: a young woman who was brought to the asylum as a result of parental concern and as a function of the family physician's inability to forestall the physical deterioration that accompanied her anorexia. Chipley's report called special attention to the behavior of a group rarely seen within the asylum: adolescent girls.[20] According to Chipley, food-refusing girls came to the asylum in a state of emaciation, always *after* treatment by their family doctor:

There is another description of cases met with by the general practitioner, but which do not ordinarily fall under the observation of our specialty [asylum superintendents] until they have so far progressed as to have ceased to be wholly mental—the digestive organs having become involved, and appearing then to be principally at fault. I allude to those cases in which a morbid desire for notoriety leads to protracted abstinence from food, in spite of the pangs of hunger, until all sustenance is refused. I have never witnessed a case of this kind except in females predisposed to hysteria.[21]

A British asylum doctor reported the same type of patient and suggested that admission to the asylum was in part a terrorizing technique. J. A. Campbell, for example, superintendent of the Garlands Asylum in Carlisle (England), told how the threat of forced feeding intimidated the adolescent patient: "Considerable numbers of girls in the hysteric state, who had refused food at home, when they were brought here, and the means and manner of giving it were explained to them, have at once given in and taken their food. I always make a point of taking such patients to see another fed with the pump."[22]

Despite the attribution of hysteria, sitophobics were not what we know as fasting girls. The sitophobe said she had no appetite or that eating distressed her, but she claimed no special powers. Neither did her parents make or supply any public pronouncements about the duration of her abstinence or her miraculous inspiration. Although sitophobes were the center of attention among close friends and relatives, they did not usually attract press coverage. Their forum was the private residence, the family, and their peers. Eating very little was their special accomplishment, a means of extracting sympathy and exerting power within a small circle of friends and associates.

Chipley railed against the sitophobic girl for seeking such attention, calling her manipulative behaviors an "attempt at imposition." He also berated her friends for their attentiveness, which, he said, further encouraged the refusal of food. Chipley believed that sitophobic behavior tied an impulse for extraordinary suffering to a desire for attention. In other words, these girls sought martyrdom: "Notoriety is the object—the poor gratification of being pitied and talked of as suffering in a manner and to an

extent which no other mortal ever endured, is the paltry reward
that lures the victim on to ruin and the grave." Chipley clearly
understood that the sitophobic girl found some moral certitude
in her denial and subsequent suffering but did not pursue the
psychology of the disorder any further. He was unequivocal,
however, in his conviction that sitophobic girls had a "desire to
excite the astonishment of the world" by abstinence from food.[23]

The unfortunate case of Miss —— demonstrated the natural
progress of sitophobia in the adolescent female. Here is Chipley's
insightful description of the patient's preoccupation with noneating:

> Of a delicate, nervous organization, [Miss ——] was a small eater,
> yet, save some disposition to moderate attacks of hysteria, she
> enjoyed good health. Unfortunately, on her return from a somewhat
> protracted absence from home, the small quantity of food consumed
> by her attracted unusual attention and remark, and awakened evi-
> dent anxiety on the part of her friends. She was not slow in per-
> ceiving that wonder and amazement grew inversely to the amount
> of food taken, and she did not fail to make herself the object of
> lively solicitude to all her numerous friends. The amount of food
> was diminished until finally she would pass whole days together
> without tasting a single morsel. To an observing eye it was evident
> that she had no more exquisite pleasure than that derived from the
> remarks of those who daily and freely discussed the wonders of her
> case in her presence, and with marked ingenuity she would manage
> to introduce the topic whenever visitors called, if it was not alluded
> to by others, without delay. After a long struggle, in spite of every
> effort to restrain her friends, and to wean her from her folly, she
> died . . . The autopsy revealed no material lesion except an extraor-
> dinary diminution in the capacity of the stomach—an effect, doubt-
> less, of the vicious habit that finally resulted in death.[24]

With organic disease eliminated as a cause of death by the
postmortem, Chipley used the case of the hysterical Miss —— to
argue that her "perverted actions [should be viewed] as evidences
of insanity." This suggestion meant that sitophobic girls should
come under the medical supervision of asylum doctors. The "vicious habit" of noneating was, from Chipley's perspective, reason
to institutionalize the sitophobe.[25] Only in the asylum could a full

arsenal of moral treatment and forced feeding be utilized to change the girl's behavior and save her life.

Chipley's attempt to expand the asylum's trade to include this type of patient was related to a social fact about sitophobic girls, that is, they came from middle-class families with sufficient resources to pay for medical services. "These cases are remarkable because they are almost peculiar to well-educated and sensible people, belonging to the higher walks of society." Calling the sitophobic daughters "high born and accomplished victims," Chipley pointed out that they enjoyed "all the advantages that wealth and station could confer."[26] (The girls were described as "delicate" and their friends as "sociable.") They were not the usual asylum clientele; consequently, Chipley found their refusal of food a particularly annoying form of profligacy.

It was the pathetic impotence of the protective parents that aroused Chipley's deepest empathy. These were good, right-minded people who were unable to moderate their daughter's extreme behavior: "The intense anxiety of a loving father, the deep indescribable agony of a devoted mother, the pallid cheeks and fast-falling tears of all who surround the couch, have no other effect on these subjects than that of incentives to carry the gross imposition to extreme lengths."[27] Unlike Evan and Hannah Jacob, the middle-class parents of a sitomaniac did not condone their daughter's behavior, finding no particular value or symbolic meaning in her rigid abstemiousness. These parents were allies of the physicians; they looked to medicine for a scientific explanation as well as day-to-day assistance in the management of a troublesome child with a willful compulsion to starve.

The fact that this kind of family and patient came within the purview of the public asylum reveals the level of desperation involved. Anxious to avoid the label of insanity and the stigma of institutionalization, most parents were extremely wary of the asylum as a place for their daughters. Whenever they could, people who aspired to middle-class respectability took their trade somewhere else—to specialists in private practice.

The asylum physician's experience with anorexia and his familiarity with forced feeding made him an appropriate person to treat the unyielding adolescent sitophobe. But for social as well as medical reasons he could not win her as a regular, paying patient, nor could he effectively cast her as insane. The girls described by William Chipley were certainly not as crazy as other food refusers within the asylum. They were not overtly delusional, they heard no voices, and they did not act indecently. Moreover, as long as emaciation did not become too extreme or threatening, a sitophobic girl could exist "on the outside," because many Victorian women and girls were notoriously poor eaters and fragility was widely cultivated.

There were other factors working against incorporation of this type of adolescent anorexia into the general lunacy trade: the bias against incarcerating the young; the stigma of institutionalization; the ability of middle-class and upper-class families to provide other more individualistic solutions, such as private "nervous" homes, spas, recuperative travel to therapeutic environments, and extended visits with relatives. The kind of youthful females who became sitophobic generally had the means (and milieu) to support their remaining outside an institution for the insane. Medical institutions—that is, hospitals without the stigma of a lunatic clientele—became an acceptable site of treatment only after severe emaciation occurred and family resources were strained. When the modern disease entity anorexia nervosa was named and identified, it recommended itself to physicians (and to families) precisely because it was a medical diagnosis that conformed to these clinical and social requirements.

Grosvenor Square Medicine

Little professional attention was paid to the existence or the description of Chipley's sitophobic girls. After 1873, as a result of two influential clinical reports—one from a famous London physician and the other from a reputable Paris neurologist—physicians began to talk about a special form of anorexia in girlhood. Until the 1920s and 1930s, however, American doctors used two terms almost interchangeably: "hysterical anorexia" (a reference to the neurological conception) and "anorexia nervosa."[28]

Anorexia nervosa might well have been called Gull's disease in that it is inextricably linked in English-language medicine to Sir William Withey Gull (1816–1890), an eminent London consultant who was an intimate of Queen Victoria and her family. Gull's power and prestige within Anglo-American medicine helped to transform a common medical symptom, lack of appetite, into a full-blown disease. For this reason our focus turns now to the London medical scene and to the professional and social circumstances that surrounded the first use of the diagnosis.

As a group, consultants such as Gull constituted a professional elite that dominated English medicine after 1860. They were fellows and members of the Royal College of Physicians and Surgeons; they were classically educated at Oxford, Cambridge, and the universities of London, Edinburgh, and Glasgow; they held posts in the large teaching hospitals, where they broadened their expertise, taught the next generation of medical men, and mingled with the aristocratic patrons who served on the hospital board. Although consultants saw poor, nonpaying patients in their hospital work, they built lucrative private consulting practices catering to the carriage trade. Not surprisingly, the intellectual authority and economic hegemony of the consultants was a source of enormous concern to other practitioners struggling for their livelihood and for professional recognition.[29]

The consultant's social advantages were buttressed by a widespread public perception that he knew more than the general practitioner about the science of medicine. (The consultant's higher fees reflected this understanding.) In fact, a central aspect of the career of the high-status doctor was publicly demonstrating what he knew, by contributing clinical findings to medical journals and participating in professional societies and associations where case histories and experiences were shared. Virtuosity as a doctor was demonstrated by successfully differentiating one disease from another; diagnostic acuity became a hallmark of success at the clinical level, making for prestige in the larger profession. This was William Withey Gull's primary accomplishment: he conceived of anorexia nervosa as a coherent disease entity distinct from starvation among the insane and unrelated to organic diseases such as tuberculosis, diabetes, or cancer. Furthermore, his disease had a very specific clientele: young women between the ages of sixteen and twenty-three.

In order to use Gull's nosology, a physician had to be clear on the question of differential diagnosis. When confronting an emaciated patient, the doctor basically had two tasks: elimination of organic disease as the cause of food refusal and starvation, and determination that the patient was not insane. In anorexia nervosa the patient's weight loss was not the result of any of the chronic wasting diseases that plagued nineteenth-century medicine. Typically, published case reports began by stating the explicit but incorrect disease the patient had been thought to have by the physician who had seen her previously (usually, a general practitioner and *not* a consultant).

The anorexia nervosa diagnosis also served to separate out the girlhood food refuser from those among the insane who would not eat. Sitophobia, the diagnosis proposed by Chipley in 1859, was a broad and imprecise subcategory of insanity in which adolescent girls were only one component. By contrast, anorexia nervosa was a discrete diagnosis associated with a specific age group and it suggested something important about the etiology of the behavior: lack of appetite was nervous (nervosa) in origin. It was evident, for example, that a patient diagnosed as having anorexia nervosa spoke of no divine commands; she heard no heavenly voices and saw no beatific visions. She was very thin primarily because she refused to eat. Thus, the nineteenth-century physician placed the girl with anorexia nervosa on "the borderline of insanity."[30] She was not crazy enough for the insane asylum, but she was too sick to remain without medical care. (In the language of contemporary psychiatry, she was neurotic rather than psychotic.)

Gull's anorexia nervosa diagnosis implied a moral or mental aberration rooted in the nervous system but exacerbated by the patient's age, her mode of life, or both. Medical notions that in the higher classes of society the adolescent female was prone to periodic bouts of hysteria underlay the diagnosis, as did the general idea that nervous disorders were themselves class based. For example, surgeon Sir Benjamin Brodie declared that he did not see hysterical conditions among females who "eat their bread in the sweat of their face."[31] Samuel Fenwick stated explicitly that anorexia nervosa was "much more common in the wealthier classes of society than amongst those who have to procure their bread by daily labor."[32]

The medical histories of the "first" British anorectics appear to confirm Fenwick's (and Chipley's) observation: the initial patients to be described by the diagnosis came from respectable, socially mobile families headed by tradesmen, artisans, civil employees, and the secondary professional classes. In other words, girls with anorexia nervosa were not themselves workers. They were drawn from families across the middle classes—from the lowest end, where social respectability was new or precarious, to more established families, with some modicum of financial security and an established social identity. In effect, these girls were privileged with some leisure even if they assisted their mother within the home.[33]

The English medical literature also reveals that these early anorectics had been seeking relief for some time, which indicates that their families had resources with which to engage medical care. Typically, the general practitioner, a local family doctor from the neighborhood or community, was the first professional to see the girl, probably in her home. Since most families sought to avoid institutionalization in a hospital or asylum, they were willing to follow many different suggestions from the general practitioner. Home remedies might include warm baths, massages, and deliberate attempts to stimulate the appetite with desirable tidbits such as delicate "sweeties" and "anchovy sandwiches."[34] In extreme cases forced feeding might be undertaken at home; in the doctor's office the patient was sometimes also subjected to the process of "faradising," stimulation with electrical shocks. Some families of a daughter who did not eat were urged to send her away from home, to a private medical facility or on a recuperative trip or visit, in the hope of restoring the appetite through a change of physical or social environment. In 1892 the daughter of a retired colonel was sent to the resort town of Brighton with two nurses because for some months she had "failed to take her food." When she returned home after nine weeks, she was still "queer in manner" and took to her bed. Within the month the young woman was sent away again to a "doctor's house in Hampshire."[35] This kind of peripatetic cure required some degree of discretionary income or else involvement in a social network where others had means enough to take in an extra person.

When the general practitioner could not stop the emaciation and the family was desperate, the next step was to seek the advice and counsel of a physician who was more expert, probably better educated, and likely to have wider clinical experience. That physician was found among the ranks of the consultants, or in some cases from among the specialists, a somewhat "lower order" of physician who built a reputation as an expert on a single disease or category of illness such as skin, eye, or throat afflictions; nervous disorders; or kidney stones.[36] Consultants and specialists, but not general practitioners, provided the bulk of contributions to the professional medical literature of the nineteenth century. Not surprisingly, then, the first diagnoses and clinical pictures of anorexia nervosa in England were presented by consulting physicians and specialists rather than by general practitioners. The specific experiences of general practitioners with individual food-refusing girls went virtually undocumented, despite the fact that general practice provided the conduit through which the patients passed into the hands of hospital consultants and specialists.

The consultants' empiricism and experience were strengthened and broadened through involvement with organizations such as the Clinical Society of London, a professional association founded in 1867 to promote exchange of the most up-to-date knowledge in both general medicine and surgery "by the collection of cases of interest, especially of such as bear upon undetermined questions in Pathology or Therapeutics." Members were nominated only by other members; the membership fee was substantial and standards of presentation had to conform to a certain protocol. At each meeting at least two clinical cases were discussed. A notice had to be filed with the association's secretary one week prior to the presentation, and all reports were expected to incorporate the following information in an established sequence: a record of the state of the patient when first observed; a statement of the personal and family history of the patient; a narrative of the illness while under observation; and a description of the patient when last seen or, in the event of a fatality, a postmortem report. To facilitate the exchange of information, every report was expected to have a similar format and to conclude with "explanatory remarks" or an "abstract." If the patient was not available, and there was no "microscopical or chemical analysis," other types of exhibitions were advised: casts, drawings, or photographs.[37]

William Withey Gull, an original member of the Clinical Society, qualified by virtue of his social status and his professional reputation. Despite modest beginnings (he was born the son of a barge owner and wharfinger in Colchester), Gull was by 1867 a "fashionable physician" in his early fifties, with an extensive private practice.[38] For over a decade he had been a consulting physician to Guy's Hospital, one of the city's renowned teaching institutions. He was also well-known among London medical men because he had been Fullerian professor of physiology at the Royal Institution from 1847 to 1849 and a joint lecturer on medicine at Guy's until 1865, when his private practice became too demanding. Most important, he was interested in how scientific knowledge could be incorporated into clinical practice. His views on this subject were valued enough so that in 1868, a year after the founding of the Clinical Society, he was asked to deliver the address in clinical medicine at the annual meeting of the British Medical Association.

In this prestigious and widely read lecture, Gull made a first preliminary reference to the disease which he would later call anorexia nervosa. The reference, however, was less than direct. As a way of illustrating general problems of differential diagnosis in abdominal disease, Gull spoke of the need to classify diseases on the basis of "cardinal facts" rather than inference. He wanted to diagnose by way of positive indicators instead of by their absence. To illustrate how negative diagnosis worked, Gull gave a number of examples including a passing reference to a nervous stomach condition—a kind of indigestion, which he called, then, hysteric apepsia: "We avoid the error of supposing mesenteric [intestinal] disease in young women emaciated to the last degree through hysteric apepsia, by our knowledge of the latter affection, and by the absence of tubercular disease elsewhere."[39]

Gull's colleagues were familiar enough with the condition to understand this single, casual reference to a genre of emaciation that at first glance might be thought to be due to tuberculosis, intestinal disease, or atrophy of the organs. The 1868 Oxford address was well received, but hysteric apepsia drew no particular attention at the time; it simply was not elaborated in any meaningful way.

Other significant happenings intervened before Gull turned his attention again to the issue of how to differentiate forms of emaciation in young women. These events marked Gull as a personage to be watched and they help to explain the sympathetic reception his diagnosis eventually received. In December 1871 Edward, the thirty-year-old heir to the British throne, contracted typhoid fever. The attention of the entire nation turned to Sandringham Palace, where the Prince of Wales lay ill. As his condition worsened, experts were called in, including William Gull and William Jenner, an associate at Guy's Hospital. (Jenner was actually an expert on the prince's disease; he had written about typhoid fever and its characteristic distinctions from typhus.)[40] Many hearts and minds were riveted on the royal bedside and the medical bulletins emanating from the team of doctors. As a supplement to scientific skills, prayers were ordered by a committee of ecclesiastical and civil authorities including Prime Minister William Gladstone. Throughout the nation, on December 10, 1871, special prayers were offered for restoration of the health of the heir. Four days later, on the tenth anniversary of the death of Victoria's husband, Prince Albert, the crisis passed and the Prince of Wales began to improve.

Naturally enough, some claimed that Edward's return to health vindicated the power of concerted, national prayer; others saw the victory against typhoid fever as proof of the power of modern medicine. In either case, William Withey Gull's performance at Sandringham marked him as a powerful "agent of mercy."

In Dr. Gull were combined energy that never tired, watchfulness that never flagged—nursing so tender, ministry so minute, that in his functions he seemed to combine the duties of physician, dispenser, valet, nurse—now arguing with the sick man [the Prince of Wales] in his delirium so softly and pleasantly that the parched lips opened to take scanty nourishment . . . now lifting the wasted body from bed to bed, now washing the worn frame with vinegar, with ever ready eye and ear and finger to mark any change and phase, to watch face and heart and pulse, and passing at times 12 or 14 hours at that bedside.[41]

Queen Victoria, impressed with the skill of the physicians who saved her son, made Gull a baronet in 1872 and later appointed him physician extraordinary to the queen and in 1887 physician in ordinary.[42]

Gull's relation to the queen and her children was professional but personal. The queen, who regarded Gull as a font of wisdom about general health, sent him numerous letters and telegrams requesting his advice (and intervention) when family members did not, in her view, rest adequately or took risks with their health. In one instance, in 1872, when the queen and her family were aboard the royal yacht *Osborne*, anchored off the Isle of Wight, Gull received a communiqué that revealed Victoria's dependence on him: "The queen has been expecting your telegram and is feeling in consequence of its not arriving very nervous."[43] The note from the *Osborne* was only one of many that showed how the queen's maternal anxieties about headaches and toothaches, dampness and cold, were soothed by Gull's professional advice. That Gull became an intimate of the royal family there is no doubt. He participated in birthday celebrations of the royal children and was invited to numerous state and private occasions.[44]

In his capacity as physician extraordinary to the queen, Gull was on retainer to the royal family but maintained a private practice as well. As Sir William, he joined the ranks of the nation's most elite doctors. In 1888 he was one of only nine doctors in the realm who held the rank of baronet. He traveled increasingly in aristocratic circles, circles that allowed, if not encouraged, the expression of literary interests—the true mark of a gentleman. According to a biographer, Gull was "fond of old and quaint literature," favoring Milton and George Herbert, but took little interest in contemporary social problems. Once, when asked what his politics were, he replied that they were the same as the queen's—"colourless." Ultimately, Gull was a conservative, even about the explanatory power of science: "To me life in all its phases seems but a revelation of more than it seems, and demonstratively so when I see that the moral law dominates the physiological laws ... I would rather believe in Moses and the Prophets than in the demonstration of science and logic as thus far exhibited."[45]

Gull's ideological conservatism, combined with his national reputation for medical excellence and closeness to "the royals," drew an affluent clientele. By 1873 he was one of the acknowledged stars of British scientific medicine with a lucrative practice operating from stylish Grosvenor Square. The *Lancet* said, "Dr. Gull is, at present . . . one of the most popular physicians in London."[46] Consequently, his decision to present case reports at the October 24th meeting of the Clinical Society provoked some real interest. If, according to procedure, Gull filed his intentions the week before, some members may have known that he intended to return to the problem of girlhood emaciation, but that he was now calling hysteric apepsia by another name: anorexia nervosa.

Misses A, B, and C

After an expression of sympathy for the passing of a colleague and a brief demonstration of a new gargling technique by a visiting French physician, Sir William read a paper of approximately 1,600 words entitled "Anorexia Hysterica."[47] The paper, which took about thirty minutes to read, was published shortly afterward as "Anorexia Nervosa (Apepsia Hysterica, Anorexia Hysterica)."

The address began with a reminder that Gull had mentioned girlhood emaciation five years before. He obviously wanted to establish his early preeminence in the discussion of this condition. In a verbal aside to his colleagues, he claimed that he appended a special note to the earlier 1868 address that said: "I have ventured to apply this term [hysteric apepsia] to the state indicated in the hope of directing attention to it." The evidence does not confirm Gull's claim that he had "staked out" the disease five years earlier as a serious, independent subject of study.[48] Given all the attention to the Jacob case in London newspapers and medical journals in 1869–1870, it is likely that Gull was ruminating about the phenomenon of anorexia and emaciation in young women and that he may even have known Robert Fowler, the London physician who visited the Welsh Fasting Girl.

By 1873 Gull was convinced that "anorexia" (lack of appetite) was a more correct term than "apepsia" (indigestion) because the food that was eaten, except in the last stages of the disease, was well digested. He admitted that a Paris neurologist, Charles Lasègue (1816–1883), had preempted his use of the term "anorexia" in an April 1873 publication, but claimed that he had thought about it earlier: "In the address at Oxford I used the term Apepsia Hysterica, but before seeing Dr. Lasègue's Paper, it had equally occurred to me that Anorexia would be more correct." Gull said virtually nothing at all about Lasègue's painstaking narrative description of the medical and mental stages of *l'anorexie hystérique*. Rather, he noted that Lasègue failed to cite Gull's 1868 address.[49] Gull was understandably cautious in his treatment of Lasègue. He could not ignore the French doctor's contribution, but he could not venerate it either without detracting from the importance of his own accomplishment. With utmost diplomacy, underwritten by professional self-interest, Sir William simultaneously set out his differences with Lasègue and embraced him as a colleague in arms.

As we shall see, the clinical descriptions of Gull and Lasègue differed enormously in emphasis. Gull's report was primarily medical, focusing on how the physician came to conclude that the condition involved "simple starvation" and no organic disease. Lasègue's commentary was psychological, outlining the mental stages through which patient and family passed in the course of the disease. Gull allowed that a "fatal termination of the malady" was possible; Lasègue, by contrast, wrote: "I have never yet seen an anorexia terminate directly in death."[50]

Gull's argument with Lasègue was not over the substance of the report or any particular medical assertion. Instead, Gull differed with Lasègue over the use of the term "hysterical," a label that technically implied a gender-specific condition. He rejected the designation "hysterical anorexia" because of its derivation from the Greek *hysteros*, meaning uterus. Lasègue's report, which treated *l'anorexie* as a "hysteria of the gastric center," was based on eight cases of women between the ages of eighteen and thirty-two; it did not mention men at all. Gull preferred "nervosa," because it implicated the central nervous system instead of the uterus and allowed that the condition could exist in males. "The subjects of this affection are mostly of the female sex, and chiefly between the ages of 16 and 23," he said, "[but] I have occasionally seen it in males at the same age."[51] (Gull never said anything more about male anorectics, nor did any other nineteenth-century writer on the subject.)

Gull's decision to abandon the term "hysterical" was also based on his uneasiness with the imprecision of the category, particularly its frequent use by neurologists. He did not, however, discard the common association between hysteria and female adolescence. Stating it somewhat differently, he wrote: "That mental states may destroy appetite is notorious, and it will be admitted that young women at the ages named [sixteen to twenty-three] are specially obnoxious to mental perversity. We might call the state hysterical without committing ourselves to the etymological value of the word, or maintaining that the subjects of it have the common symptoms of hysteria."[52] Ultimately, Sir William offered his French competitor a scholarly olive branch. He told his London audience that the real value of Lasègue's earlier paper on *l'anorexie hystérique* was that it constituted an independent verification of the same malady.[53]

Anxious to avoid the ambiguity and confusion that accompanied the hysteria diagnosis, Gull sought to establish the characteristics of a new disease entity based on positive medical indicators. For him the integrity of anorexia nervosa as an independent disease was substantiated in the medical process of differential diagnosis. Whenever an emaciated girl was brought to him, Gull performed the same diagnostic tasks. He looked first to determine the existence of disease or lesions in the chest or abdomen. Once tuberculosis and intestinal disease were eliminated, attention was paid to vital functions. Gull maintained that the diagnosis of anorexia nervosa could almost always be made on the basis of severe emaciation combined with observation of the pulse and breathing. (In such patients both were depressed and body temperature was slightly below normal.) Moreover, the catamenia (menses) failed to appear, part of a general lowering of the vital functions.

Gull attributed the anorectic's alleged lack of appetite to a morbid (diseased) mental state and not to gastric disorder of any kind. As to the specific cause of the mental state that destroyed the appetite, Gull made only a single statement that suggested his underlying sympathies for neurology. He said in a letter to a provincial general practitioner that he thought anorexia nervosa to be "essentially a failure of the powers of the gastric branches of the pneumogastric [vagus] nerve." Gull never pursued the neurological explanation further and tended to speak about anorexia nervosa as a "perversion of the will." Patients with anorexia nervosa "complained of no pain, nor indeed of any malaise, but were often restless and wayward."[54]

Gull presented three cases, all of young women between the ages of sixteen and twenty-three, who had been referred to him through general practitioners;[55] he had treated each on a private basis without resort to hospitalization of any kind. Along with the case studies, Gull exhibited a set of before-and-after photographs of Misses A, B, and C. "Before" showed the gaunt and doleful patient as she appeared at the period of her emaciation; "after" showed the patient in a normal state, with a certain roundness of face, as a result of her medical treatment.

In each of his case reports Gull focused on medical symptoms and eschewed the discussion of moral (mental) causes. The first of his 1873 cases, Miss A, came to Sir William's attention through a general practitioner and apothecary, Kelson Wright, who had a practice in Brixton-Rise, south of the Thames River.[56] Seventeen-year-old Miss A was severely emaciated: at 5 feet 5 inches she weighed only 82 pounds. Apparently Wright treated her perplexing lack of appetite with a variety of tonics, which he probably sold to her: preparations of cinchona, bichloride of mercury, syrups of the iodide of iron, and citrate of quinine. These medicines seemed to have no perceptible effect, for the hyperactive girl persisted in eating only tiny amounts of a very limited range of things. (Gull observed that Miss A had "complete anorexia for animal food, and almost complete anorexia for everything else.") Of her psychological state Gull said only: "There was some peevishness of temper, and a feeling of jealousy. No account could be given of the exciting cause."

Eighteen-year-old Miss B was brought to Sir William's private offices as a case of "latent tubercule." Sick and emaciated as she was, the supposedly tubercular girl craved physical activity, causing her mother to wonder why "she is never tired." On the basis of earlier medical advice, Miss B had spent two winters in southern Europe trying to rehabilitate herself. Gull disapproved of this particular therapeutic tactic and regarded the girl's continued emaciation as proof of its ineffectiveness. On trips such as these, he wrote, "willful patients are often allowed to drift their own way into a state of extreme exhaustion, when it might have been prevented by placing them under different moral conditions." Gull realized as soon as he saw Miss B that she did not have tuberculosis: her emaciation was too extreme, she had not menstruated in two years, and her pulse and respiration were nearly identical to Miss A.

Sir William saw fifteen-year-old Miss C as a referral from William Anderson, a doctor from Richmond who was an Edinburgh University graduate with some publications of his own.[57] Gull wrote a collegial letter to Anderson, explaining his diagnosis and citing his own work: "The case appears to be an extreme instance of what I have proposed to call 'Apepsia hysterica' or 'Anorexia nervosa.' (See 'Address on Medicine at Oxford,' 1868.)" Miss C shared physical characteristics with each of the other patients but she was also described as "obstinate." Dr. Anderson told Sir William that she "used to be a nice, plump, good natured little girl. Believe me . . ."

The photos of Misses A, B, and C captured the spirit of Dr. Anderson's comment. In their "before," or "sick," portraiture, each of the anorexic girls looked somewhat sullen; Misses A and B, in particular, had their heads turned, glancing downward, and their eyes and features were a bit off center. Miss C was unquestionably emaciated, and her accentuated jawline and profile were reminiscent of a willful young horse. In all of the "before" pictures there was a look of derangement, a look that was not present in the "after" portraiture, where the girls looked tranquil, pleasant, and ordinary. In their healthy state, each of the girls was more elaborately adorned with the accoutrements of middle-class femininity: cameos, earrings, hair ribbons, and curls. They assumed the demeanor proper to young women of their role and station and lost the look of dour petulance that Gull believed characterized the anorectic.

As therapy, Gull was insistent that medicines and tonics were really of no avail. "I do not at present prescribe medicines," he wrote, "because the nursing and the food are more important than anything else." In his view anorexic patients required a nourishing diet of milk, cream, soup, eggs, fish, and chicken to be administered at two-hour intervals by a trained nurse, when and if family resources made the nurse possible. Heavy clothing and "warm bed rest" along with external heat applied to the spine with a hot water bottle aided the digestive problems that accompanied severe inanition.

In order for Gull's nutritional program to be successful, the patient had to be willing to ingest small amounts of food and submit to those who supervised her. Although Gull never discussed his actual conversations with anorectics, he did suggest that both moral control of the patient and a change in her domestic relations were essential to a cure. Because he regarded the patient to be of "unsound mind," she forfeited her autonomy with respect to the issue of eating. Gull explained that "the inclination of the patient must be in no way consulted." Only medical concerns should govern her regimen, not the girl's fretfulness over being forced to eat or her parents' desire to avoid a scene. As a physician, Gull argued that he could not pander to the patient's perverse compulsion: "It is not unusual for the medical attendant to say, in reply to the anxious solicitude of the parents, 'Let her do as she likes. Don't force food.' Formerly I thought such advice admissible and proper, but larger experience has shown plainly the danger of allowing the starvation process to go on."

The best way to achieve the moral authority that a cure required was to separate a patient from her home environment. Gull said quite baldly that "relations and friends [are] generally the worst attendants." In the 1873 report Sir William made no systematic recommendations on how this new environment was to be achieved; it was not clear if home care by a doctor and a professional nurse was the best solution or if patients should be sent away to a medical facility. The existing historical evidence suggests that solutions were, of necessity, ad hoc and individualistic. Miss C, for example, became "plump and rosy as of yore" after spending a few months at Shanklin, on the Isle of Wight, with a trained nurse. In contrast, Miss A was monitored at home for two years by Sir William himself, until her "health was good" and she weighed 128 pounds.

Gull was essentially optimistic about the potential of moral as opposed to medical therapy: "The medical treatment probably need not be considered as contributing much to the recovery." Although he admitted to having seen death from anorexia nervosa, he asserted that however frustrating the situation was, "none of these cases . . . are really hopeless whilst life exists; and for the most part, the prognosis may be considered favorable." Gull's willingness to generalize about outcome and cure was based on his familiarity with the syndrome. "Such cases not unfrequently come before me," he said.

Gull's colleagues at the Clinical Society had enough experience with the disease to respond in the discussion period with examples of their own. Of the eight physicians who made substantive comments after the presentation, six stated explicitly that they had seen or treated what Gull called anorexia nervosa. One doctor described a case of some duration where the girl's "absolute loathing for food" eventually caused her to resemble a "dried mummy [rather] than a living being." Life was sustained by the physician's administration of "essence of meat" mixed with brandy and disguised as medicine. By way of indicating a general familiarity with this condition, the doctors also made reference to the Welsh Fasting Girl. One physician noted that Sarah Jacob was reportedly "restless and sleepless," much like a victim of anorexia nervosa.[58]

The doctors' discussion of Gull's lecture and photographs also showed that most medical men were conversant with the older idea that anorexia could result from a localized nervous affection. One member of the audience observed that "twenty years ago these cases [anorectics] used to be sent to Mr. [Morrell] MacKenzie," a noted specialist in the diseases of the throat.[59] Most of the commentators seemed to absorb Gull's central message that the anorexia in anorexia nervosa was essentially a mental rather than a medical condition. Still, because of the nature of the report, Gull's colleagues raised questions about why there was an aversion to food, whether or not the disease constituted insanity, and how anorexia nervosa should be managed. One physician who regarded the condition as a form of "autointoxication" spoke of girls who made food "horrible" to themselves by raising the "disgusting image" of "putrid cat pudding" [stuffed cat intestines] each time they were supposed to eat. Symes Thompson, who found it hard to "draw the line between such cases and insanity," admitted that he sent one food-refusing young woman to an asylum. There, under the proper moral treatment, she recovered; but after her release, she starved herself to death.[60] How should a doctor respond to this strange and potentially dangerous nervous condition? One member asked if forced feeding were not justifiable and appropriate, given the mental origin of anorexia nervosa; another doctor confirmed the importance of "altering surroundings" and told how, in two instances, his patients were "moved to another house."[61]

Sir William's response to the observations of his colleagues was selective and short. To the doctor who reported success with removing patients from their domestic environments, Gull said practically and simply, "We could not always send these patients from home."[62] Certainly some families would have neither the inclination nor the means to relocate their daughters. (Gull's next published report on anorexia nervosa, in 1888, involved a trained nurse from Guy's Hospital who was sent into the girl's home for two months in order to establish a nutritional and moral regimen.) Gull said nothing in reply to the questions about forced feeding or self-induced repugnance for food. What did provoke an answer from him was the question about where anorexia nervosa stood in relation to hysteria and insanity. Gull answered succinctly that there was "no great amount of hysteria [in anorexia nervosa] but it could hardly be called insanity" either.[63] This was a reply that fit Sir William's basic purpose: to define anorexia nervosa as an independent disease to be treated outside the mental asylum.

5 · Love and Food in the Bourgeois Family

By the late nineteenth century, middle-class families were distinguished by their declining size and the way in which they nurtured their children. Increasingly, middle-class sons and daughters in the United States, England, and France lived with their parents until they married (typically in their early twenties) and moved to a home of their own. This period of dependency, generally known as adolescence, distinguished the middle class from the working class and the poor, who of necessity lived and labored outside the natal home, even in childhood. As a result of the intensification of family life (that is, fewer people and longer residency), middle-class children received more parental attention and closer scrutiny. In this environment middle-class children became "emotionally priceless" at the same time as they became economically useless.[1]

Young women were perceived as reaping the greatest benefits from the protections provided by this middle-class Christian family style. In the child-centered nuclear family mothers and daughters were proudly and symbolically set apart from market activity and wage labor of any kind. Domestic production slowed; women and girls in this class could buy (rather than make) the things they needed and desired. Those able to spend adolescence and young adulthood in this environment were considered safe from the characteristic pitfalls of their age group—premature romances and sexual exploitation. Medical men encouraged girls to delay marriage until their early twenties on the grounds that pelvic development was incomplete until then. It was also said that girls

who did not work and lived at home with their mothers and *True Womanhood*
fathers were less likely to be tarnished by the ways of the world.[2]

The middle-class economic umbrella did in fact constitute a form of protection from early marriage and from the exigencies of laboring outside the home. Middle-class English girls were not swept out of the home by precocious marriages aimed at effecting the union of grand estates (as was frequently the case with the landed gentry); neither were middle-class girls forced by chronic scarcity to leave their parents and siblings prematurely for dependency as a wife or for domestic service in another domicile.[3] In effect, young women from the middle classes in the United States, England, and France enjoyed a period of prolonged dependency in which their parents, if so inclined, might lavish affection and energy on them.

The bourgeoisie was self-congratulatory about what this situation (along with ample money) implied for girls. Few stopped to consider that the haven that sheltered young women from the heartless world had its own set of problems.[4] In fact, there was little recognition of the ways in which prolonged dependency and intensification of parent-child relations could generate their own psychopathologies.

For this reason Charles Lasègue's 1873 description of *l'anorexie hystérique* is an important document in the history of childhood and the family as well as in the history of medicine.[5] It was Lasègue, not William Gull, who provided the first real glimpse of the pressurized family environment in anorexia nervosa. Unlike Gull, who hoped to isolate a new disease, Lasègue was part of an influential group in early French psychiatry—the *médecins-alienistes*—who were interested in delineating each of the symptomatic groups under the broad rubric of hysteria. By 1873 Lasègue was chairman of clinical medicine at La Pitié Hospital, coeditor of the *Archives générales de médecine* (a leading French journal), and author of at least two articles on hysterical disorders.[6] *L'anorexie hystérique* was, in his view, a "hysteria of the gastric center," a form of hysterical localization in keeping with the general digestive disturbances, curious appetite, and "mutism" that doctors observed in hysterical patients.[7] With respect to the issue of classification, Lasègue was derivative in that he followed the neurologists. But in the matter of clinical observation and social description, Lasègue's paper stands out as an original and insightful psychiatric contribution.

Unlike Gull, who concentrated on the strictly medical aspects of differential diagnosis, Lasègue provided some entrée into the private world of middle-class families and their relationships with their daughters. Even though his portrait was rooted in the specific texture of French social life, the outlines and perspective are clear and they point in an important direction. The prolongation of dependency seemed to add to the intensity of parental love and set the stage for anorexia nervosa in middle-class daughters. Among the bourgeoisie, adolescent girls who refused to eat had the power to disrupt their families. A girl who declined the food provided by her family became the focus of conversation and concern; her appetite, her diet, and her body became a preoccupation in the child-centered family.

In anticipation of what we now call "family system's theory," Lasègue wrote: "It must not cause surprise to find me thus always placing in parallel the morbid [diseased] condition of the hysterical subject and the preoccupations of those who surround her. These two circumstances are intimately connected, and we should acquire an erroneous idea of the disease by confining ourselves to an examination of the patient." Lasègue's emphasis on family interactions in *l'anorexie hystérique* was based on his experiences in private practice, treating the families of the Paris bourgeoisie. Throughout his report the family was omnipresent, providing an illuminating backdrop for the emotional struggle over eating. Lasègue's attention to his patient's relations with her family and friends confirmed what Gull's work only suggested: that anorexic women came from families willing and able to expend emotional and financial resources on them. Lasègue was the first nineteenth-century physician to suggest that food refusal constituted a form of intrafamilial conflict between the maturing girl and her parents.

A deep sensitivity to food and its meanings also underlay Lasègue's astute clinical portrait of the anorectic and her family. Lasègue was, after all, a member of the French bourgeoisie, a class notable for its commitment to the importance of cuisine and eating. For the French, cuisine had great import; the unexplained

rejection of attractive foods was a decidedly strange and provocative act. Lasègue marveled, "I have seen [an anorectic] chewing
morsels of rhubarb whom no consideration would have induced
to taste a cutlet." In effect, it took a Frenchman, convinced of the
manifold delights of the palate, to suggest the basic connection
between love and food in the making of anorexia nervosa.

The Three Stages of L'anorexie

According to Lasègue, *l'anorexie hystérique* typically began between the ages of fifteen and twenty as the result of some "emotional cause" which the patient might either "avow or conceal."
The exact nature of these precipitating emotional stresses was
hard to ascertain, because physicians at this point in time recorded
little direct testimony from their patients. Lasègue always supposed that they were connected to "some real or imaginary marriage proposal" or to "a violence done to some sympathy, or to
some more or less conscient desire." In effect, Lasègue was relating
the onset of anorexia nervosa to a broad set of frustrations that
we would link with the transition to adulthood: inappropriate
romantic expectations, blocked educational or social opportunities, struggles with parents. The natural course of the disease was
never less than eighteen to twenty-four months but it evolved in
three distinct stages, each with a set of characteristic medical and
emotional developments.

In stage 1, the young woman began to express a general uneasiness after eating. These complaints were largely somatic: "vague
sensations of fullness" or "suffering after commencement of the
repast." Always attentive to the medical dimensions of the situation, Lasègue noted that the pain had some special characteristics:
it was sudden and unrelated to the type of food eaten, and it was
generally unaccompanied by either vomiting or any impairment
of intestinal functions (except habitual constipation). "Gradually,
she reduces her food," Lasègue wrote, "furnishing pretexts sometimes in a headache, sometimes in a temporary distaste, and sometimes in the fear of a recurrence of pain after eating." Days turned
into weeks, yet the patient's anorexia continued. "Meal after meal
is discontinued . . . and almost always some article of diet is

successively suppressed, whether this be bread, meat or certain vegetables—sometimes one alimentary substance being replaced by another, for which an exclusive predilection may be manifested for weeks together." When the food repertoire was reduced to almost nothing, Lasègue said "The disease is now declared."

Surprisingly, in stage 1 the patient's general health remained satisfactory. Despite the fact that she ate less than one-tenth of a normal diet, there was no emaciation. The slow process of inanition was, however, accompanied by observable hyperactivity. Lasègue wrote of this phase: "[The] abstinence tends to increase the aptitude for movement. The patient feels more light and active, rides on horseback, receives and pays visits, and is able to pursue a fatiguing life in the world." Lasègue's typical anorexic patient was a leisured young woman who pointed to her social calendar as proof that she was really quite well and that abstinence from food constituted a sound personal policy, no matter how upsetting it might be to her parents. Although she was characteristically "docile" about taking medicine from a physician, she was obstinate about not eating meals at home.

Despite the lack of any overt illness and the girl's consistent activity, the family obviously disliked and feared the behavior pattern emerging in stage 1. Family dining, a centerpiece of middle-class French life, was inevitably altered if one member of the group consistently refused to eat despite the coaxing of others. In stage 1 most parents tried to entice the food-refusing girl into eating by either (1) offering highly desirable or favorite foods in the hope of activating the appetite or (2) asserting that eating, as opposed to noneating, was an expression of filial love. Lasègue's observations of the difficulties surrounding eating suggest that the frustration of French parents was intense and that some vacillated between spoiling and punishing the girl. Usually the parents pushed for compromises, but they were rendered ineffective by the patient's staunch resistance to anything more than token cooperation. The painful interactions of parents and anorexic daughters in stage 1 was described by Lasègue:

The family has but two methods at its service which it always exhausts—entreaties and menaces—and which both serve as a touchstone. The delicacies of the table are multiplied in the hope of

[margin handwritten note: make problem worse / food = acceptance]

stimulating the appetite; but the more solicitude increases, the more the appetite diminishes. The patient disdainfully tastes the new viands, and after having thus shown her willingness, holds herself absolved from any obligation to do more. She is besought, as a favor, and *as a sovereign proof of affection,* to consent to add even an additional mouthful to what she has taken; but this *excess of insistence begets the excess of resistance.* (Italics added.)

Lasègue obviously understood the manner in which the middle-class French reverence for cuisine fueled the manipulative politics of anorexia nervosa. The parents hoped to coax their child back to normalcy through the presentation of gifts in the form of irresistible foods.[8] Middle-class French mothers and their cooks catered to the individual tastes of the patient, usually to no avail; delectable creations viewed with relish by the normal had no effect on the impassivity of the anorectic. Sometimes, in order to demonstrate her good intent, and to acknowledge that the culinary gift was not entirely without merit, the girl allowed herself a single taste of the proffered food, but she did not relent in her underlying commitment to starvation. Even the acknowledged delicacies of the bourgeois French table could not persuade her to eat.

At this point anxious parents sought to induce guilt for non-eating by making eating an act of love, a "sovereign proof of affection." If she loved her parents, the girl was told, she would abandon her compulsion to refuse food and begin normal alimentation. For Lasègue the fact that she did not respond affirmatively to this provocative proposition signified that the mental perversion was firmly in place. In stage 1, Lasègue advised that a "prudent course" for the doctor was "to observe, to keep silent, and to remember that when voluntary inanition dates from several weeks it has become a pathological condition, having a long course to run."[9]

In stage 2, the physician remained in the background as the patient's mental state intensified and her anorexia became the "sole object of preoccupation and conversation." Distressed families of girls in this stage spoke "mournfully . . . all day and to the first comer . . . of the girl's food."[10] The patient was "surrounded by a kind of atmosphere from which there [was] no escape . . . Friends join[ed] counsel with relatives, each contributing to the common stock."[11] Undoubtedly, the disease was partially structured by the young woman's social milieu. "By the force of sentiments as much as by the necessities caused by new sufferings, the hysterical subject has been constituted really a sick person, no longer taking part in the free movements of common life."

Because the anorectic was the center of attention, her malaise hardened, resulting, said Lasègue, in a form of "pathological contentment" with her situation: "Not only does she not sigh for recovery, but she is not ill-pleased with her condition." In stage 2, reports of physical discomfort after eating stopped; the anorectic, in fact, believed that her food refusal was working a cure. Consequently, in this stage a patient typically agreed to join her family at meals if she set the terms. She would come to the table "on the condition that she [would be] allowed to take only what she wishe[d]." She sat there, visible but abstemious, and allegedly indifferent to the quality, quantity, or attractiveness of the fare her family provided.

Lasègue likened the "satisfied assurance" of the stage 2 anorectic to the "obstinacy of the insane" and marveled at the "inexhaustible optimism" that led the girl to believe that she could continue to refuse indefinitely all but the tiniest morsels of food. Lasègue captured the shift from stage 1 to stage 2 in the patient's own words. He said that in the initial weeks of the disease he repeatedly heard the monotonous formula, "I cannot eat because I suffer." But in stage 2 the patient ritualistically explained that she did not need to eat: "I do not suffer, and must then be well." Both parents and physicians warned the increasingly thin young woman that her refusal of food could lead to serious illness or death. The patient with anorexia nervosa did not heed such warnings and ignored those physical changes that were already apparent: in stage 2 menstruation was becoming "irregular or insufficient," and chronic constipation no longer responded to common purgatives.

In stage 3, the physical deterioration of the patient became explicit, generating fear among her family and friends. Emaciation, debility, and anemia all began to appear. Lasègue described a spectrum of additional physiological consequences: amenorrhea, chronic thirst, dry and pale skin, unremitting constipation, atrophied stomach, anemia, vertigo, and fainting. The patient was spending more and more time alone, lying down, because exercise of any kind was now "laborious." "The appearance of these signs," wrote Lasègue, "the import of which can escape no one, redoubles anxieties, and the relatives and friends begin to regard the case as desperate." If to this point families had not sought experienced medical personnel, most now did so. Significantly, the patient began to be influenced by the fear that was in the air. The observable dismay and terror of family and friends led the patient to consider that she could die. "The young girl begins to be anxious from the sad appearance of those who surround her, and for the first time her self-satisfied indifference receives a shock."

At this juncture the physician was able to enter the case and assume his proper role as expert and moral authority. Lasègue painted the prospects of the stage 3 patient this way:

> Two courses are now open . . . She either is so yielding as to become obedient without restriction, which is rare; or she submits with a semi-docility, with the evident hope that she will avert the peril [of death] without renouncing her ideas and perhaps the interest that her malady has inspired. The second tendency, which is by far the more common, vastly complicates the situation.

Lasègue never detailed the specifics of his moral or nutritional treatment of anorectics; rather, he mentioned how hard it was to reestablish regular functioning in an atrophied stomach.[12] (Reportedly, he had seen some former victims of anorexia nervosa who were still not eating "like other people" even after a decade.) Change came slowly, he said, and by "successive starts." Although he personally had never seen death from anorexia nervosa, he was aware of the possibility; therefore, familial anxieties were "well-founded" and medical "perplexities" justified. *L'anorexie hystérique* was not, after all, an exotic syndrome. Among the French bourgeoisie, at least, Charles Lasègue found the recalcitrant food-refusing girl "too often observed to be a mere exceptional occurrence."[13]

The fact that the food refuser was almost always a girl made the phenomenon and the parental response even more interesting. If we conceptualize anorexia nervosa as a set of continuing inter-actions that involve parent as well as child, food offering as well as food refusal, then the diagnosis made a statement about the willingness of middle-class parents to commit emotional and fi-nancial resources to adolescent daughters. Because anorexic girls were not ignored or sloughed off as superfluous children, the emergence of the diagnosis confirmed the breakdown of patriar-chalism in its most extreme form: daughters as well as sons were asserting emotional and economic claims on the late-nineteenth-century family.

But daughters sacrifice their health for it.

I disagree; anorexics are responding to patriarchy by becoming the "perfect woman"

A Middle-Class Psychopathology

In nineteenth-century middle-class society, parents gave gifts of a material nature to their children as an expression of their love and as a concomitant to their social status.[14] In this very funda-mental way love and one of the most basic gifts—food—were intimately connected. Children who refused to eat constituted an affront to their parents as well as a danger to themselves. The work of Charles Lasègue, more than that of any other nineteenth-century doctor, captured the unhappy rhythm of repeated offer-ings and refusals that signaled the breakdown of reciprocity be-tween parents and their anorexic daughter. In this context an-orexia nervosa can be seen for what it is: a striking dysfunction in the bourgeois family system.

What was the intrafamilial struggle in anorexia nervosa all about? Why did parental insistence beget resistance rather than compliance? What kind of emotional leverage or power did the stubborn noneater have over her family and friends? What issues posed potential emotional problems for the "first generation" of anorectics? The nature of the nineteenth-century bourgeois family, in particular the role of adolescent daughters, was the key. The shape and texture of Victorian domestic life, including the pattern of nurturance, demonstrate the relation of family form and values to the behavioral pattern in anorexia nervosa.

Lasègue's 1873 description of anorexia nervosa, along with other nineteenth-century medical reports, suggested that confused or unfulfilled expectation in the domain of courtship was a common precipitating agent in the mental disorders of adolescent women. (Lasègue specified "real or imaginary marriage project[s]" in the etiology of the disease.) To view this common problem as the momentary by-product of a particular male's rejection is to miss the point. In many families pressures to marry were sufficiently intense to generate unhappiness and provoke hostile behaviors.[15] Both the love and the social ambition of middle-class parents could make adolescence a difficult time for daughters.

Although marriage was delayed, it was not "out of mind" for parents or daughters. It was the backdrop against which most young women played out their future; the fact that it was oftentimes beyond their control made the subject of marriage (to say nothing of the actual prospect) a source of emotional stress. Because the match reflected on the family, middle-class girls were under considerable scrutiny in their peer relations and many experienced intense pressures associated with becoming a "proper" kind of woman and making an appropriate if not advantageous marriage. Although middle-class girlhood was often idealized (especially in America), many understood the pressures incumbent upon this particular stage of life: "I do not think that girlhood is always such a very happy time; at least not to thoughtful girls."[16]

Ambitious parents surely understood that by marrying well, at an appropriate moment, a daughter, while she did not carry the family name, might be an important instrument of family aspirations—particularly in a burgeoning middle-class society. The forms of wealth and status for this class were more diverse than simple inheritance of land, as in marriages of the upper class. Good daughters at least considered how a marriage might affect or enhance the family's position. As a result, marriage probably loomed large in the life of a dutiful middle-class daughter: it was the event for which she was continually being prepared, and a desirable outcome depended on the ability of the parents and the girl to work together, that is, to state clearly what each wanted or to read each other's heart and mind. Good will between parents and their daughters was essential for a happy resolution. In the very best scenario, love and economic aspiration were joined; but we know this was not always accomplished.[17] In the context of marital expectations, a daughter's refusal to eat was a provocative rejection of both the family's aspirations and their good will toward her. All of the family's plans for her future (and theirs) could be stymied by her peculiar and unpleasant alimentary nihilism.

In an era when domestic food consumption was increasing and culinary standards were escalating, refusing to eat must have been an unabashedly antisocial act.[18] Family meals assumed enormous importance in the bourgeois milieu, in the United States as well as in France. The ambience of the meal symbolized the spirit and values of the family: "Simple, healthy food, exquisitely prepared, and served upon shining dishes and brilliant silverware, with snowy napkins, and glistening goblets, a gentle blessing, and cheerful conversation, embrace the sweetest communions and the happiest moments of life." Among the middle class it seems that eating correctly was emerging as a new morality, one that set its members apart from the working class. A neatly set table, one American author wrote, "inspires" in a way "we cannot feel when dining from rough boards."[19] Given that a large proportion of social time centered around the table, an anorectic's annoying refusal was probably endured at least two or three times a day. In fact, anorexic behavior was antithetical to the very ideal of bourgeois eating. "Heated discussion and quarrels, fretfulness and sullen taciturnity while eating, are as unwholesome as they are unchristian."[20]

Clinical reports suggest that anorexic behavior seemed to be most difficult for middle-class mothers, probably because of their significant investment in making family meals both attractive and pleasant.[21] But there were other reasons: for one thing, Victorian mothers, rather than fathers, assumed primary responsibility for helping their daughters develop a suitable social identity and moral character. This maternal involvement was reflected in the popularity of late-nineteenth-century advice books, which depicted mothers as the best guide for helping a girl traverse the difficulties of puberty and adolescence. Much of the advice to mothers centered on the hygiene of puberty: how girls should eat and exercise, how they should bathe and fix their hair, and what they should be told about menstruation and adult heterosexuality.[22] By the late nineteenth century the bourgeois mother was no longer even a midwife to her daughter in childbirth. She gave that role to professional medicine and became, instead, a midwife to her daughter's social persona. Because she was so actively engaged in managing her daughter's physical growth, appearance, and moral development, the middle-class mother had a significant investment in how her daughter fared in the marriage market. A daughter was, after all, an extension of the mother. To see her consistently refuse food was hurtful and frustrating indeed.

Chodorow separation individuation

Above and beyond the specific anxieties generated by marital pressure, the Victorian family milieu in America and in Western Europe harbored a mélange of other tensions and problems that constituted emotional preconditions for the emergence of anorexia nervosa. As love replaced authority as the cement of family relations, the new edifice developed a particular set of structural problems. Middle-class family life and the ideology of unreserved love began to generate its own set of emotional disorders.

For example, possessiveness was definitely a problem in Victorian family life.[23] Where love between parents and children was the prevailing and avowed ethic, there was always the risk of excess. Where love became suffocating or manipulative, individuation and separation from the family could become extremely painful, if not impossible. Increased intimacy with children, a concomitant to the ethic of family love, could also lead to debilitating forms of psychological interdependence, for parents as well as for children.

In the context of increased intimacy, adolescent privacy was especially problematic. Parents and their sexually maturing children had to maneuver over what constituted an appropriate degree of privacy. Middle-class girls, for example, almost always had their own rooms or shared them with sisters, but they had greater difficulty establishing autonomous psychic space.[24] The well-known penchant of adolescent girls for novel reading was an expression of their need for imaginative freedom, yet many parents and educators in this era decried both the hours girls "wasted" in reading and the effusive emotions these romantic idylls seemed to generate. Some parents recognized that their daughters needed channels for expressing emotions so they encouraged private diary keeping. But some of the same parents who gave lovely marbled diaries as gifts also monitored their use and restricted their content.[25] Because mothers and daughters were supposed to be especially close, some daughters may have been subjected to socially acceptable (but privately intolerable) forms of possessive behavior that rankled and allowed little room for independent growth. Since emotional freedom was not a common prerogative of the Victorian adolescent girl, it seems reasonable to assert that unhappiness was likely to be expressed in nonverbal forms of behavior. One such behavior was refusal of food.

The use of noneating as a form of expression was not, however, unique to the child. As corporal punishment declined as a technique in the control of children, new forms of emotional or moral discipline took the place of the rod, the slipper, and the leather thong. In the middle-class home of late-nineteenth-century Britain, for example, food was the "favorite method" of punishment "other than beating."[26] Because food was readily available, it constituted a resource that could be manipulated by both parent and child. In effect, each generation could use food and appetite against the other.

This was particularly true in the treatment of young children, who were routinely sent to bed without supper or refused a special sweet because they had been "bad." Denial of food was an easy, accessible parental weapon against the misbehaving child. Middle-class parents prided themselves on providing ample food for their children. Yet when a child's behavior required it, they chose to let the child go unfed, that is, with the appetite unfulfilled. This disciplinary strategy was in keeping with a conception of the appetite as a representation of the child's will. "An almost universal tenet, was that [Victorian] children should never be allowed to ask for anything, or to express a preference, but simply to eat what was set before them."[27]

At the same time, food was used to express love in the bourgeois household. Offering attractive and ample food was the particular responsibility and pleasure of middle-class wives and mothers. "Every grandmother shows her affection," wrote George and Susan Everett in 1875, "by loading the plate and urging us to eat."[28] If a child's appetite was a naughty expression of will that must not be catered to, it was also an expression of loving reciprocity and healthy engagement with its mother, the primary feeder. In America the feeding of middle-class children, from infancy on, was a maternal concern that was considered inappropriate to delegate to wet nurses, domestics, or governesses.[29] Family meals were expected to be a time of instructive and engaging conversation. "Ideas are the choicest spices and flavors at table," wrote one domestic adviser.[30] Children and young adults were not expected to direct or dominate the dinner-table conversation, but instead to be attentive and answer when questions were directed to them. Participation was expected on both a gustatory and a verbal level.

When an adolescent daughter became sullen and chronically refused food at table, the behavior was therefore very threatening and confusing. On the one hand, the girl was perceived as willfully manipulating her appetite as a younger child might do. Because parents did not want to encourage this behavior, they often refused at first to indulge the favorite tastes or caprices of their daughter. As emaciation became visible and the girl looked sick, many violated the canon of prudent child rearing and put aside their moral objections to pampering the appetite. Eventually they begged their daughter to eat whatever she liked—but eat she must, "as a sovereign proof of affection" for them. From the parents' perspective, a return to eating was a confirmation of filial love.

The efficacy of food refusal as an emotional tactic within the family depended on food's being plentiful, pleasing, and connected to love. Anorexia nervosa required a certain standard of family provisioning and a regularity of fare for the girl's rejection of food to have any meaning. Where food was eaten simply to assuage hunger, where it had only minimal aesthetic and symbolic messages, or where the girl had to provide her own nourishment, refusal of food was not particularly noteworthy or troublesome. In contrast, the patient with anorexia nervosa was surrounded by a provident, if not indulgent, family that was distressed by her refusal of their largesse.

In an environment such as this, where love and food were easily conflated, some troubled young women found it effective to stop eating. Refusing food at the family dinner table was a silent but potent form of expression that fit within the Victorian conception of decorum at table. Refusing to eat was not as confrontational as yelling, having a tantrum, or throwing things; refusing to eat expressed emotional hostility without being flamboyant. Refusing to eat had the advantage of being ambiguous. If a girl repeatedly claimed lack of appetite, she might indeed be ill and therefore entitled to special treatment and favors.

Anorexia nervosa was an intense form of nonverbal discourse that honored the emotional guidelines governing the middle-class Victorian family. In her own way, the anorectic respected what historian Peter Gay called "the great bourgeois compromise between the need for reserve and the capacity for emotion."[31] Food refusal, while an emotionally charged behavior, was also discreet, quiet, and ladylike, in keeping with the Victorian notion that women were expected to "carry reserve further than the male."[32] The unhappy adolescent girl, who was in all other ways a dutiful daughter, chose food refusal from within the symptom repertoire available to her. Precisely because she was not a lunatic, she selected a behavior that she knew had some efficacy within her own family. Middle-class parents, especially mothers, were predictable in their responses: they consistently offered more food and more love in the face of the girl's compulsion to starve. To have anorexia nervosa, the adolescent girl had to be privileged both emotionally and materially by her family.

6 · Therapeutic Intervention

American and British doctors were familiar with William Gull's "new" disease. Samuel Wilks (1824–1911), a well-respected pathologist and consultant at Guy's Hospital, said that he had seen at least three "good examples" of anorexia nervosa, one of which he described as "the thinnest person I have ever seen." James Barnes Adams, a surgeon with offices on Harley Street (London's medical row), welcomed Gull's 1873 report because it was so relevant, "especially among those [of us] whose duty it is daily to minister to such cases." For metropolitan practitioners in both Britain and the United States, anorexia nervosa was a familiar and fascinating phenomenon. According to William Smoult Playfair (1836–1903), a prominent obstetrician with experience in the treatment of nervous diseases, "the particular type Sir William Gull describes is . . . [a] very common occurrence." Playfair was so interested in the disease that he compiled a scrapbook of patients. In 1888 he wrote, "I possess a whole album of photographs which would cap those which Sir William has engraved [published]."[1]

Medical journals after 1873 were peppered with articles and letters based on experiences with anorexia nervosa in private practice and in hospitals. In these, doctors substantiated the pattern of physical symptoms described by William Gull. Physicians agreed almost unanimously on the medical characteristics: in addition to lack of appetite and emaciation, the most significant physical markers were amenorrhea, low body temperature, and hyperactivity. Doctors described anorectics who leaped and danced in their bedrooms before daybreak, some who did somersaults in bed, and others who were caught up in a frenzied pattern of good works: "A young woman thus afflicted [with anorexia nervosa], her clothes scarcely hanging together on her anatomy . . . this wan creature, whose daily food might lie on a crown piece, will be busy with mother's meetings, with little sister's frocks, with university extension, and with what else of unselfish effort, yet on what funds God only knows."[2] The fact that the emaciated anorectic was so active was taken to mean that she suffered from a moral (mental) rather than an organic illness.

Victorian physicians, who explained symptoms by reference to personality traits believed to be characteristic of the patient type, attributed hyperactivity in anorexia nervosa to the basic perversity of the female adolescent. They reasoned that the perpetual movement of the patient was a conscious strategy to discredit the assertions of parents and doctors that food was necessary for the maintenance of physical strength. The anorectic (like the fasting girl) made a false claim that she did not need to eat. From the physician's perspective she was desperately trying to "assert her good health."[3] Anorexic hyperactivity was, then, an expression of the latent spitefulness of adolescent women.

Because the etiology was unknown, the published literature on anorexia nervosa concentrated on treatment of the primary symptom (noneating) rather than its cause. Explanations of the cause fell into some fairly predictable categories: a few doctors, usually neurologists, advocated strictly somatic interpretations (that lack of appetite and digestive power arose from the failure of the gastric nerves); many suggested emotional or nervous upset (that lack of appetite was brought on by a particular incident or unpleasantness in the girl's personal life); a small number proposed broad-ranging cultural explanations (that lack of appetite reflected the pressures of the modern age and were linked to new aspirations on the part of girls).

But the most prevalent and widely held nineteenth-century explanation of anorexia nervosa rested on the idea that the patient refused to eat in order to attract attention. This craving for sympathy was regarded as a basic characteristic of hysterical behavior in females of all ages. (Robert Fowler explained Sarah Jacob in these terms; William Hammond did the same in the case of Mollie Fancher.) Samuel Gee stated the principle explicitly: "[Anorexia nervosa] seems to arise from a morbid excess of that craving for sympathy which is common to all mankind, as is especially strong in the female sex."[4]

Victorian physicians faulted families, as well as girls, for their complicity in the behavior. In anorexia nervosa the family was portrayed as weak, pandering to the demands of a spoiled adolescent daughter. Thomas Stretch Dowse said that his patient "had been allowed to do nearly as she liked"; William Smoult Playfair spoke of "injudicious sympathy" of the parents; Lockhardt Stephens described the anorectic as the "spoilt child in the family"; Timothy McGillicuddy called the mother and father "indulgent"; Charles Féré told of parents who "submit themselves to all her caprices"; Samuel Gee hoped to redirect all the "solicitude of the family" away from the girl; and Clifford Allbutt lamented the ineffectiveness of the parents in their domestic environment: "At meal times her mother may cry, her father may storm, her friends may banter [but] the cheerful reply never fails, that she has eaten amply."[5] Physicians were observing what Lasègue was the first to describe—a family that allowed emotional demands to be expressed around issues of food and appetite.

The failure of parents to assert their moral authority was presented in a nearly formulaic way. In the face of their daughter's persistent rejection of food, mothers typically cried and fathers characteristically raised their voice or uttered threats. The principle that the family responded incorrectly to the girl's perverse behavior superseded any consideration of the idea that the family made her so unhappy that she could not eat. No attention was paid to the patient's unconscious or to the unstated meanings of food; neither was the anorectic cast as depressed or melancholic.[6] In general, it was assumed that families able to provide necessities, as well as leisure, protection, and guidance, met all the legitimate needs of their daughters.

Medical concentration on the parents' lack of moral authority did not entirely obscure the current of hostility that bubbled beneath the surface. One early clinical report did state clearly that the anorexic girl "would never speak to her mother except in tones of the greatest violence."[7] Rather than intervene in such a charged situation, the majority of physicians chose pragmatically to remove the patient with anorexia nervosa from her home—that is, they advocated what is today called a parentectomy.[8]

Most doctors concurred that "the first thing to be done is to secure the confidence of the patient's friends, and to persuade them to allow her to be put under the care of strangers, away from home."[9] This model of treatment came principally from the French and the Americans, namely Jean-Martin Charcot (1825–1893) and Silas Weir Mitchell (1829–1914). In designing therapy for hysteria in "young and marriageable girls," Charcot, a noted Parisian psychiatrist and director of the Salpêtrière, argued that isolation was always a "most efficacious" treatment. In handling the case of a girl with *l'anorexie hystérique*, Charcot spoke harshly to the parents who placed their emaciated daughter in a hydrotherapeutic (water cure) establishment but refused to leave her there alone. ("They were resolved not to be separated from their child.") In a "blunt remonstrance" to the parents, Charcot told them that in order to help their daughter they "should go away, or pretend to go away . . . as quickly as possible." Eventually, when isolation was established, the results were "rapid" and "marvellous."[10] Mitchell, an American neurologist, known for his advocacy and development of cures for female nervous disorders that involved total seclusion, bed rest, a skim-milk diet, and massage, figured prominently in the British debate over how to treat anorexia nervosa.[11] British doctors referred consistently to the success of the so-called Mitchell method.

Doctors gave nearly uniform endorsement to the idea that removal from the domestic environment was a necessary first step in the process of returning the emaciated girl to health.[12] From as far afield as Australia, a physician wrote that the "best chances of recovery rest . . . on her removal from home sympathy and influences . . . I persuaded the parents," he said, "to send her to Port Eliot, and there in the house of a stranger she rapidly recovered." The same doctor reported that in another case an eighteen-year-old instantaneously recovered from anorexia nervosa while "her parents went to the Melbourne Exhibition, leaving [her] at home with the servants."[13] Few cases were actually quite that simple. The question of where the girl should go was complicated and related, naturally enough, to the family's financial resources and personal proclivities. Institutions for the insane were inappropriate; the anorectic was by definition not a lunatic. Parents might threaten their daughters with the prospect of commitment, but they did not generally follow through.

The physicians' sense that the home environment was implicated in anorexia nervosa, coupled with the middle-class bias against institutionalization, contributed to many ad hoc, highly individualistic therapies: sending an anorexic girl to visit a sympathetic aunt; proposing a recuperative sea voyage with an older sister, adult friend, or nurse; traveling to a scenic lake or mountain district where the air was pure and invigorating; or going to live with a simple farm family in a bucolic setting. Only when these strategies failed were middle-class families willing to consider the spectrum of available institutional options. Above and beyond lunatic asylums and charity hospitals, families with money to spend might place an anorexic daughter in a private asylum, "hysterical home," cottage hospital, or water-cure establishment. All apparently did some business in the care and treatment of anorexia nervosa.[14]

Unfortunately, none of these therapeutic options were systematically documented, so we know almost nothing of their success or failure. We know only that they were costly and that they were tried by a small number of desperate families whose starving daughters eventually came to the attention of consultants and specialists. On the advice of experts such as William Gull, families who would not ordinarily have allowed their daughters to enter public hospitals did exactly that—because the doctors were convincing and the high cost of private hysterical homes was beyond their reach.

At least one consultant, John Ogle, had reservations about the general medical hospital as a place for treating hysterical young women. Ogle found fault with the wards in places like St. George's (where he was a clinical consultant), because they had no program of "congenial inspiring pursuits and means of diversion." Ogle preferred "some retreat" with "suitable modes of entertainment . . . fresh air; and . . . scenes of country life."[15] In treating anorexia nervosa, as in treating hysteria, Ogle firmly believed that young women profited from moral as well as medical therapy.

Throughout the 1880s and 1890s doctors discussed the issue of what constituted the preferred treatment for anorexia nervosa. While nearly all favored the so-called parentectomy, there was disagreement about where the patient should be situated. In general, the debate over treatment reflected the intraprofessional rivalries that characterized Anglo-American medicine. Different kinds of physicians favored treatment locations and stratagems that reflected their own self-interest as well as the economic resources of their clientele.

In the interest of demonstrating how well they managed anorexia nervosa in their own particular medical setting, nineteenth-century physicians created a notably optimistic clinical literature. Until 1895, published reports on anorexia nervosa described only successful cures; no case of anorexia nervosa was reported to be either chronic or fatal. Medical claims to quick and complete recovery were underscored by pictures that showed anorexic patients transformed from emaciation to health, "plump and rosy as of yore."[16] The optimistic tone of the medical literature was a function of the exigencies of life in the Victorian medical world. In order to compete for the trade in anorexia nervosa, doctors had to demonstrate their efficacy to their colleagues as well as to the world at large.

The Question of Treatment

Thomas Stretch Dowse, a specialist with an appointment at the relatively new Hospital for Epilepsy and Paralysis, was the first British physician to publish on anorexia nervosa in the journals after Gull's 1873 report. Dowse sought to confirm Gull's identification, and he hoped to imitate the consultant's success. His 1881 article, which appeared in one of the less prestigious medical journals of the city, told the story of an emaciated and "sullen" fourteen-year-old (identified as A.T.) whose father threatened to place her in the County Hospital at Colchester near her home. The mother had, in desperation, "used an enema to her"—that is, she attempted to administer a nutritive enema—but it caused enormous pain. When A.T. expressed a wish to go to London to the home of her married brother and his wife, the local doctor and the parents agreed, although the girl was so severely emaciated that she had to be "supported and lifted out of various conveyances" en route.[17]

In London her brother and sister-in-law "tried what a little firmer treatment could do." In other words, they proceeded to force-feed the girl on their own. This resulted, not surprisingly, in a violent and unpleasant struggle that brought A.T. to the floor. Once the patient was hospitalized, Dowse, in conjunction with an authoritative nurse, had only to threaten forced feeding and the girl began eating. Dowse clearly meant to imply that the moral authority of doctors was greater than that of any family or kin. Outside the family, the girl's appetite returned. Just as Sir William had done, Dowse displayed engravings of his patient before she began treatment and then two months later, when she was cured.

Dowse's article made an important and largely self-promotional point. By building fear of domestic reverberations in anorexia nervosa, Dowse suggested that the condition required medical intervention. But the form of that intervention need not be restricted to elite consulting physicians such as Sir William Gull. The published case of A.T. proved that more accessible doctors (those who asked lower fees) working in smaller, specialized hospitals (such as the sixty-bed Hospital for Epilepsy and Paralysis) were equally appropriate resources for the management of anorexic young women. In effect, Dowse argued that Sir William, the high-status consultants, and the teaching hospitals ought not monopolize the trade in anorexia nervosa.

In March 1888 Gull published a second clinical report on the disease, which included a striking engraving, taken from a photograph, of the wasted, nude torso of Miss K.R. The report was really nothing more than a compilation of notes describing the case of a fourteen-year-old brought to him by the medical officer of the Petersfield Cottage Hospital but cured in her own home through a dietary regimen enforced by a trained nurse.[18] It did not incorporate Lasègue's notion of stages in the disease; it did not pay more than rudimentary attention to the nature of the family environment; it did not describe the nature or substance of the curative process. It did illustrate, however, in dramatic visual form, the speedy success of his therapeutic method. Miss K.R. went from the brink of death to genuine health in short order.

Gull explained: "The case was so extreme that had it not been photographed and accurately engraved, some assurance would have been necessary that the appearances were not exaggerated, or even caricatured, which they were not."[19] As in his 1873 report, Sir William had a point to make in selecting the visual image: in his April 1887 engraving, the patient's hair was cropped short and close to her head in a manner reminiscent of a medieval ascetic; her eyes were cast in a faraway gaze; and her narrow lips were set tightly together. By June, less than two months later, the same patient had remarkably long, luxuriant hair and her expression was decidedly different. Restored to health by Sir William, the fourteen-year-old from Petersfield emerged as an attractive young woman with a sensitive half-smile on her face. The smile conveyed the message that anorexic perversity had passed and equanimity reigned. Medical accolades were surely due the physician who could effect such a startling transformation.

The memorable engraving, combined with the fact that Gull had been paralyzed by a stroke in the months before his March publication, drew unusual attention to his 1888 article, thereby contributing to the further identification of his name with the independent disease he sought to promote. An editorial in the *Lancet* proclaimed great "satisfaction that Sir William Gull is so far recovered as to have directed the publication of the case of anorexia nervosa, which, with very striking illustrations, appeared in our impression of last week. The brevity and pithiness of Sir William's account of the case are happy proof that his keen clinical perceptions have suffered no abatement."[20] What the *Lancet* did not say was that Gull was so incapacitated by this time that he had closed his private practice.[21]

By 1888 Anglo-American interest in anorexia nervosa ran high as a result of Gull's status as one of medicine's elder statesmen. Despite enthusiasm for the man, Gull's conception of anorexia nervosa as an independent disease did not hold—even though the name he gave the syndrome did. Because of the contemporary medical emphasis on organ systems, anorexia nervosa was generally presented in Anglo-American textbooks as Gull's "discovery," but it was cast as a stomach or gastrointestinal disorder of hysteria in keeping with Lasègue's analysis.[22] (Anorexia nervosa was most often discussed in the context of how hysteria impaired visceral functions such as respiration and digestion.) Girls admitted to general hospitals suffering from emaciation without organic cause were acknowledged to have Gull's disease, but doctors still wrote "hysterical anorexia" on their charts. Thus, in spite of its professional association with a famous physician who deliberately sought to separate it from hysteria, anorexia nervosa continued to be conceptualized by most doctors as a variant of hysterical behavior.

[handwritten margin note: The two are often compared]

Gull did have his critics, even among his peers. According to William Smoult Playfair, Gull's identification and analysis of anorexia nervosa was naive. Immediately after Gull's second report, Playfair raised strenuous objections to Gull's assertion that anorexia nervosa was an independent disease. Playfair explained deferentially that while he too took pleasure in "seeing Sir William's honoured name appearing [again] in connexion with medical work," he could not agree with Gull's analysis or his treatment. According to Playfair, Gull took a simplistic view of a complicated functional disorder, that is, a disease for which no gross pathology or organic cause could be found. "The point I would particularly insist upon," Playfair wrote, "is that the excessive disgust for food, which is so striking a feature, is only one of many coexisting indications of a profound alteration of the nervous system."[23] Playfair categorically dismissed the idea that anorexia, or lack of appetite, was the disease's primary symptom. Moreover, he argued that the disorder was usually not cured by the simple introduction of nursing care, as Gull had suggested in the case of the girl from Petersfield.

Playfair regarded anorexia nervosa as a variant of neurasthenia, a functional nervous disorder first named in 1869 by American neurologist George Beard, a supporting actor in the Fancher drama, and characterized by profound physical and mental exhaustion. Neurasthenia meant "nervous exhaustion" and the name was supposed to convey a deficiency of nervous energy.

Proponents of the diagnosis regarded it as a new disease generated by nineteenth-century industrialization and a mode of life associated with advanced technology, scientific progress, and the emancipation of women. The diverse symptoms of neurasthenia included sick headache, dyspepsia, bad dreams and insomnia, heart palpitations, uterine sensitivity, impotence, neuralgia, ringing in the ears, and flat or unaccented voice. (Even Beard himself regarded neurasthenia as subjective and called its symptoms "slippery, fleeting, and vague.")[24] To this cauldron of varied ingredients Playfair sought to add lack of appetite: "In spite of the objections that have been made to it [neurasthenia], it seems to me to describe the essential nature of the disease as well as any other that has been suggested."[25]

Playfair, a distinguished obstetrician who delivered the children of royalty and peers, was the author of a book on *Systematic Treatment of Nervous Prostration and Hysteria* and the collector of the album of anorexic photographs that allegedly rivaled Sir William's engravings. Because of his interest in nervous diseases, Playfair was well acquainted with the work of Beard and the phenomenon of neurasthenia. He was also alert to the fact that the same debility that was immobilizing the Americans was "alive and well" in Britain. In fact, he regarded anorexia in girlhood as a "very common occurrence": it is "one type only of the multiform functional neuroses . . . that are the despair of the profession, which are daily increasing in frequency, in this age of culture, over-strain, and pressure."[26] Playfair suggested that Gull's disease, anorexia nervosa, was really a juvenile form of neurasthenia precipitated by almost any stressful life event—domestic bereavement, money loss, disappointment in love, excessive or unwise doctoring—in combination with the new social pressures.

The pressures Playfair singled out for emphasis were part and parcel of the argument that neurasthenia was caused by too much civilization, as well as a telling indicator of his social agenda for women. "I have seen many instances [of anorexia nervosa] in young girls which have followed severe study for some of the higher examinations for women now so much in vogue."[27] The idea that intellectual work and advanced schooling precipitated anorexia nervosa was related to influential medical and social theories about the consequences of higher education for the health of Victorian girls and the well-being of society. Between 1860 and 1880, in Britain and in the United States, the first postsecondary institutions for women students opened their doors, attracting the eager daughters of families who had both the money to put them there and some degree of commitment to the progressive idea that women were worth educating. On both sides of the Atlantic the public debated the "woman question," while doctors railed against the social and medical effects of educating them.[28]

Playfair's position on the education of women was not anomalous. In fact, his thinking was representative of many of the best minds in the medical profession. In 1884, for example, T. S. Clouston, the highly regarded superintendent of the Edinburgh asylum, spoke for the value to society of women's traditional roles; he asked, "Why should we spoil a good mother by making an ordinary grammarian?"[29] Clouston, like many others, assumed that women's intellectual contributions would be, at best, mediocre. In the United States Edward H. Clarke (1820–1877), professor of medicine at Harvard, fought actively against higher education for young women because he believed that the "complicated apparatus peculiar to the female" needed time and ease to develop, free from the drain of intellectual activity.

In the view of these ovarian determinists, female adolescence should be a quiet time, filled with consistent monitoring by an inspirational mother, healthful but limited physical exercise, and prudent, nonstimulating sociability. In his well-known book, *Sex in Education*, which appeared in the same year as the anorexia nervosa diagnosis, Edward Clarke presented a set of case studies, allegedly drawn from clinical practice, of adolescent students whose "catamenial function," ovarian development, and general health were ruined by inattention to the special demands of their new "periodicity."[30] Clarke and others condemned higher education for women as a form of excess which, they claimed, depleted the nerve energy required for reproduction. It led not only to an increasing number of functional disorders but to infertility. Amenorrhea in anorexia nervosa was exactly the kind of morbid physical consequence that doctors such as Clarke and Playfair linked to intellectual activity.

Unlike Sir William, Playfair admitted that anorexia nervosa was a complicated disorder with no easy cure. In his published reports of the disease Gull advocated hiring a trained nurse who, under the direction of a doctor, would enforce a dietary regimen within the girl's home. The nurse was a factotum for the doctor; she represented his moral authority within the distressed household. The type of nurse who did this work most effectively was described as "trained," "firm," and "persuasive"—suggesting that physicians had a clear sense of what constituted appropriate professional and personal credentials in their support staff.[31] Yet home nursing was never widely advocated by physicians in the treatment of anorexia nervosa. Home nursing was costly and difficult to arrange. It was a problematic undertaking to hire a suitable full-time private-duty nurse, that is, a woman who understood her medical and social relationship to both the belabored family and the doctor. In addition, doctors did not want to suggest that simply by employing a nurse one could obtain the same medical and moral benefits that came with engaging a doctor.

Playfair openly challenged Gull's assertion that rest, feeding, and home nursing brought renewed health. According to Playfair, Gull had been lucky in handling the case from Petersfield:

> It is true that his case recovered under the care of a good nurse, by a happy chance, but it is to be noted that it occurred in a child of fourteen who had been ill for less than a year, and who was not the hardened neurotic sinner so often met with. I assert that not one case in twenty could be cured in this way, and the proof of it is that in nearly every case the plan has been already tried and failed, sometimes under the supervision of a whole phalanx of medical men. Absolute rest, massage, and the abundant over-feeding which comes so easily under their influence, are no doubt valuable adjuncts in the case, but without isolation they will almost certainly fail. With it [isolation] the cure of these cases is reduced to as great a certainty as anything medical can be.[32]

The commitment to isolation represented implicit acceptance of the role of the family and the girl's social milieu in generating anorexia nervosa. Isolation was advocated by the same people who cast anorexia nervosa as a form of neurasthenia, William Smoult Playfair being a case in point. For doctors who conceived of anorexia nervosa as a form of neurasthenia in the "junior miss," the model for treatment came essentially from the United States— particularly from a therapeutic treatment associated with Silas Weir Mitchell, who was unanimously elected to the presidency of the American Neurological Association in 1874.

In *Fat and Blood: And How to Make Them* Mitchell argued that seclusion was the sine qua non in the treatment of serious nervous disorders: "Once separate the patient from the moral and physical surroundings which have become part of her life of sickness, and you will have made a change which will be in itself beneficial, and will enormously aid in the treatment which is to follow." Mitchell explained that while "this step is not essential in such cases as are merely anaemic and feeble and thin owing to distinct [medical] causes," seclusion was the proper treatment for that "large and troublesome" class of "thin-blooded emotional women" who make "weak health" a "cherished habit." Mitchell reasoned that seclusion was the only sensible way around what he regarded as the manipulative politics of female invalidism:

> There is often no success possible until we have broken up the whole daily drama of the sick-room, with its little selfishnesses and its craving for sympathy and indulgence . . . A hysterical girl is, as Wendell Holmes has said in his decisive phrase, a vampire who sucks the blood of the healthy people about her; and I may add that pretty surely where there is one hysterical girl there will be soon or late two sick women.[33]

Because the girl with anorexia nervosa seemed so very much like the patients Mitchell described, his treatment was embraced by many physicians. Removed from family and friends, it was agreed that the girl should experience "a combination of entire rest and of excessive feeding, made possible by passive exercise obtained through steady use of massage and electricity."[34] In her isolation the young woman saw no one but her doctor and nurse; moreover, she was expected to remain totally prone, submit to vigorous bodily massage for at least an hour a day, and eschew reading or writing because of their stimulative effects. As Mitchell described it, "The only action allowed is that needed to clean the teeth."[35] While many young women undoubtedly underwent a regimen of absolute isolation, others experienced the cure in moderation. These patients were separated from their families but assigned to wards in hospital settings where there were other patients and hospital staff, as well as visitors. Real isolation required intensive private care, an expense not every family could afford.

Mitchell's name and his method of seclusion and feeding were widely known and imitated in Britain and in the United States, suggesting an important process of cross-fertilization in the Anglo-American medical world. (*Fat and Blood* was published simultaneously in Philadelphia and London.) Physicians from as far afield as Australia wrote to the journals that in cases of anorexia nervosa "Dr. Mitchell's treatment of hysteria" seemed appropriate. William Osler said explicitly that while anorexia nervosa looked "alarming," patients "treated by Weir Mitchell's method" might recover "in a remarkable way." In a 1904 medical discussion among West London physicians, one participant stated that "the Weir Mitchell treatment affords the greatest success"—and none of his colleagues sought to disagree.[36] What the British called the Mitchell method was the cutting edge in the clinical treatment of anorexia nervosa.

There were, however, a few significant expressions of disagreement from physicians who regarded isolation as a too-costly, inappropriate, and potentially dangerous form of therapeutic intervention. In April 1888 Andrew Scott Myrtle, a provincial doctor from Harrogate, wrote a cantankerous letter to the *Lancet* taking issue with Playfair's assertion that Gull's cure was a fluke and that anorexia nervosa required total seclusion of the patient, according to the Mitchell method. Wrote Myrtle: "All I can say is, I have never failed ultimately in seeing health established in every case of anorexia nervosa without isolation, and above all, without the aid of that most fashionable, and in a very great number of cases most unnecessary, though systematic, piece of humbug—massage. I allude to the 'knotted muscles,' 'the blocked vessels,' 'contracted sinews,' 'thickened nerves and oiless joints,' so readily discovered by the fingers of both male and female rubbers." In effect, Myrtle believed modern medicine was making too much of what was really just nervous dyspepsia. "Besides," he wrote, "isolation means a lot of money; it is not everyone who can afford to enter a so-called 'home' and purchase health according to its tariff."[37]

The efficacy of the "home" to which the anorectic was sent was also the subject of some criticism. Dennis De Berdt Hovell, who had a surgery in Cavendish Square and a connection to London Hospital, raised questions about the type of medicine being practiced in the small, private hysterical homes, where physicians were not well trained. De Berdt Hovell published on the subjects of hysteria and neurasthenia and saw some anorectics in his practice. He reported that patients came to him for advice—after stays at these places—"certainly not cured, but indignant on the one hand and humiliated on the other."[38]

The allusion to humiliation in the hysterical home may be a reference to indignities suffered in the process of forced feeding. Threats of forced feeding were very useful in asylum practice, although consulting physicians of the very highest status—such as Gull and Playfair—did not admit to ever employing them. They liked to think that their moral authority would always prevail. Published clinical reports from doctors of lesser status, however, reveal that forced feeding was not uncommon in cases of anorexia nervosa. And clinical case reports from the lunatic asylums and from public hospitals indicate that the practice was a fairly regular response to patients who refused food for any length of time. In public hospitals, orders merely were written that if the patient continued to refuse her food, she must be tube-fed. Surely, the medical entrepreneurs who ran the private asylums turned to the same procedures when they faced an intractable patient whose parents were paying handsomely to see her weight increase.

De Berdt Hovell's argument with what he snidely called "the presiding medical genius" of the hysterical home was actually wider than the specific charge that patients in seclusion were humiliated. As a consulting physician to a major London hospital, De Berdt Hovell understood that the Mitchell method generated business for the private madhouses, a type of institution he did not admire. He preferred to treat anorectics in a medical as opposed to a psychiatric facility. As a result, he suggested that it was unfair (and possibly unsafe) for parents to send the anorexic girl away from home simply because she was perverse or willful.

In so doing, De Berdt Hovell argued that Gull and others were throwing "the blame on the patient." This kind of unsympathetic treatment, he said, inevitably created what Playfair called the "hardened neurotic sinner." In contrast, De Berdt Hovell wrote, "my directions to this class of patient are to do daily as much as their strength admits, and not to attempt more; to be content with the little they are able to do, and not to fret because they cannot accomplish more; and to apply to me directly [when] they get into any trouble or difficulty."[39] Anorectics who were severely emaciated should be "lifted and encouraged" through the quiet sympathy and disinterested guidance of professional men who were expert in the medical management of these cases. It was absolutely critical that girls with anorexia nervosa not be treated with "censure and neglect," that is, banishment to a disreputable medical facility and the severities of the Mitchell method. Nonetheless, the fact of the matter was that at this point in time the private hysterical home was the treatment of choice. Being a patient in a specialist or general hospital was simply not part of middle-class culture in England or America until quite late in the century. Because a public hospital was about as unthinkable as the workhouse or the poorhouse, only a few desperate parents ever sent their anorexic daughters to them.

At the Hospital

Adding flesh to the emaciated frame of the food refuser was the nineteenth-century physician's primary responsibility and challenge. In the treatment of anorexia nervosa, medical success was measured in weight gain. This symptom-reduction approach prevailed in the few published reports from general and cottage hospitals.

Little time was spent in exploring the question of motivation or etiology. In this regard Gull was a model for the profession. Once it was determined through differential diagnosis that the patient had no organic reason to refuse food, then the medical course was set. She must be fed consistently and abundantly, either of her own volition or by some other means. Medical efforts focused on construction and maintenance of a "plethoric" or superabundant diet. When a reasonable weight was attained, the patient was declared cured without further investigation of why she had stopped eating. In effect, the doctor was first and foremost a nutritional manager.

The case of Eva Williams, age nineteen, demonstrates the Victorian doctor's role in the management and cure of anorexia nervosa. Eva was admitted to London Hospital's Rachel ward in January 1897 weighing 78 pounds. The girl was not happy about her confinement. One of six children in a comfortable middle-class family from Bow, Eva had "never done work of any kind." Before her admission to London Hospital, she spent a number of months at Eastbourne, a resort, seeking to restore her appetite and health. Williams was under the care of Stephen MacKenzie, a well-regarded consultant to London Hospital who lectured in the medical college and was a fellow of the Royal College of Physicians. (MacKenzie was a son of the distinguished throat specialist Morrell MacKenzie, who two decades before had treated cases of globus hystericus.)[40] In the Rachel ward, Eva was separated from her family but was not isolated. At least a dozen other children, all girls, were part of her hospital environment.

When MacKenzie and his clinical clerk took the girl's history, they discovered that she "went off her food" over a year before, complaining of indigestion, pain after eating, and flatulence. The girl told the doctors she had no appetite and spoke of persistent constipation. She had not menstruated for over two years. A check of her heart, lungs, abdomen, tongue, teeth, throat, blood, and urine revealed no disease or abnormalities of any kind. There was no evidence of vertigo, headaches, paralysis, neuralgia, or tremor, and her family had no relevant history of nervous or organic disease. In fact, the patient felt "quite well and strong" until the onset of her current illness. The only signs of that illness were the patient's mental state ("she is somewhat depressed") and her visible wasting: "The patient states that three years ago she weighed 10 stone [140 pounds]. Now she weighs 5 stone 8 lbs. [78 pounds]. Her chest, ankles, wrists, and hands show considerable wasting. Breasts do not show marked wasting. Ribs and clavicle stand out prominently. There is also considerable muscular wasting as shown in intravenous spaces." Given that anorexia and emaciation were her only symptoms, MacKenzie wrote the diagnosis, "hysterical anorexia."[41]

During the first week in the hospital the girl ate next to nothing and lost 3 more pounds within days. Obviously, separation from her family was not enough to induce normal eating. A rigorous dietary regimen was instituted. Dr. MacKenzie ordered the following treatment to be continued each day: "Massage after which a warm bath and then food, the nourishment gradually to be increased. If patient objects to food it is to be forced by means of stomach pump." The girl's diet basically included ample portions of fish, milk, eggs, bread, and vegetables. On a typical day she was either persuaded, cajoled, or forced to take the following:

Early in the morning—an egg, a round of toast, and cocoa made with a half-pint of milk
About 10 A.M.—more toast and more milk
At noon—fish, green vegetables, and pudding
At 3 P.M.—an egg and another cup of hot milk
At 4 P.M.—a cup of coffee and two pieces of toast
At 7:30 P.M.—some toast and jelly with a cup of hot milk

The nurses' reports indicate that there was little struggle once MacKenzie and the hospital staff began to enforce a regimen. Eva Williams was compliant in the strange, professional atmosphere of the hospital and in the care of an authoritative doctor. (A fourteen-year-old French anorectic, in much the same state as Eva, told her doctor, "When I saw that you were determined to be master, I was afraid, and in spite of my repugnance I tried to eat, and I was able to, little by little.")[42] By February 2, Eva Williams had gained 4 pounds; by February 8, she had gained another 5. New items were gradually added to her diet: butter, minced oysters, fish soufflés, omelets, and some mincemeat. In the following weeks her weight gain slowed but there were never any losses. The record reveals that she took her own food and appeared to "feel stronger and sleep well." On March 3, 1897—

after a hospital stay of only seven weeks—Eva Williams was discharged, cured. She was returned to her family after having gained 14 pounds.

MacKenzie's notes on the Williams case reveal that he concentrated on the patient's weight gain and gave little attention to what we would call the psychology of anorexia nervosa. Described only as "intelligent" and "somewhat depressed," Eva Williams apparently would not say anything more than that it hurt her to eat. MacKenzie never reported the substance of any conversation he had with the patient, but he did make the following notation about information obtained secondhand: "She gives no reason for her abstaining from food but one of her friends states that she refuses to take food on account of her mothers [*sic*] talking to her about being so fat." This bit of information about Williams and her mother, information suggesting that the girl's body was an issue between them, elicited no particular response from Dr. MacKenzie, who continued to focus his examinations on the issue of the girl's somatic complaints and her weight gain. When Eva Williams weighed 92 pounds she was discharged, probably without reference to the tensions with her mother. Why fatness was an issue was left totally unexplained.

In a landmark case in 1895, a physician in a cottage hospital who attempted to perform the parentectomy was unsuccessful and the patient died.[43] The doctor, Lockhardt Stephens (1858–1940), had trained as a surgeon at Guy's Hospital before becoming chief medical officer of the Emsworth Cottage Hospital near Bristol. Cottage hospitals were designed to be homelike; their architecture and interior decoration were intended to be reminiscent of the domicile of a "well-to-do working man or a small farmer."[44] As a general principle, cottage hospitals distinguished themselves from larger medical facilities by their informal style, especially the easy access of families to patients. Emsworth was a typical cottage hospital with six regular beds and one emergency bed.

Stephens reported the case of a sixteen-year-old schoolgirl who remained at home until her emaciation became so severe and dangerous that she had to be hospitalized. "As the girl was under no control whatever at home I advised her parents to allow her to come into the Cottage Hospital on the distinct understanding and promise that whatever treatment was thought necessary should be carried out."[45] The patient, the only daughter among six children, was admitted to Emsworth in March 1888, and she died less than a month later despite the vigorous efforts of Stephens and his staff. Neither the doctor's moral authority nor the medical armamentarium provided a means for arresting her refusal of food and the consequences of starvation.

The Bristol schoolgirl was anorexic for over ten months prior to admission. According to reports from family and friends, the onset of her behavior was quite sudden. She had been a "remarkably well-made, plump, and healthy looking girl, full of spirits and eager to attract the notice of her friends, which she did to a considerable degree, becoming a favorite with her teachers and others."[46] Then, for "no apparent cause," this sociable and well-behaved youngster began to show a reluctance to "take the same food and at the ordinary meal times as the rest of the family." This disinclination soon became habit, upsetting both the routine and the tenor of family life. The parents were incapable of changing her behavior.

According to Stephens, the family indisputably failed to establish control over the girl. The mother was identified as the problematic parent, and Stephens used her not only as a justification for seeking complete authority in the case but ultimately as an explanation for medical failure. Described as "very excitable and quite under the influence of the patient," the mother was told that she must not visit the girl at Emsworth, since a cure demanded an in-hospital version of the Mitchell method. Stephens insisted on this, even though easy visitation was one of the guidelines of the cottage hospitals.

In the hospital the girl was kept immobile in bed with her "limbs and body bandaged in cotton wool," a technique for elevating the body temperature and restricting activity. Despite her protestations, she was fed pulverized food every four hours. Apparently after a few days the girl became quite resentful, "sullen," and "fretful," "crying out for her mother." "In spite of [medical] advice to the contrary," the nervous mother commenced daily visits to the hospital. For Stephens the return of the mother to Emsworth marked the beginning of the end. "From this point she [the patient] began to lose the little ground we had gained; she took very small quantities of food and resorted to every conceivable trick to avoid swallowing it, although she would take it in her mouth."[47] With the mother on the scene, the doctor claimed that he was unable to establish the proper moral environment to effect a cure.

At the end of the third week of treatment, the early-morning nurse noted that the patient was incredibly weak, so weak that she could not even swallow liquids. Within hours she was in a position of "extreme helplessness, the eyes were fixed, the pupils dilated and insensitive." Respiration slowed, the extremities became cold and clammy, and the breath odious. Hypodermic injections of brandy were given every ten minutes and a heroic effort was made to keep the patient warm. The nurses applied hot flannels to the stomach and hot-water bottles to the feet, hands, armpits, and torso. The last food the girl ever took was ten ounces of milk, "as hot as could be bourne in the mouth," administered through an esophageal tube.

The death of the Bristol schoolgirl was of sufficient interest for Stephens to call in a photographer to capture a likeness of his 5-foot-4-inch, 49-pound patient. Although medical photography was not commonplace, Victorian physicians put great value on visual representations of pathology.[48] Because a photograph could provide an objective record of disease that verbal accounts could not, Stephens felt the need to document the reality of death from anorexia nervosa.

Although Stephens wanted a realistic, scientific picture of the girl's emaciation, he chose to construct the record in a way that honored convention and Victorian aesthetics. At her death, the girl would surely have been wrapped in clothing and blankets in order to maintain her body temperature. For the purposes of the picture, however, Stephens had the body undressed and draped. A sheet, placed in such a way as to discreetly cover her genitals but leave her breasts and protruding hipbones exposed, indicates some level of contrivance and attention to Victorian proprieties. Genitalia were simply not shown in the photographic medium.

But the Victorians did take pleasure from beauty in the nude, particularly soft, opalescent, womanly flesh and the budding bodies of young women on the brink of their sexual potential.[49] In contrast, Stephens' 1895 photograph showed a stark, horrifying image of a wasted adolescent body whose unfulfilled sexual and reproductive potential was symbolized in the prominence of her only subcutaneous fat, rounded and full breasts. Devoid of eroticism, the angular torso and tortured eyes of the Bristol schoolgirl provided compelling testimony to the destructive power of anorexia nervosa.

Lockhardt Stephens' attempt to establish isolation failed unambiguously. Perhaps for this reason he waited nearly seven years to publish the report and the engravings taken from the original 1888 photograph. In the competitive world of British medicine, Stephens' article constituted a public admission that he was unable to establish the kind of moral environment that the patient required. For a nineteenth-century physician this was a critical lapse. It was a particularly difficult admission given that the patient was an adolescent female. (The report of death may also have been taken as a negative reflection on the efficacy of cottage hospitals.)

In truth, Stephens had little to say that was original about the physical symptoms, etiology, or treatment of patients with anorexia nervosa. The report from Emsworth merely confirmed what Victorian medicine already knew: that anorexic girls appeared to come from families that spoiled them in unspecified ways, and that a cure was often effected by separating the girl from the influence of her family. The death of the Bristol schoolgirl did, however, increase medical awareness of the danger of the disorder.

After two decades of clinical experience with the disease many questions were still unanswered. Unlike infectious diseases caused by particular microorganisms, anorexia nervosa had no specific etiological agent. As Gull and Lasègue described it, anorexia nervosa was defined primarily in terms of a behavior (noneating) accompanied by a set of physical symptoms related to the behavior (low body temperature, amenorrhea, hyperactivity). Such a definition would inevitably create problems, because both behavior and symptoms can vary. Consequently, ever since its "discovery" there has been great latitude in the use of the diagnosis as well as continuing speculation about the etiology. What finally emerges as striking about anorexia nervosa in the nineteenth century is that for all the therapeutic attention paid to alleviating the primary symptom, medical men never sought to explain, from the girl's perspective, why she did not eat.

7 · The Appetite as Voice

The symptoms of disease never exist in a cultural vacuum. Even in a strictly biomedical illness, patient responses to physical discomfort and pain are structured in part by who the patient is, the nature of the care giver, and the ideas and values at work in that society. Similarly, in mental illness, basic forms of cognitive and emotional disorientation are expressed in behavioral aberrations that mirror the deep preoccupations of a particular culture. For this reason a history of anorexia nervosa must consider the ways in which different societies create their own symptom repertoires and how the changing cultural context gives meaning to a symptom such as noneating.[1]

In this chapter I suggest a link between the emergence of anorexia nervosa in the nineteenth century and the cultural predispositions of that era. Just as the incidence of anorexia nervosa today is related to powerful contemporary messages about body image and dieting, there is a cultural context—albeit a somewhat different one—that helps to explain the Victorian anorectic. Again, this is not to say that cultural ideas directly cause the disease. At the outset I acknowledged the etiological complexities and the limitations of historical study; anorexia nervosa is a multidetermined disorder that involves individual biological and psychological factors as well as environmental influences. As a historian, I cannot resolve the problem of causation nor can I chart individual psychopathologies. Historical study does, however, illuminate the larger meanings of food and eating in Victorian society and in that process posits a certain set of cultural preoccupations that had particular impact on adolescent women among the bourgeoisie. In effect, by supplying something of the female "food vocabulary" of a distant era, I hope to explain how there could have been anorexia nervosa before there was Twiggy.

The medical literature of the nineteenth century provides few clues to the meaning of anorexic behavior in that period. Physicians reported the characteristic cry of the anorectic as "I will not eat," but they rarely provided the text of the critical subordinate clause, "I will not eat because . . ." The medical literature supplied few accounts by Victorian anorectics, *in their own words*, of why they refused their food and why they deprived their bodies as they did. The Victorian anorectic's understanding of her own behavior remains something of a mystery.

Victorian anorectics did present somatic complaints about gastric discomfort and difficulty in swallowing. Because nineteenth-century doctors emphasized physical diagnosis and somatic treatment, they probably reinforced presentations of this type of distress.[2] Parents also found it easier to accept physical rather than emotional reasons as an explanation of their daughter's emaciation and food-refusing behavior. Yet in cases of anorexia nervosa, biomedical reasons for noneating were quickly undercut, since the diagnosis itself meant that there was no organic disease. Most physicians avoided explanations of etiology and concentrated instead on curing the primary symptoms, noneating and emaciation.

Among the few careful medical reports that include any discussion of motivation is Stephen MacKenzie's 1895 account of his anorexic patient's refusing her food "on account of her mother talking to her about being so fat." A decade earlier Jean-Martin Charcot discovered a rose-colored ribbon wound tightly around the waist of a patient with anorexia nervosa. Questioning revealed the girl's preoccupation with the size of her body: the ribbon was a measure that her waist was not to exceed. Max Wallet's 1895 discussion of two cases of anorexia nervosa suggested the same theme and implicated peers. A seventeen-year-old refused her food because of a "fear of being seen as a bit heavy," and a fifteen-year-old stopped eating when she "got the idea that she was too fat after seeing her friends forcing themselves to lose weight."[3]

These behaviors were likely to be dismissed by physicians as the flirtatious "coquetries" and simpleminded "scruples" of female adolescence.[4] In effect, nineteenth-century medicine did not relate anorexia nervosa to the cultural milieu that surrounded the Victorian girl. The ideas of Victorian women and girls about appetite, food, and eating, as well as the cultural categories of fat and thin, were not mentioned as contributing to the disease. Only in the twentieth century has medicine come to understand that society plays a role in shaping the form of psychological disorders and that behavior and physical symptoms are related to cultural systems. Throughout the nineteenth century most doctors gave and accepted formulaic explanations of anorexia nervosa (for example, their patients "craved sympathy" or experienced a "perversion of the will") without providing any substantive discussion of why appetite and food were at issue. These explanations said more about the doctors' general views on adolescence, gender, and hysteria than they did about the specific mentality of patients with anorexia nervosa.

Given the attention paid to anorexia nervosa in late-nineteenth-century Anglo-American medicine, the failure of physicians to document the anorectic's explanations, however mundane or bizarre they might have been, is a provocative omission. This lapse raises a number of questions about the state of doctor-patient relations and the history of diagnostic and therapeutic techniques in the late nineteenth century. What were the dynamics of doctor, patient, and mother within the Victorian examining room? What expectations did the doctor have of his young female patients? A sensitivity to the relationship between culture and symptomatologies prompts additional questions. What motivated young women in the late nineteenth century to persistently refuse food in the face of familial coaxing and professional medical supervision? What role did food and eating play in female identity in the Victorian era?

In the Examining Room

By the 1870s physical examinations included visual observation and manual manipulation of the body, combined with a few rudimentary tests of body temperature, blood, and urine. Because manual examinations were a progressive innovation done only by better-trained physicians, some patients were probably still unfamiliar and uneasy with the latest information-gathering techniques: listening to the body through a stethoscope, manipulation of the body parts, and tactile probing of the body. In cases involving young women, professionally knowledgeable and socially correct doctors did the examination in the presence of the girl's mother as well as a clinical clerk. The clerk recorded information while the physician listened to, poked, and thumped the patient, who remained partially dressed in her underclothing.[5]

The nineteenth-century physician's new faith in the verifiable external signs and sounds of illness shaped the interaction in the examining room. The doctor was more interested in what the body revealed than in anything the patient had to say about her illness. Educated physicians came to regard the process of history taking as secondary to the process of physical examination. Doctors were assured that patient accounts of illness were more often than not prejudiced, ignorant, and unreliable; personal and family narratives were rarely objective and they almost always revealed the ignorance of lay people about medical phenomena. In this atmosphere of suspicion about all patient accounts, volatile adolescent girls were considered particularly unreliable informants.[6]

As a consequence, the professionally correct doctor turned to the girl's mother, in her authoritative role as parent, for information about the patient's medical history and current symptoms. Social convention supported this strategy; as long as an unmarried girl resided at home, her parents unquestionably had authority over her. Consequently, the doctor, who was in the employ of the parents, dealt with the young woman as a child. In the Victorian examining room, the mother was not only a monitor of the physical examination of her daughter's body but a check on the substance of the conversation between doctor and patient.

In this scenario, which assumes that doctor, mother, and patient all played out their expected social roles, the examining room reproduced the situation in the home. The doctor and the mother were the primary conversants; again, two adults, a male and a female, were focused on the girl's wasting body and her refusal of food. Again, she was told that she ought to eat. Her response, shaped by the nature of the medical investigation and parental expectations, was to say that she could not—eating hurt in some vague, nonspecific way. When the examination showed no organic problem to sustain this interpretation, the doctor made his diagnosis: anorexia nervosa.

It is unlikely that the doctor ever dismissed the mother and tried to see the patient alone in order to search out what was troubling the girl and causing her to refuse food. Propriety worked against such a scenario, as did the conception of the patient as a dependent person and the doctor's lack of interest in girlish narratives. Adolescent patients must have sensed the doctors' disinterest in their point of view. A recovered anorexic told her physician that, during treatment, "I saw that you wished to shut me up."[7]

In an era that valued demure behavior in all women, it is not inconceivable that the anorexic girl honored social conventions by respecting her mother's authority and keeping silent. It is also possible that the partially dressed young woman was so embarrassed by her situation and so intimidated by her doctor that she could not speak. Another explanation, culled directly from the medical record, suggests that the patient responded to questions in a diffident manner. Published case reports repeatedly said that girls with anorexia nervosa were "sullen," "sly," and "peevish," implying that they were as parsimonious with their words as with their food.[8] Refusal to sustain conversation with either one's parents or one's doctor went hand in hand with refusal to eat. The anorexic girl used both her appetite and her body as a substitute for rhetorical behavior.

When the doctor had ascertained that the patient had no physical reason not to eat, his forbearance might ebb. At that point an authoritarian regimen of overfeeding, weighing, and isolation was usually instituted. This regimen became the primary basis of the doctor's relationship with his patient. Conversation, when it occurred, centered on the amount of food taken and weight and strength gained. Both doctor and patient acted as if the girl's illness was strictly physical (rather than emotional), despite the fact that differential diagnosis established exactly the opposite.

The physician maintained an exclusive focus on the issue of the girl's body and her need to add flesh. To do otherwise was to pander to the sympathies of a hysterical adolescent.

Anorexic patients did sometimes talk to less authoritative female medical personnel and to their peers. Although the evidence is undeniably scanty, a few examples reveal that the Victorian anorectic shared aspects of her compulsion to starve with individuals she perceived as less threatening and more sympathetic than the doctor. If she did not speak to them directly about why she refused her food, she left telltale pieces of evidence that provided some explanation of her behavior. This evidence was rarely uncovered by the supervising doctor.

For example, ward nurses and nursing nuns were in close and intimate contact with patients—feeding them regularly, washing their bodies, and supervising their waking hours. In the 1890s a French physician ousted a high-strung mother from the home where her anorexic daughter was being treated and sent in a nun, *une religieuse*, to care for the emaciated fifteen-year-old. At first, the "new attitude of her caretakers" terrified the girl and she became even more recalcitrant about eating and said that she wished to die. After three months of an enforced dietary regimen of arrowroot, bread, eggs, and beef tea, the girl left the recuperative home "fat" and capable of a normal, active life. At discharge the nun disclosed that she had in her possession a series of letters written by the former patient, which "constituted a peculiarly interesting witness from the point of view of causation of her malady." The letters, addressed to an older male relative, disclosed that the patient's food refusal was generated by her romantic and "singular passion" for this man who, in the young girl's presence, had explicitly admired another woman who was "extremely lean." In the effort to please him, the girl began to starve herself, walk excessively, and lace herself very tightly. Yet she never once told her doctor about her passion for her relative or her desire to be thin.[9]

The nurse functioned as detective in another case involving a twenty-year-old at St. George's Hospital in London. None of the consulting doctors could find an organic reason why their hysterical patient refused to eat, but they continued to work diligently to ease the stomach pains of which she complained. The nurse on the ward, however, regarded the girl as a malingerer and told the doctors, "On December 6th, whilst the girl was apparently suffering . . . the Queen [Victoria] passed the hospital, on her way to open Blackfriar's Bridge; [the girl] rose in bed to watch her out of the window, having been thought utterly unable to move, owing to pain." On yet another occasion, when friends were admitted for hospital visiting hours, the nurse found the supposedly debilitated girl "sitting up in bed, trying on a new coloured frock."

This same patient, who told the doctors that she could not and would not eat, engaged in surreptitious relationships with other patients in order to get bits of their food, which she would eat on the sly. The nurse at St. George's Hospital found a note from the girl indicating that she did eat secretly:

> My dear Mrs. Evans — I was very sorry you should take the trouble of cutting me such a nice peice [sic] of bread and butter yesterday. I would of taken it, but all of them saw you send it, and they would of made enough to have talked about, but I should be very glad if you will cut me a nice peice [sic] of crust and put it in a peice [sic] of paper and send it or else bring it, so as they do not see it, for they all watch me very much.[10]

The nurse's information on this patient provided no real explanation of why the girl would not eat in the presence of her caretakers, but it did confirm the physician's belief that hysterical adolescents were by definition deceptive. This attitude surely affected the doctors' interactions with anorexic patients. If it was assumed that the patient was by nature duplicitous, then any explanation she gave would be suspect.

Sensing the doctor's loyalties to her parents and his suspicious attitude toward her, the anorectic usually chose not to disclose her private preoccupations to an unsympathetic male authority figure. When she spoke, it was almost always of bodily ills: pain after eating, a sour stomach, difficulty in swallowing, flatulence. Deference, fear, and anger all combined to keep her essentially mute. When her bodily preoccupations were rooted in ideas that the doctor might find childish, inappropriate, or distasteful, her silence became confirmed. Furthermore, there was always the distinct possibility of misunderstanding or embarrassment when girls told personal things to men or boys. The bourgeois world of the nineteenth century was still very much sex segregated.[11] Consequently, enormous emotional risks were involved in baring one's soul to the doctor. Most adult men did not understand the language of girlhood sentiment and knew neither its vocabulary nor its symbols. The silence of the Victorian anorectic was in keeping with her provocative resort to symbolic rather than rhetorical behavior.

The Irrational Appetite

In the late nineteenth century, adolescent girls demonstrated an array of health problems that involved eating and appetite disturbances. These problems lent confusion rather than clarity to the process of making the diagnosis for anorexia nervosa. In effect, there was a wide spectrum of "picky eating" and food refusal, ranging from the normative to the pathological. Anorexia nervosa was the extreme—but it was not altogether alien, given the range of behaviors that doctors saw in adolescent female patients. As one astute twentieth-century physician wrote about the origins of anorexia nervosa in the era of William Gull, "the conditions of life were well staged for such a disturbance."[12]

The health of young women was definitely influenced by a general female fashion for sickness and debility.[13] The sickly wives and daughters of the bourgeoisie provided the medical profession with a ready clientele. In Victorian society unhappy women (and men) had to employ physical complaints in order to be permitted to take on the privileged "sick role." Because the most prevalent diseases in this period were those that involved "wasting," it is no wonder that becoming thin, through noneating, became a focal symptom. Wasting was in style.

Among women, invalidism and scanty eating commonly accompanied each other. The partnership was familiar enough to become the subject of a satirical novel. In *The Female Sufferer; or, Chapters from Life's Comedy*, Augustus Hoppin satirized the indolent existence of an upper-class invalid who, while ever so ill, managed to run a vigorous social life from her sick chamber. The stylized eating of this "nervous exhaustionist" was central to the author's portrait. Delicate foods such as "tidbits of fruit and jelly," "a snip of a roll," "a wren's leg on toast," were taken only to "appease the cravings of her exhausted nerves"—but not because she was hungry. At times, however, the debilitated patient would become voracious for "dainty" items such as wedding cake, peaches and cream, and freshly cut melon. According to Hoppin, another characteristic type among female sufferers was the woman supposedly perishing of starvation or "pining away." "Well! dying of inanition is doing something, isn't it?" asked one of the admirers who surrounded the sick couch. Another replied, "Inanition being merely action begun, demands too much exertion for [the lady] to finish."[14]

Adolescent girls simply followed and imitated the behavioral styles of adult women. As a consequence, mothers were urged to take action against their daughters' fondness for wasting and debility. In *Eve's Daughters; or, Common Sense for Maid, Wife, and Mother*, Marion Harland told parents:

> Show no charity to the faded frippery of sentiment that prates over romantic sickliness. Inculcate a fine scorn for the desire to exchange her present excellent health for the estate of the pale, drooping, human-flower damsel; the taste that covets the "fascination" of lingering consumption; the "sensation" of early decease induced by the rupture of a blood-vessel over a laced handkerchief held firmly to her lily mouth by agonized parent or distracted lover. All this is bathos and vulgarity . . . Bid her leave such balderdash to the pretender to ladyhood, the low-minded *parvenu*, who, because foibles are more readily imitated than virtues, and tricks than graces, copies the mistakes of her superiors in breeding and sense, and is persuaded that she has learned "how to do it."[15]

Harland, an American, called the "cultivation of fragility" a "national curse."

Of the conditions that affected girls most frequently, dyspepsia and chlorosis both incorporated peculiar eating and both could be confused with anorexia nervosa. Dyspepsia, a form of chronic indigestion with discomfort after eating, was widespread in middle-class adults and in their daughters. Physicians saw the adolescent dyspeptic frequently; advice writers suggested how she should be managed at home; health reformers used her existence to argue for changes in the American diet; and even novelists considered her enough of a fixture on the domestic scene to include her in their portraits of social life.[16] The dyspeptic had no particular organic problem; her stomach was simply so sensitive that it precluded normal eating. Whereas dyspeptic women could be extremely thin, some, according to doctors' reports, were corpulent. Yet dyspepsia sometimes looked much like anorexia nervosa. For example, a physician described his young dyspeptic patients as persons "who enter upon a strict regimen which they follow only too well. By auto-observation and auto-suggestion, by constantly noticing and classifying their foods, and rejecting all kinds that they think they cannot digest, they finally manage to live on an incredibly small amount."[17]

Chlorosis, a form of anemia named for the greenish tinge that allegedly marked the skin of the patient, was the characteristic malady of the Victorian adolescent girl. Although chlorosis was never precisely defined and differentiated, it was unequivocally regarded as a disease of girlhood rather than boyhood. Its symptoms included lack of energy, shortness of breath, dyspepsia, headaches, and capricious or scanty appetite; sometimes the menses stopped. Chlorotic girls tended to lose some weight as a result of poor eating and aversion to specific foods, particularly meat.[18] (Today iron-deficiency anemia corresponds to the older diagnosis of chlorosis.)

Doctors of the Victorian era fostered the notion that all adolescent girls were potentially chlorotic: "Every girl passes as it were through the outer court of chlorosis in her progress from youth to maturity . . . Perhaps, no girl escapes it altogether."[19] In contrast to anorexia nervosa, treatment for this popular disease was relatively easy: large doses of iron salts and a period of rest at home. As a result, parents were not afraid of chlorosis. In fact, it was accepted as a normal part of adolescent development. Many doctors and families were also fond of tonics to stimulate the appetite, restore the blush to the cheek, and cure latent consumption. "Young Girls Fading Away" was the headline of a well-known advertisement for Dr. William's Pink Pills for Pale People, a medicine aimed at the chlorotic market.[20] A vast amount of patent medicine was sold to families that assumed chlorosis in an adolescent whenever her energy, spirits, or appetite waned. In cases that were eventually diagnosed as anorexia nervosa, the patient in the earliest stages may well have been regarded as dyspeptic or chlorotic. Because clinical descriptions of the confirmed dyspeptic, the chlorotic, and the anorectic had many features in common, we must assume that the diagnoses occasionally overlapped.[21]

Taken together, these conditions suggest that young women presented unusual eating and diminished appetite more often than any other group in the population. Apparently, it was relatively normal for a Victorian girl to develop poor appetite and skip her meals, "affect daintiness" and eat only sweets, or express strong food preferences and dislikes.[22] A popular women's magazine told its readership that in adolescence "digestive problems are common, the appetite is fickle, and evidences of poor nourishment abound."[23] Between 1850 and 1900 the most frequent warning issued to parents of girls had to do with forestalling the development of idiosyncracies, irregularities, or strange whims of appetite because these were precursors of disease as well as signs of questionable moral character.

Ideas about female physiology and sexual development underlay the physician's expectations and his clinical treatment. Doctors believed that women were prone to gastric disorders because of the superior sensitivity of the female digestive system. Using the machine metaphor that was popular in describing bodily functions, they likened a man's stomach to a quartz-crushing machine that required coarse, solid food. By contrast, the mechanisms of a woman's stomach could be ruined if fed the same materials. The female digestive apparatus required foods that were soft, light, and liquid.[24] (Dyspepsia in women could result from the choice of inappropriate foods that required considerable chewing and digestion.)

To the physician's mind, a young woman caught up in the process of sexual maturation was subject to vagaries of appetite and peculiar cravings. "The rapid expansion of the passions and the mind often renders the tastes and appetite capricious," wrote a midcentury physician.[25] Therefore, even normal sexual development had the potential to create a disequilibrium that could lead to irregular eating such as the kind reported in dyspepsia and chlorosis. But physicians reported on eating behavior that was far more bizarre. In fact, the adolescent female with "morbid cravings" was a stock figure in the medical and advice literature of the Victorian period. Stories circulated of "craving damsels" who were "trash-eaters, oatmeal-chewers, pipe-chompers, chalk-lickers, wax-nibblers, coal-scratchers, wall-peelers, and gravel-diggers." The clinical literature also provided a list of "foods" that some adolescent girls allegedly craved: chalk, cinders, magnesia, slate pencils, plaster, charcoal, earth, spiders, and bugs.[26] Modern medicine associates iron-deficiency anemia with eating nonnutritive items, such as pica. For the Victorian physician, nonnutritive eating constituted proof of the fact that the adolescent girl was essentially out of control and that the process of sexual maturation could generate voracious and dangerous appetites.

In this context physicians asserted that even normal adolescent girls had a penchant for highly flavored and stimulating foods. A reputable Baltimore physician, for example, described three girl-friends who constantly carried with them boxes of pepper and salt, taking the condiments as if they were snuff.[27] The story was meant to imply that the girls were slaves of their bodily appetites. Throughout the medical and advice literature an active appetite or an appetite for particular foods was used as a trope for dangerous sexuality. Mary Wood-Allen warned young readers that the girl who masturbated "will manifest an unnatural appetite, sometime desiring mustard, pepper, vinegar and spices, cloves, clay, salt, chalk, charcoal, etc."[28]

Because appetite was regarded as a barometer of sexuality, both mothers and daughters were concerned about its expression and its control. It was incumbent upon the mother to train the appetite of the daughter so that it represented only the highest moral and aesthetic sensibilities. A good mother was expected to manage this situation before it escalated into a medical or social problem. Marion Harland's Mamie, the prototypical adolescent, developed at puberty "morbid cravings of appetite and suffered after eating things that never disagreed with her before." Mamie's mother was cautioned about the possibility that a disturbance of appetite could precipitate an adolescent decline. Mothers were urged to be vigilant: "If Mamie has not a rational appetite, create a digestive conscious [*sic*] that may serve her instead." Mothers were expected to educate, if not tame, their adolescent daughter's propensity for "sweetmeats, bonbons, and summer drinks" as well as for "stimulating foods such as black pepper and vinegar pickle."[29] "Inflammatory foods" such as condiments and acids, thought to be favored by the tumultuous female adolescent, were strictly prohibited by judicious mothers. Adolescent girls were expressly cautioned against coffee, tea, and chocolate; salted meats and spices; warm bread and pastry; confectionery; nuts and raisins; and, of course, alcohol.[30] These sorts of foods stimulated the sensual rather than the moral nature of the girl.

No food (other than alcohol) caused Victorian women and girls greater moral anxiety than meat. The flesh of animals was considered a heat-producing food that stimulated production of blood and fat as well as passion. Doctors and patients shared a common conception of meat as a food that stimulated sexual development and activity. For example, Lucien Warner, a popular medical writer, suggested that meat eating in adolescence could actually accelerate the development of the breasts and other sex characteristics; at the same time, a restriction on the carnivorous aspects of the diet could moderate premature or rampant sexuality as well as overabundant menstrual flow. "If there is any tendency to precocity in menstruation, or if the system is very robust and plethoric, the supply of meat should be quite limited. If, on the other hand, the girl is of sluggish temperament and the menses are tardy in appearance, the supply of meat should be especially generous."[31] Meat eating in excess was linked to adolescent insanity and to nymphomania.[32] A stimulative diet of meat and condiments was recommended only for those girls whose development of the passions seemed, somehow, "deficient."

By all reports adolescent girls ate very little meat, a practice that certainly contributed to chlorosis or iron-deficiency anemia. In fact, many openly disdained meat without being necessarily committed to the ideological principles of the health reformers who espoused vegetarianism.[33] Meat avoidance, therefore, is the most apt term for this pattern of behavior. According to E. Lloyd

Jones, adolescent girls "are fond of biscuits, potatoes, etc. while they avoid meat on most occasions, and when they do eat meat, they prefer the burnt outside portion." Another doctor confirmed the same problem in a dialogue between himself and a patient. "Oh, I like pies and preserves but I can't bear meat," the young woman reportedly told the family physician. A "disgust for meat in any form" characterized many of the adolescent female patients of a Pennsylvania practitioner of this period.[34]

When it became necessary to eat meat (say, if prescribed by a doctor), it was an event worthy of note. For many, meat eating was endured for its healing qualities but despised as a moral and aesthetic act. For example, eighteen-year-old Nellie Browne wrote to tell her mother that a delicate classmate [Laura] had, like her own sister Alice, been forced to change her eating habits:

> I am very sorry to hear Alice has been so sick. Tell her she must eat meat if she wishes to get well. Laura eats meat *three* times a day.—She says she cannot go without it.—If Laura *can* eat *meat, I am sure Alice can*. If Laura needs it *three* times a day, Alice needs it *six*. (Italics in original.)[35]

After acknowledging the "common distaste for meat" among his adolescent patients, Clifford Allbutt wrote, "Girls will say the entry of a dish of hot meat into the room makes them feel sick."[36]

The repugnance for fatty animal flesh among Victorian adolescents ultimately had a larger cultural significance. Meat avoidance was tied to cultural notions of sexuality and decorum as well as to medical ideas about the digestive delicacy of the female stomach. Carnality at table was avoided by many who made sexual purity an axiom. Proper women, especially sexually maturing girls, adopted this orientation with the result that meat became taboo. Contemporary descriptions reveal that some young women may well have been phobic about meat eating because of its associations:

> There is the common illustration which every one meets a thousand times in a lifetime, of the girl whose stomach rebels at the very thought of fat meat. The mother tries persuasion and entreaty and threats and penalties. But nothing can overcome the artistic development in the girl's nature which makes her revolt at the bare idea of putting the fat piece of a dead animal between her lips.[37]

In this milieu food was obviously more than a source of nutrition or a means of curbing hunger; it was an integral part of individual identity. For women in particular, how one ate spoke to issues of basic character.

"A Woman Should Never Be Seen Eating"

In Victorian society food and femininity were linked in such a way as to promote restrictive eating among privileged adolescent women. Bourgeois society generated anxieties about food and eating—especially among women. Where food was plentiful and domesticity venerated, eating became a highly charged emotional and social undertaking. Displays of appetite were particularly difficult for young women who understood appetite to be both a sign of sexuality and an indication of lack of self-restraint. Eating was important because food was an analogue of the self. Food choice was a form of self-expression, made according to cultural and social ideas as well as physiological requirements. As the anthropologist Claude Lévi-Strauss put it, things must be "not only good to eat, but also good to think."[38]

Female discomfort with food, as well as with the act of eating, was a pervasive subtext of Victorian popular culture.[39] The naturalness of eating was especially problematic among upwardly mobile, middle-class women who were preoccupied with establishing their own good taste.[40] Food and eating presented obvious difficulties because they implied digestion and defecation, as well as sexuality. A doctor explained that one of his anorexic patients "refused to eat for fear that, during her digestion, her face should grow red and appear less pleasant in the eyes of a professor whose lectures she attended after her meals."[41] A woman who ate inevitably had to urinate and move her bowels. Concern about these bodily indelicacies explains why constipation was incorporated into the ideal of Victorian femininity. (It was almost always a symptom in anorexia nervosa.) Some women "boasted that the calls of Nature upon them averaged but one or two demands per week."[42]

Food and eating were connected to other unpleasantries that reflected the self-identity of middle-class women. Many women, for good reason, connected food with work and drudgery. Food preparation was a time-consuming and exhausting job in the middle-class household, where families no longer ate from a common soup pot. Instead, meals were served as individual dishes in a sequence of courses. Women of real means and position were able to remove themselves from food preparation almost entirely by turning over the arduous daily work to cooks, bakers, scullery and serving maids, and butlers. Middle-class women, however, could not achieve the same distance from food.[43]

Advice books admonished women "not to be ashamed of the kitchen," but many still sought to separate themselves from both food and the working-class women they hired to do the preparation and cooking. A few women felt the need to make alienation from food a centerpiece of their identity. A young "lady teacher," for example, "regard[ed] it as unbecoming her position to know anything about dinner before the hour for eating arrived . . . [She was] ashamed of domestic work, and graduate[d] her pupils with a similar sense of false propriety."[44] Similarly, in the 1880s in Rochester, New York, a schoolgirl was chastised by her aunt for describing (with relish) in her diary the foods she had eaten during the preceding two weeks.[45]

Food was to be feared because it was connected to gluttony and to physical ugliness. In advice books such as the 1875 *Health Fragments; or, Steps toward a True Life* women were cautioned to be careful about what and how much they ate. Authors George and Susan Everett enjoined: "Coarse, gross, and gluttonous habits of life degrade the physical appearance. You will rarely be disappointed in supposing that a lucid, self-respectful lady is very careful of the food which forms her body and tints her cheeks." Sarah Josepha Hale, the influential editor of *Godey's Lady's Book* and an arbiter of American domestic manners, warned women that it was always vulgar to load the plate.[46]

Careful, abstemious eating was presented as insurance against ugliness and loss of love. Girls in particular were told: "Keep a great watch over your appetite. Don't always take the nicest things you see, but be frugal and plain in your tastes."[47] Young women were told directly that "gross eaters" not only developed thick skin but had prominent blemishes and broken blood vessels on the nose. Gluttony also robbed the eyes of their intensity and caused the lips to thicken, crack, and lose their red color. "The glutton's mouth may remind us of cod-fish—never of kisses." A woman with a rosebud mouth was expected to have an "ethereal appetite." A story circulated that Madam von Stein "lost Goethe's love by gross habits of eating sausages and drinking strong coffee, which destroyed her beauty." Women such as von Stein, who indulged in the pleasures of the appetite, were said to develop "a certain unspiritual or superanimal expression" that conveyed their base instincts. "[We] have never met true refinement in the person of a gross eater," wrote the Everetts.[48]

Indulgence in foods that were considered stimulating or inflammatory served not only as an emblem of unchecked sensuality but sometimes as a sign of social aggression. Women who ate meat could be regarded as acting out of place; they were assuming a male prerogative. In *Daniel Deronda* (1876) George Eliot described a group of local gentry, all men, who came together after a hunt to take their meal apart from the women. As they ate, the men took turns telling stories about the "epicurism of the ladies, who had somehow been reported to show a revolting masculine judgement in venison." Female eating was a source of titillation to men precisely because they understood eating to be a trope for sexuality. Furthermore, women who asked baldly for venison were aggressive if not insatiable. What most bothered the local gentry was the women's effrontery to "ask . . . for the fat—a proof of the frightful rate at which corruption might go in women, but for severe social restraint."[49]

Because food and eating carried such complex meanings, manners at the table became an important aspect of a woman's social persona. In their use of certain kinds of conventions, nineteenth-century novelists captured the crucial importance of food and eating in the milieu of middle-class women. Because they understood the middle-class reverence for the family meal, writers such as Jane Austen and Anthony Trollope saw the meal as an arena for potential individual and collective embarrassment. These novelists provided numerous examples of young women whose lives and fortunes hung on the issue of dinner-table decorum. For example, in Austen's *Mansfield Park* (1814) the heroine, Fanny

Price, was horrified at the prospect of having her well-bred suitor eat with her family and "see all their deficiencies." Fanny was concerned not only about her family's lower standard of cookery, but about her sister's mortifying tendency to eat "without restraint." In Trollope's *Ralph the Heir* (1871) the family of Mr. Neefit, a tradesman, invited Ralph Newton, a gentleman, to their family table after some degree of preparation and nervousness on the part of the wife and daughter. Newton, who was halfheartedly courting the daughter at the request of her socially ambitious father, ultimately concluded that the young woman was attractive enough but the roughness of her father was unbearable. He found particularly galling the manner in which Mr. Neefit ate his shrimp.[50] Manners at table were often a dead giveaway of one's true social origins. This convention for marking the social distance between the classes was utilized by Mark Twain in the famous scene in *The Prince and the Pauper* (1881) where the prince's impersonator drinks from his fingerbowl.[51]

Women's anxieties about how to eat in genteel fashion were widespread and conveyed by novelists in a number of different ways. In Elizabeth Gaskell's *Cranford* (1853), the middle-class ladies of the town were made uncomfortable by the presentation of foods that were difficult to eat—in this case, peas and oranges. One woman "sighed over her delicate young peas [but] left them on one side of her plate untasted" rather than attempt to stab them or risk dropping them between the two prongs of her fork. She knew that she could not do "the ungenteel thing"—shoveling them with her knife. So, too, oranges presented difficulties for the decorous middle-class women of Cranford:

> When oranges came in, a curious proceeding was gone through. Miss Jenkyns did not like to cut the fruit; for, as she observed, the juice all ran out nobody knew where; sucking (only I think she used some more recondite word) was in fact the only way of enjoying oranges; but then there was the unpleasant association with a ceremony frequently gone through by little babies; and so, after dessert, in orange season, Miss Jenkyns and Miss Matty used to rise up, possess themselves each of an orange in silence, and withdraw to the privacy of their own rooms to indulge in sucking oranges.[52]

In fact, secret eating was not unknown among those who subscribed

to the absurd dictum that "a woman should never be seen eating."[53] This statement, attributed by George Eliot to the famed
poet Lord Byron, was the ultimate embodiment of Victorian imperatives about food and gender.

*chauvinist
pig!!)*

Over and over again, in all of the popular literature of the
Victorian period, good women distanced themselves from the act
of eating with disclaimers that pronounced their disinterest in
anything but the aesthetics of food. "It's very little I eat myself,"
a proper Trollopian hostess explained, "but I do like to see things
nice."[54] Apparently, Victorian girls adopted the aesthetic sensibilities of their mothers, displaying extraordinary interest in the
appearance and color of their food, in the effect of fine china and
linen, and in agreeable surroundings. A 1904 study of the psychology of foods in adolescence reported that boys most valued
companionship at table, whereas girls emphasized "ceremony"
and "appointments."[55] Attention to the aesthetics of eating
seemed to minimize the negative implications of participating in
the gustatory and digestive process.

But Victorian women avoided connections to food for a number
of other reasons. The woman who put soul over body was the
ideal of Victorian femininity. The genteel woman responded not
to the lower senses of taste and smell but to the highest senses—
sight and hearing—which were used for moral and aesthetic purposes.[56] One of the most convincing demonstrations of a spiritual
orientation was a thin body—that is, a physique that symbolized
rejection of all carnal appetites. To be hungry, in any sense, was
a social faux pas. Denial became a form of moral certitude and
refusal of attractive foods a means for advancing in the moral
hierarchy.

Appetite, then, was a barometer of a woman's moral state.
Control of eating was eminently desirable, if not necessary. Where
control was lacking, young women were subject to derision. "The
girl who openly enjoys bread-and-butter, milk, beefsteak and potatoes, and thrives thereby, is the object of many a covert sneer,
or even overt jest, even in these sensible days and among sensible
people."[57] Given the intensity of concern about control of appetite, it is not surprising that some women found strong attraction
in cultural figures whose biographies exemplified the triumph of
spirit over flesh. Two figures representing the Romantic and me-

dieval traditions became especially relevant to how young women thought about these issues: Lord Byron and Catherine of Siena. Both spoke to the moral desirability of being thin.

Known to the Victorian reading public as the author of the immensely popular epic poems *Childe Harold* and *Don Juan*, Lord Byron (1788–1824) remained an important cultural figure whose life and work stood, even as late as the third quarter of the century, as a symbol of the power of the Romantic movement.[58] Young women who shared the Romantic sensibility found Byron's poetry inspirational. *Childe Harold*, which detailed a youth's struggle for meaning, spoke to the inner reaches of the soul and helped its readers transcend the "tawdry world." For many, such as Trollope's Lizzie Eustace, Byron was "the boy poet who understood it all."[59]

Although Byron's tempestuous love life served to titillate some and revolt others, the poet's struggles with the relation of his body to his mind were of enormous interest to women. Byron starved his body in order to keep his brain clear. He existed on biscuits and soda water for days and took no animal food. According to memoirs written by acquaintances, the poet had a "horror of fat"; to his mind, fat symbolized lethargy, dullness, and stupidity. Byron feared that if he ate normally he would lose his creativity. Only through abstinence could his mind exercise and improve. In short, Byron was a model of exquisite slenderness and his sensibilities about fat were embraced by legions of young women.[60]

Adults, especially physicians, lamented Byron's influence on youthful Victorians. In addition to encouraging melancholia and emotional volatility, Byronism had consequence for the eating habits of girls. In Britain "the dread of being fat weigh[ed] like an incubus" on Romantic youngsters who consumed vinegar "to produce thinness" and swallowed rice "to cause the complexion to become paler."[61] According to American George Beard, "our young ladies live all their growing girlhood in semi-starvation" because of a fear of "incurring the horror of disciples of Lord Byron."[62] Byronic youth, in imitation of their idol, disparaged fat of any kind, a practice which advice writers found detrimental to their good health. "If plump, [the girl] berates herself as a criminal against refinement and aesthetic taste; and prays in good or bad earnest, for a spell of illness to pull her down."[63] Other doctors

besides Beard spoke of the popular Romantic association between
scanty eating, a slim body, and "delicacy of mind." Beard, however, did not let the blame for modern eating habits rest entirely
on the Romantics. He decried the influence of Calvinist doctrine
as well. Cultivated people, he said, eat too little because of the
old belief that "satiety is a conviction of sin."[64]

Women attuned to the higher senses did find inspiration for
their abstemious eating in the austerities of medieval Catholics—
particularly Catherine of Siena. Although Protestant Victorian
writers presented Catherine's asceticism as a dangerous form of
self-mortification, there was also widespread admiration for the
spiritual intensity that drove her fasts. Victorian writers used the
biography of Saint Catherine to demonstrate how selfhood could
be lost to a higher moral or spiritual purpose. This message was
considered particularly relevant to girls, in that self-love was supposed to be a distinguishing characteristic of the female adolescent.[65] Saint Catherine's biography was included in inspirational
books for girls, and two prominent women of the period demonstrated serious interest in her life. Josephine Butler, an articulate
English feminist, published a full-length biography in 1879; and
Vida Scudder, a Wellesley College professor of English and a
Christian socialist, published her letters in 1895.[66] Because she
provided a vivid demonstration of a woman who placed spiritual
over bodily concerns, Catherine of Siena was of enormous interest
to Anglo-American women.

This lingering ascetic imperative did not go unnoticed by one
of the period's most astute observers of religious behavior, William James. In *The Varieties of Religious Experience* the Harvard
philosopher and psychologist noted quite correctly that old religious habits of "misery" and "morbidness" had fallen into dis-
repute. Those who pursued "hard and painful" austerities were
regarded, in the modern era, as "abnormal." Yet James noted
that young women were the most likely to remain tied to the
dying tradition of religious asceticism. Although he understood
that ascetic behavior had many sources (what he called "diverse
psychological levels"), he did mark girls as the group most likely
to embrace "saintliness." "We all have some friend," James wrote,
"perhaps more often feminine than masculine, and young than

old, whose soul is of this blue-sky tint, whose affinities are rather with flowers and birds and all enchanting innocencies than with dark human passions."[67] Girls seemed to be the most interested in the tenets of what James called saintliness: conquering the ordinary desires of the flesh, establishing purity, and taking pleasure in sacrifice.[68]

Those who were ascetic in girlhood tried to act as well as look like saints. In *The Morgesons* (1862) Veronica, an adolescent invalid and dyspeptic, defined her saintliness through a diet of tea and dry toast. She cropped her hair short in the manner of a penitent; constantly washed her hands with lavender water, as if she were taking a ritual absolution; and on her bedroom wall hung a picture of the martyred Saint Cecilia with white roses in her hair.[69] Although Veronica was a Protestant, she revered Saint Cecilia for her spirituality. Many novelists linked asceticism to physical beauty as well as to spiritual perfection. In short, beautiful women were often "saintlike," a relationship that implied the inverse as well—the "saintlike" were beautiful. Trollope, for example, described a young gentleman who "declared to himself at once that she was the most lovely young woman he had ever seen. She had dark eyes, and perfect eyebrows, and a face which, either for colour or lines of beauty, might have been taken for a model for any female saint or martyr."[70]

By the last decades of the nineteenth century, a thin body symbolized more than just sublimity of mind and purity of soul. Slimness in women was also a sign of social status. This phenomenon, noted by Thorstein Veblen in *The Theory of the Leisure Class*, heralded the demise of the traditional view that girth in a woman signaled prosperity in a man. Rather, the reverse was true: a thin, frail woman was a symbol of status and an object of beauty precisely because she was unfit for productive (or reproductive) work. Body image rather than body function became a paramount concern.[71] According to Veblen, a thin woman signified the idle idyll of the leisured classes.

By the turn of the twentieth century, elite society already preferred its women thin and frail as a symbol of their social distance from the working classes. Consequently, women with social aspirations adopted the rule of slenderness and its related dicta about parsimonious appetite and delicate food. Through restrictive eating and restrictive clothing (that is, the corset), women changed their bodies in the name of gentility.

Women of means were the first to diet to constrain their appetite, and they began to do so before the sexual and fashion revolutions of the 1920s and the 1960s. In the 1890s Veblen noted that privileged women "[took] thought to alter their persons, so as to conform more nearly to the instructed taste of the time."[72] In effect, Veblen documented the existence of a critical gender and class imperative born of social stratification. In bourgeois society it became incumbent upon women to control their appetite in order to encode their body with the correct social messages.[73] Appetite became less of a biological drive and more of a social and emotional instrument.

Historical evidence suggests that many women managed their food and their appetite in response to the notion that sturdiness in women implied low status, a lack of gentility, and even vulgarity. Eating less rather than more became a preferred pattern for those who were status conscious. The pressure to be thin in order to appear genteel came from many quarters, including parents. "The mother, also, would look upon the sturdy frame and ruddy cheeks as tokens of vulgarity."[74] Recall that Eva Williams, admitted to London Hospital in 1895 for treatment of anorexia nervosa, told friends that it was her mother who complained about her rotundity.

A controlled appetite and ill health were twin vehicles to elevated womanhood. Advice to parents about the care of adolescent daughters regularly included the observation that young women ate scantily because they denigrated health and fat for their declassé associations. In 1863 Hester Pendleton, an American writer on the role of heredity in human growth, lamented the fact that the natural development of young women was being affected by these popular ideas. "So perverted are the tastes of some persons," Pendleton wrote, "that delicacy of constitution is considered a badge of aristocracy, and daughters would feel themselves deprecated by too robust health."[75] Health in this case meant a sturdy body, a problem for those who cultivated the fashion of refined femininity. One writer felt compelled to assert: "Bodily health is never pertinently termed 'rude.' It is not coarse to eat heartily, sleep well, and to feel the life throbbing joyously in heart and limb."[76]

Consequently, to have it insinuated or said that a woman was robust constituted an insult. This convention was captured by Anthony Trollope in *Can You Forgive Her?* (1864). After a late-night walk on the grounds of the Palliser estate, the novel's genteel but impoverished young heroine, Alice Vavasour, was criticized by a male guest for her insensitivity to the physical delicacy of her walking companion and host, Lady Glencora Palliser. The youthful and beautiful Lady Glencora caught cold from the midnight romp, but Alice did not. The critical gentleman immediately caught the social implications of the fact that Alice was *not* unwell from the escapade, and he used her health against her: "Alice knew that she was being accused of being robust . . . but she bore it in silence. Ploughboys and milkmaids are robust, and the accusation was a heavy one."[77] The same associations were relevant thirty years later in the lives of middle-class American girls. Marion Harland observed that the typical young woman "would be disgraced in her own opinion and lost caste with her refined mates, were she to eat like a ploughboy."[78]

In the effort to set themselves apart from plowboys and milkmaids—that is, working and rural youth—middle-class daughters chose to pursue a body configuration that was small, slim, and essentially decorative. By eating only tiny amounts of food, young women could disassociate themselves from sexuality and fecundity and they could achieve an unambiguous class identity. The thin body not only implied asexuality and an elevated social address, it was also an expression of intelligence, sensitivity, and morality. Through control of appetite Victorian girls found a way of expressing a complex of emotional, aesthetic, and class sensibilities.

By 1900 the imperative to be thin was pervasive, particularly among affluent female adolescents. Albutt wrote in 1905, "Many young women, as their frames develop, fall into a panic fear of obesity, and not only cut down on their food, but swallow vinegar and other alleged antidotes to fatness."[79] The phenomenon of adolescent food restriction was so widespread that an advice writer told mothers, "It is a circumstance at once fortunate and notable if [your daughter] does not take the notion into her pulpy brain that a healthy appetite for good substantial food is 'not a bit nice,' 'quite too awfully vulgar you know.'"[80]

Because food was a common resource in the middle-class household, it was available for manipulation. Middle-class girls, rather than boys, turned to food as a symbolic language, because the culture made an important connection between food and femininity and because girls' options for self-expression outside the family were limited by parental concern and social convention. In addition, doctors and parents expected adolescent girls to be finicky and restrictive about their food. Young women searching for an idiom in which to say things about themselves focused on food and the body. Some middle-class girls, then as now, became preoccupied with expressing an ideal of female perfection and moral superiority through denial of appetite. The popularity of food restriction or dieting, even among normal girls, suggests that in bourgeois society appetite was (and is) an important voice in the identity of a woman. In this context anorexia nervosa was born.

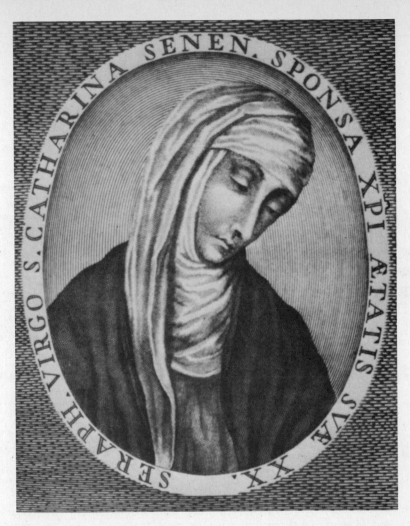

Fasting was one facet of the penitential program that absorbed religious women in the Middle Ages. Like many other female ascetics, Saint Catherine of Siena ate little normal food and allegedly existed on a spoonful of herbs each day. *Frontispiece to Edmund Garratt Gardner,* Saint Catherine of Siena *(New York: E. P. Dutton, 1907).*

ANN MOORE,

THE FASTING WOMAN OF TUTBURY.

THERE is living in the village of TUTBURY, in Staffordshire, a woman named ANN MOORE, whose extraordinary and perpetual abstinence from food, has, for a considerable time been the subject of much wonder and attention :—the following is a concise statement of her case.

ANN MOORE had been in a declining state of health for many years previous to her first attack of anorexy, which she believes to have been occasioned by her attendance on a diseased boy, whose loathsome complaint produced that effect on her imagination, which caused an habitual disinclination for all kind of food.

FOR some time, this remarkable case was treated as an imposition, until humanity prompted some of her neighbours to represent her distressing state of existence to the neighbouring gentlemen of the medical profession, and others; who, to satisfy themselves and the public, instituted an examination of the truth of her case, which terminated in proving the facts here stated.

"ON the 14th of April, 1807, she took to her bed for a continuance. In the latter end of June following, she eat a few black currants, being the last substance she swallowed. From that time until the examination was instituted, she occasionally took a tea spoonful of water or tea, without sugar or milk; but it occasioned such extreme pain in swallowing, that she was advised by the medical attendant, to refrain from taking any more. For the space of *sixteen* days she was strictly watched, under the direction of MR. ROBERT TAYLOR, Member of the Royal College of Surgeons, London, and every method adopted, for detecting the supposed imposition. But the watch ended in proving, that she existed for *thirteen* days, without aliment of any kind, either liquid or solid; at the end of which time, she was better in health than when the examination was established." For the period of *several years* from the time above stated, she has been in the same recumbent state of existence, without the support of nutriment of any kind.

THE state of her physical powers, is extremely weak and emaciated; the body resembling a human skeleton, more than a living subject; her legs are drawn up in a contracted form, and are quite useless. Her countenance is handsome, and her face has not that emaciated appearance to which her body is reduced, but retains the character of apparent health.

SHE seldom sleeps, and the position in which she usually sits in her bed, is that in which she is represented in a drawing, taken from life, by MR. LINCELL, and engraved by ANTHONY CARDON, Esq., which portrays her exactly as she was soon after the watch had ended. She is able to read with the aid of glasses, and has the Bible generally on the bed before her, which she calls her "best companion." She seems free from superstition, and endures her sufferings with a serenity of mind, that characterizes the Christian in a state of patient and pious resignation.

HER readiness to satisfy any inquiries that visitors think proper to make, gives to every one an opportunity of investigating particulars, and ascertaining facts already given to the public. The curious in physiology, or anatomical detail, may be gratified with the particulars of her case by referring to the Medical and Physical Journals, which contain several accounts by medical gentlemen who have examined her.

PRINTED BY T. WAYTE, HIGH-STREET, BURTON, 1811.

By the seventeenth and eighteenth centuries, claims to miraculously inspired lack of appetite generated skepticism as well as awe. At the turn of the nineteenth century, Ann Moore's "anorexy" stimulated public discussion among English clergymen, doctors, and local villagers. Moore's claim that she ate nothing at all was eventually proved fraudulent by examiners who sought to demonstrate that prolonged abstinence could be understood as something other than miraculous.

1812 broadside, "Ann Moore, The Fasting Woman of Tutbury," printed by T. Wayte in James Ward, Some Account of Mary Thomas of Tanyralt . . . and of Ann Moore . . . of Tutbury *(London, 1813); courtesy of the Wellcome Institute Library, London.*

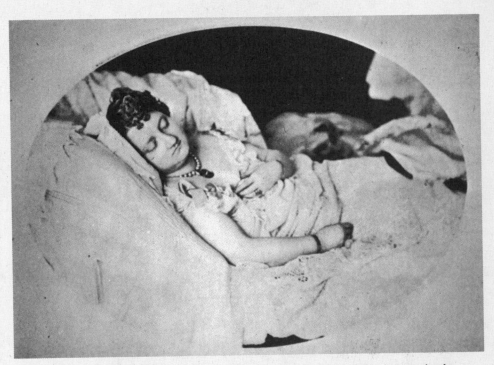

Brooklyn's Mollie Fancher was one of the famous fasting girls who caught the attention of newspaper audiences in Britain and the United States in the late 1860s and 1870s. Many believed that the fasting girls actually lived without eating. Sophisticated doctors, however, insisted that prolonged abstinence from food was impossible without death and regarded the fasting girls as either fraudulent or hysterical. Men of science found Fancher's case particularly annoying because she claimed to be clairvoyant as well as absolutely abstemious. *Frontispiece from Abram Dailey,* Mollie Fancher: The Brooklyn Enigma *(Brooklyn, 1894).*

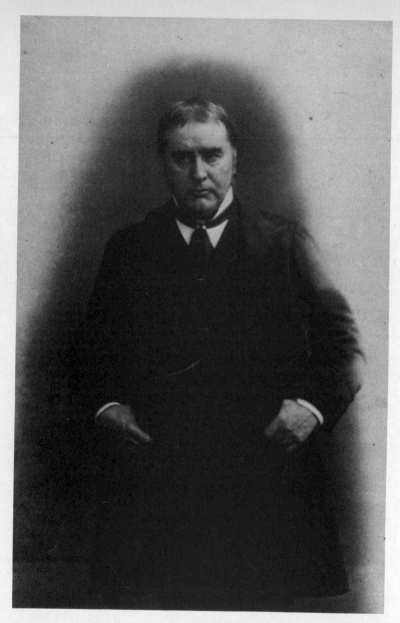

Sir William Withey Gull, elite London physician and medical adviser to the family of Queen Victoria, named and identified anorexia nervosa in 1873. Gull was never particularly interested in the mental state of anorexic patients, but he did provide physicians with a reliable way to differentiate emaciation in anorexia nervosa from emaciation in other "wasting diseases" or biomedical conditions. *Photograph of Sir William Withey Gull, M.D., by Elliot and Fry; courtesy of the Wellcome Institute Library, London.*

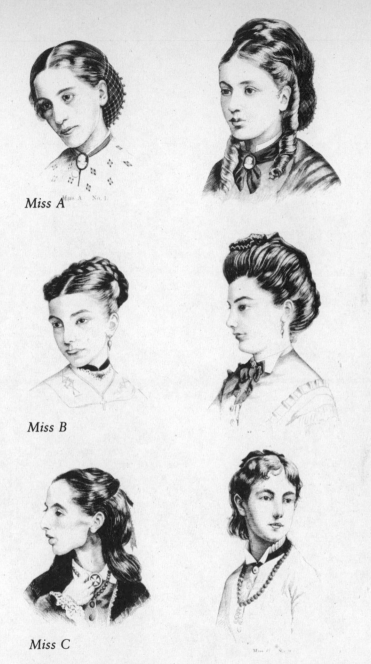

Miss A

Miss B

Miss C

Gull's first anorexic patients were young women, between the ages of sixteen and twenty-four, from reputable families with some economic resources. Gull advised rest, regular feeding, and, where possible, removal from the family environment.

Engravings from Gull's first clinical case report, Transactions of the Clinical Society of London 7 (1874), 22–28.

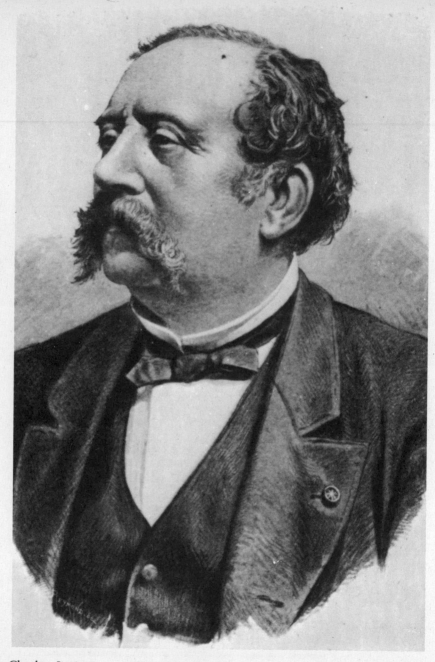

Charles Lasègue, a well-known French physician, identified and described *l'anorexie hystérique* a few months before William Gull published his report. The two doctors agreed that most anorectics were adolescent girls. Lasègue was more interested than Gull in the psychology of the disorder and the manner in which families responded to their daughter's refusal to eat.

Lithograph portrait of Charles Lasègue, M.D., from Corlieu, Centenaire *(1896); courtesy of the Wellcome Institute Library, London.*

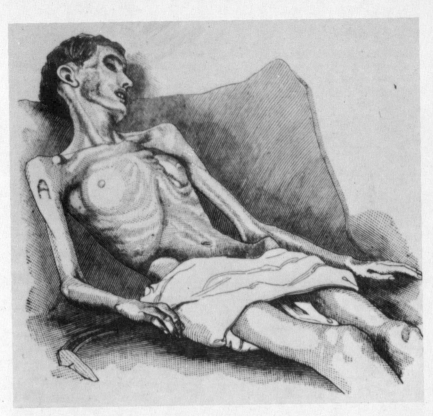

Late-nineteenth-century doctors developed a number of specialized techniques for treating anorectics. For example, in 1895 *Lancet* reported the case of a sixteen-year-old Bristol schoolgirl. In the hospital, the 5-foot-4-inch patient was kept immobile in her bed by wrapping her limbs and body in cotton wool, a method for elevating body temperature and restricting activity. She was fed pulverized food every four hours. The attending physician attempted to keep her family, particularly her mother, away from the girl. Despite these efforts, the patient died at 49 pounds, the first reported death from the modern disorder in English-language medicine.
Lancet *(January 5, 1895), 31.*

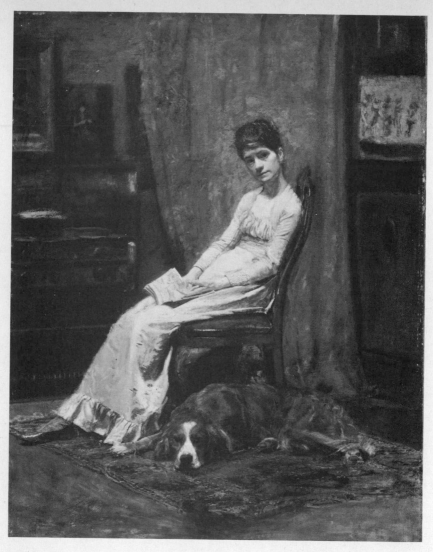

In Victorian society how and what one ate were important indications of female character for middle-class and upper-class women. The slim body and languishing posture of this young woman, painted by Thomas Eakins in 1885, epitomized the Victorian ideal of femininity. In the minds of privileged young women, fragility and debility were linked to a spirituality that transcended the need for food.

Thomas Eakins, Portrait of a Lady with a Setter Dog (1885) *from the Metropolitan Museum of Art, Fletcher Fund, 1933, New York.*

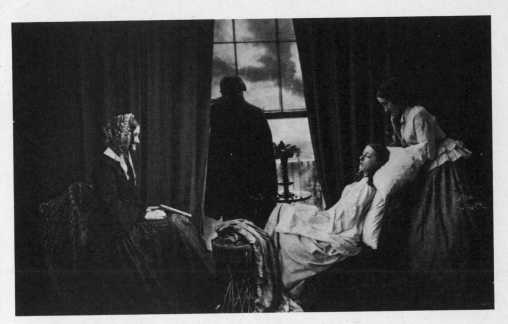

Many Victorian women, especially adolescent girls, suffered from appetite disorders and sensitive stomachs as well as consumption and tuberculosis. Frightened by emaciation and the prospect of death, bourgeois parents turned to professional medicine for assistance in a painful and confusing family ordeal. *Henry Peach Robinson,* Fading Away *(1858); courtesy of the International Museum of Photography, George Eastman House, Rochester, N.Y.*

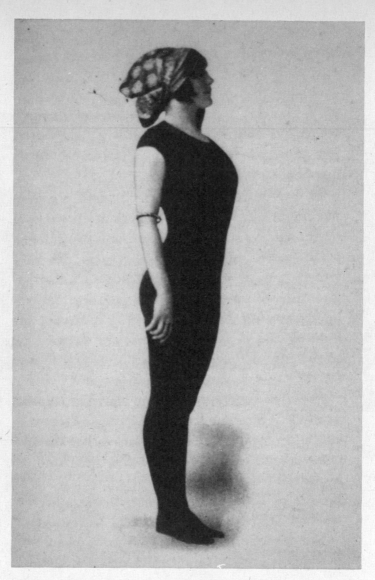

In the 1920s a svelte female figure became the ultimate symbol of heterosexual interest and success. Annette Kellerman, swimmer and early movie star, advocated female athleticism and the primacy of the body. Kellerman proclaimed the figure even more essential than the face in the definition of feminine good looks.
Annette Kellerman, Physical Beauty *(New York, 1918).*

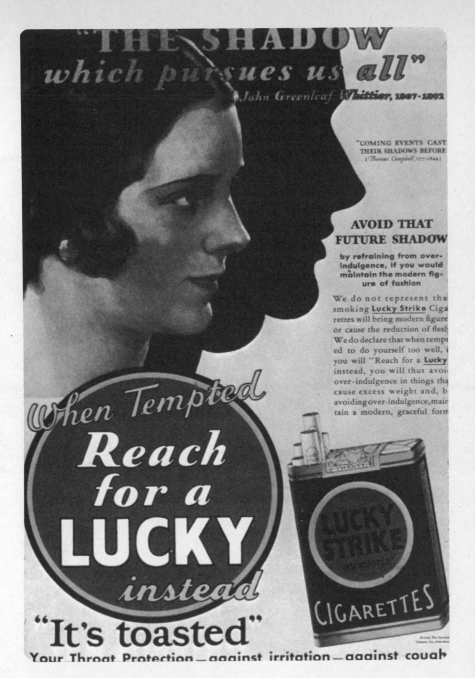

Over the years, as the imperatives for female dieting intensified, women were sold many products—including cigarettes—to help them become or remain slim. Despite the barrage of warnings to the general public by the 1980s, today's teenage girls are the fastest-growing market for cigarettes, precisely because they regard smoking as an aid to appetite control.
Literary Digest *(April 5, 1930).*

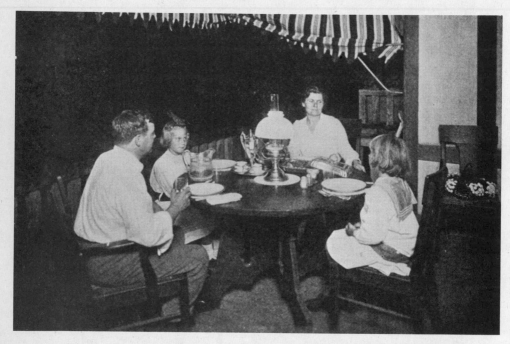

As food and eating moved to the heart of middle-class domesticity in the nineteenth century, the dinner table became an arena for many of the problems as well as the pleasures of family life. In the early twentieth century, home economists made it woman's responsibility to manage, even preside over, family meals. In essence, she determined the welfare of the family.

Frontispiece from Mary Swartz Rose, Feeding the Family *(New York, 1916).*

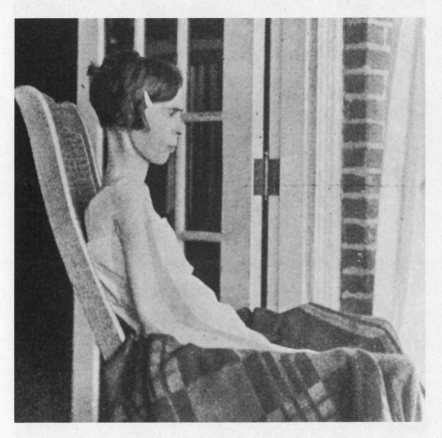

By the 1930s there were three essential techniques in the management of anorexia nervosa: change of environment, forced feeding, and psychotherapy. Severe cases were generally treated in private psychiatric hospitals. The young woman shown here was a patient in a New Hampshire hospital; this is the first published photo of an anorectic in an American medical journal.
Reprinted by permission of the New England Journal of Medicine *207 (October 5, 1932), 613–617.*

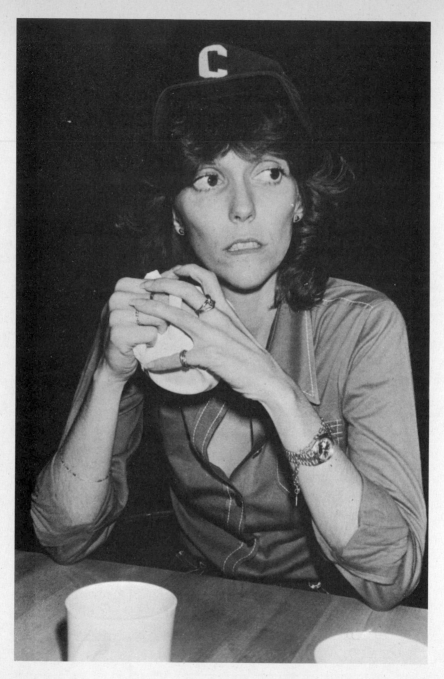

In January 1983 thirty-two-year-old popular singer Karen Carpenter died as a result of complications of anorexia nervosa. Her tragic death generated a great deal of interest in the disorder and made anorexia nervosa well-known among the American public. Phrases such as "You look anorexic" have become common parlance and are used by many outside the medical profession, especially women, to comment on one another's bodies.
© B. Schiffman, Gamma-Liaison.

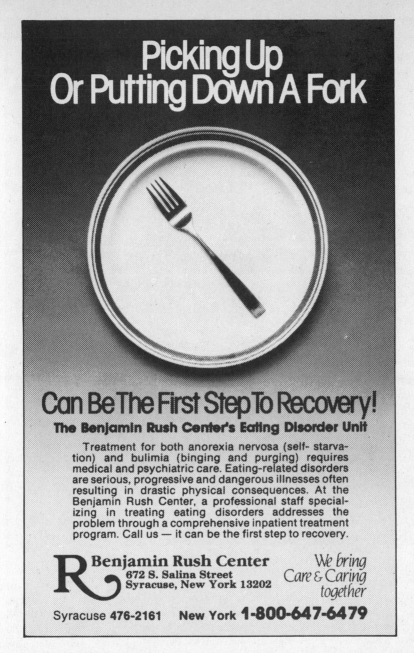
In response to the recent increase in anorexia nervosa and bulimia, there has been an explosion of professional interest in eating disorders as well as a growing number of therapeutic options for sufferers. In the 1980s patients and their families can choose among outpatient and inpatient facilities in a variety of settings both public and private. Special eating-disorder clinics—such as the Benjamin Rush Center in Syracuse—provide a functional way to organize comprehensive medical and psychiatric treatment within a single medical institution. *Courtesy of the Benjamin Rush Center, Syracuse, N.Y.*

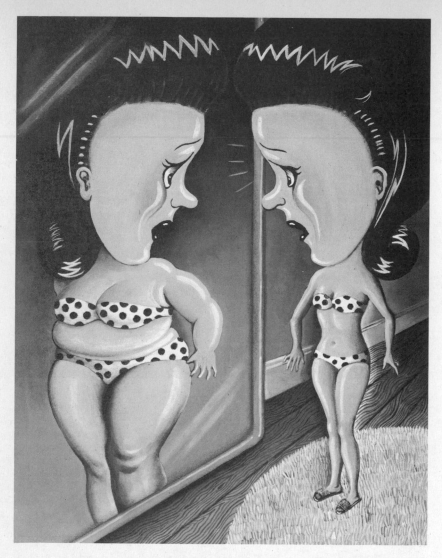

This image, drawn by Sheba Ross for *Ms.*, became the symbol of anorexia nervosa and has been repeated with many variations in publications about the disorder. In reality, the image of the thin woman who sees herself as fat captures the predicament of most American women of the middle and upper classes. Among women aged eighteen to thirty-five, 75 percent regard themselves as fat even though only 25 percent are overweight. Psychological and cultural studies confirm that weight is women's "normative obsession" and that American society is obesophobic.

Sheba Ross, Ms. (October 1983); courtesy of Nina Sklansky.

8 · Hormones and Psychotherapy

In the twentieth century the treatment of anorexia nervosa changed to incorporate new medical theories and developments. Because nineteenth-century medicine had not resolved the problem of etiology, the twentieth century was characterized by a multiplicity of treatment strategies that reflected new developments within both medical and psychiatric practice. At the time of World War I, patients with anorexia nervosa were still subject to frequent high-calorie feedings (à la William Gull) but they were also likely to receive—either orally or by injection—hormonal extracts that were intended to effect the metabolism of food and stimulate the appetite. By World War II, physicians were taking vaginal smears from anorexic patients, administering synthetic estrogen in order to stimulate menstrual functioning, and probing the psyche for ideas about sexuality.

In the period 1900–1940, treatment of anorexic patients followed two distinct and largely isolated models of research and practice, the biological and the psychoanalytic. In the 1930s, the psychosomatic movement provided an appealing (but for the most part unsuccessful) effort to join the two. Among psychiatrists, psychosomatic medicine held out the promise of increasing the authority of the specialty by uncovering the mysterious links between mental and biological factors in the generation of disease. Although twentieth-century treatment of anorexia nervosa evolved from these particular medical models (biological, psychoanalytic, and psychosomatic), the situation was rarely as neat as the categories suggest. In fact, most physicians were eclectic and few held to a purely somatic or psychotherapeutic approach.

Because of the diversity of therapeutic strategies, there has also been confusion about the use of anorexia nervosa as a clinical classification. The diagnosis was used by twentieth-century clinicians to designate diverse patient types and not just the classic adolescent or young adult woman who refused to eat. These new anorectics included emaciated adults with thyroid conditions, very young children with failed appetites, and adult schizophrenics whose refusal of food was a secondary feature of their illness.[1] The enlargement of the classification evolved primarily because of psychiatry's tendency to base its nosology on external behavioral symptoms (such as refusing food) rather than on a specific etiology. Moreover, because symptoms are always subject to medical interpretation and reevaluation, disease definitions will inevitably vary and so will the nature of the patient group. In the twentieth century there has been significant fluidity in the use of the term "anorexia nervosa," and the diagnosis has been used to cover a number of different kinds of patients. My primary focus here, however, will be on the evolution of treatment strategies used with adolescent and young adult women who continue to be the primary constituency for the disease.

Organ Juices

Scientific and medical discoveries in the 1890s set the stage for a new kind of treatment of anorexia nervosa based on a biological model. In the last decade of the nineteenth century French and Anglo-American doctors experimented with organotherapy, a generalized form of treatment rooted in the principle that disease resulted from the removal or dysfunction of secreting organs or glands. Organotherapists such as the French physiologist and neurologist C. E. Brown-Séquard (1817–1914) were particularly interested in the therapeutic potential of "organ juices" derived from these glands. They proposed that all sorts of diseases and conditions (including aging) could be treated with liquid extracts taken from the tissues of appropriate animal or human organs. Late-nineteenth-century organotherapy followed a "simple" research formula: remove the gland, record the specific function lost, match the symptoms with a known disease, restore the function with either organ grafts or extracts.[2]

In 1891 a widely known clinical experiment with "thyroid juice" in the treatment of myxedema took place. George R. Murray, a British pathologist, demonstrated that loss of thyroid function in humans could be remedied by injections of liquid extracted from the thyroid of sheep.[3] (Persons with myxedema develop thickened dry skin, coarse hair, intolerance to cold, slowed metabolism and heart rate, as well as mental changes such as depression.) Murray suggested further physiological research on "internal secretions" and their role in general metabolism, as well as distinctions between the ductless glands (the thyroid, the pituitary, and the suprarenal bodies) and glands with ducts (the liver, the pancreas, and the kidney).[4] His success also stimulated further experimentation with the clinical efficacy of extracts of animal tissue. Many physicians believed, for example, that diabetes might be cured by the simple administration of pancreatic juice before or after meals. Juices extracted from the testes, sex glands, kidney, pancreas, pituitary, adrenal, and vascular glands were all considered by physicians as therapeutic agents in specific diseases. As a result, many endocrine preparations were placed on the market by entrepreneurs interested in the commercial application of organotherapy. In 1905 Ernest Starling, Jodrell Professor of Physiology at University College, London, introduced the term "hormone" to designate the chemical messengers carried in the blood. Increasingly, the isolation of individual hormones became a major focus in the expanding field of endocrinology.[5]

Recognition of the importance of hormones and their potential clinical utility transformed the treatment of anorexia nervosa. In addition to prescribing glandular extracts as therapy for specific diseases, American and British physicians used hormones as a tool of diagnosis in diseases whose etiology was unknown but whose pathology was correlated with a particular organ. The evidence suggests that doctors were more apt to use these extracts in the treatment of women. According to George Corner, an endocrinologist and historian of the field, early-twentieth-century clinical practice included the testing of many "ill-defined extracts on hysterical women and cachexic girls."[6] The story of how anorexia nervosa was linked to both pituitary and thyroid dysfunction provides a case in point.

In 1914 Morris Simmonds, a pathologist at the University of Hamburg, published a clinical description of a form of emaciation or pituitary cachexia due to destruction of the anterior lobe of the pituitary. Simmonds' discovery, observed at autopsy, was a result of the new interest in glands, and it was made possible through recent advances in microscopy.[7] In clinical practice, however, Simmonds' disease was problematic because the diagnosis in life was always uncertain. Still, the concept that the condition originated in the pathology of a gland made Simmonds' disease a favored diagnosis in cases of unexplained emaciation.

Following the strategies outlined in organotherapy, pituitary extract was given to patients with extreme weight loss, whether or not they showed other signs of pituitary failure. Physicians noted that patients with anorexia nervosa and those with Simmonds' disease shared a set of common symptoms. Obviously, when a high-calorie diet produced weight gain in a patient with unexplained emaciation, the condition was probably not the result of a pituitary deficiency. Still, for the next thirty years medical practitioners struggled with the clinical differentiation of Simmonds' disease, a relatively rare pituitary insufficiency, and anorexia nervosa. Finally, in 1942, a summary of the world literature on Simmonds' disease concluded that of 595 reported cases, only 101 were proved through pathological evidence. Many supposed cases of Simmonds' disease were actually misdiagnosed anorexia nervosa; and many emaciated young women were treated with pituitary extracts even though they demonstrated no particular glandular insufficiency.[8]

In the period between the two world wars thyroid insufficiency also was implicated in anorexia nervosa. In 1930 physician John Mayo Berkman (1898–1978), a nephew of William J. Mayo and Charles H. Mayo, founders of the nation's first and largest group practice, reported on a decade's worth of clinical experience with the disease at the Mayo Clinic in Rochester, Minnesota.[9] Because it was the medical mecca of the Midwest, the Mayo Clinic attracted patients from far and wide, many of whom had already tried unsuccessfully to find relief for unexplained emaciation and an unwillingness to eat.

Letters written to Mayo Clinic doctors reveal that cases of prolonged starvation were extremely troublesome and that families sought a more efficacious cure and a more precise diagnosis. In 1920 a real estate man from Marathon, Iowa, wrote the "Doctors Mayo" about his fifteen-year-old daughter who dropped out of high school because of weakness engendered by a weight loss of 30 pounds: "My daughter has a very bad stomach, and a great deal I am sure is caused by the stomach, she is very nervous and cross at times, just cant control herself, and at other times is much better. I have called in servel Doctors, and they now tell me that its just a case of Histeria . . . Could you suggest what to do for this truble?" In 1929 a widowed mother from Attica, Indiana, wrote about her only child who would soon be diagnosed as an anorectic in the Mayo hospital: "I have a daughter fifteen years old [who] had been going down for about five months [She] has entirely lost her appetite only eats a little when forced. I have been doctoring with some of the best doctors around here. They all pronounce it anemia . . . [She] seems to have good strength but nothing will produce an appetite. Do you think if I could bring her out to you that you could do anything for her?" Following his sister's admission to the hospital for treatment for anorexia nervosa, an attentive brother wrote the doctor nearly every week: "Would you please let me know whether she is gaining or not?"[10]

Because of their understanding of the relation of the thyroid to body weight, Mayo Clinic physicians defined and treated anorexia nervosa as if it were a general metabolic disorder. They found it in a broad constituency that included men as well as women and the old as well as the young. The Mayo doctors' notion that anorexia nervosa designated a wide category of metabolic dysfunction was reflected in the language of their case notes which often reported that a patient had "*an* anorexia nervosa." (Italics added.)

Technological innovation underwrote the medical focus on the thyroid gland. By the time of World War I doctors were able to measure the functioning of the thyroid through the use of a portable respiration apparatus developed by Francis Gano Benedict (1870–1915), director of the Boston Nutrition Laboratory and an expert in the field of animal calorimetry.[11] Consequently, in cases of anorexia nervosa the doctor's first order of business was to establish a basal metabolism rate (BMR). If the BMR fell outside the normal range of −15 percent to +5 percent, thyroid extract was prescribed, at a dosage determined by the rate of thyroid insufficiency. Mayo doctors found the BMR to be reduced (rather than elevated) in many of their emaciated patients as a secondary consequence of undernutrition and emaciation. John Mayo Berkman reasoned that in cases of anorexia nervosa a low BMR "acts as somewhat of a protective mechanism, for if the metabolism remained normal these patients would eventually go on to death . . ."[12]

On the basis of their understanding of the relationship between thyroid insufficiency and a low BMR, Mayo Clinic doctors recommended replacement therapy—specifically, the administration of thyroxin or desiccated thyroid.[13] In anorexic patients, however, the problem was that if metabolic activity increased as a result of hormonal extracts, weight loss could become even more severe. Consequently, physicians had to practice two parallel forms of intervention, one new and one old: administration of thyroid hormones combined with a steady regimen of increased nourishment. The combination of the two was absolutely critical and the model of treatment essentially mechanistic. The physician's task was to maintain a balance between the body's energy expenditure and its nutritional intake.

A Mayo doctor explained the situation to the anxious parents of a Terre Haute student whose weight fell below 100 pounds:

[Your daughter] has a condition we designate as an anorexia nervosa. In this condition the patient loses appetite, probably from nervous causes, and the food is gradually burned more and more slowly in the tissues of the body. The best method that we have at present is to increase the rate of burning the food by the administration of thyroid. In order to do this properly it is necessary to keep the patient under observation so we can determine the exact dose of thyroid necessary to hold the rate of burning food at the proper level. This procedure is well underway in your daughter's case although it is impossible to tell what we are going to get out of it at present.[14]

The balancing act was not easily accomplished nor were the results predictable. "We cannot say what our success in management of the case will be," an honest clinician told the parents of an anorexic girl who was taking thyroid extract.[15]

In general, patients with anorexia nervosa were kept in the hospital for a minimum of two to three weeks in order to monitor the thyroid rate and food intake. When and if the BMR was brought up to normal and substantial weight gain occurred, patients were either discharged to their own homes or to residences in the city of Rochester where their eating was put under the day-to-day supervision of a professional dietitian in one of the Mayo's special "diet kitchens." In some cases the metabolic therapy worked. A pleased father wrote to his daughter's physician after she returned home, "Emma is sure doing fine now, she eats good, and is getting fleshy."[16]

Other patients were discharged with only minimal weight gain and marginal improvement in the BMR. A twenty-year-old from Parkville, Missouri, for example, left the Mayo Clinic when she weighed just over 100 pounds and her BMR had been elevated from −18 percent (on admission) to −4 percent (on dismissal). Unfortunately, after her return home the girl's loss of appetite continued and her weight dropped to less than 80 pounds. Unable or unwilling to return to the Minnesota clinic, doctor and patient began a lengthy correspondence in which the doctor proposed reinstituting thyroid therapy and discussed where the proper hormonal extract could be obtained in the patient's hometown.[17]

Mayo doctors were forthright about their inability to provide a definitive explanation of anorexia nervosa. They were also circumspect about the outcome of thyroid replacement therapy, recommending it to parents as merely the best available option: "We felt the elevation of the basal metabolism offered her more than any other procedure which we could suggest."[18] Although Mayo doctors remained faithful to the biological model of disease and eschewed psychological treatment in favor of medical intervention, they also acknowledged the role of "psychic disturbance" or "nervous causes" in anorexia nervosa. Nonetheless, of the 117 cases reviewed by Berkman, only a handful received any kind of psychiatric treatment.

Throughout the 1920s and well into the 1930s, many physicians favored endocrinologic rather than psychotherapeutic modes of treatment in anorexia nervosa. Their faith in endocrinology led them to experiment in anorexia nervosa treatment (as in the treatment of other mental disorders) with natural and synthetic hormones such as insulin, antuitrin, and estrogen.[19] By 1936, however, some doctors were skeptical. John Ryle, an eminent British practitioner and professor of medicine at Cambridge University, observed that "physicians subject to the lure of endocrinology" had failed to find the cause of anorexia nervosa in either "deficiency or disharmony of the internal secretions." Ryle wrote: "There is no justification, in my belief, for employing thyroid . . . or for giving insulin to promote appetite and help in the utilization of ingested carbohydrates. Nor should there be any justification for the use of ovarian hormones." For Ryle anorexia nervosa was preeminently a "disturbance of the mind" accompanied by prolonged starvation and nothing more.[20]

In the United States also, the dominance of endocrinology was in question. A study of anorexia nervosa in the 1939 *Journal of the American Medical Association* concluded: "There is no specific endocrine therapy for this condition, but these patients being of hysterical nature will often respond temporarily to the suggestion that goes with confident administration of a special extract. Actually such treatment should be avoided because permanent results are more likely to be obtained if no artificial aids are employed."[21] By 1940 explanations that "blamed" the thyroid, ovaries, pituitary, or pancreas were less than satisfactory because anorexia nervosa was being reconstructed as a "psychologic disorder" by mid-twentieth-century psychiatry.

The Discovery of Sexuality

Although most asylum doctors in the nineteenth century realized that the unhappy, the melancholic, and the insane often stopped eating, they made little attempt to study the psychological meaning of such a symptom. Despite clinical notations that intense emotions were implicated in anorexia nervosa, most physicians clung tenaciously to physical treatment. In fact, until the advent of dynamic psychiatry, a late-nineteenth-century mode of treatment that emphasized the individual and the process by which mental disease developed, few clinicians were interested in explanations of behavior that incorporated early childhood or adolescent experiences. In effect, dynamic psychiatry turned medical attention to developmental explanations.

Beginning in the last decade of the nineteenth century, practitioners of dynamic psychiatry made increasing use of the life history of individual patients and focused their attention on uncovering the emotional or psychogenic sources of nervous disease.[22] Among the leading practitioners of the new field, Sigmund Freud (1856–1939) and Pierre Janet (1859–1947) had the greatest impact on the understanding and treatment of anorexia nervosa. In somewhat different but essentially related ways, Freud and Janet were the first to link loss of appetite to sexuality.

Freud, who attempted to systematize the study of the unconscious, suggested a specific psychodynamic mechanism in the etiology of anorexia nervosa. In 1895 he wrote, "The famous anorexia nervosa of . . . young girls seems to me . . . to be a melancholia where sexuality is undeveloped."[23] Anorexia nervosa received only a passing reference in the corpus of Freud's work, but his brief analysis of the condition was indicative of his larger theory and it had a powerful influence on subsequent generations of doctors and patients. Although he classified the disease in a conventional way, as a "nutritional neurosis," Freud posed the important conceptual question that had not been asked before: What does the anorectic's lack of appetite *mean*?

Freud's revolutionary emphasis on the individual's infantile past made the appetite for food, the first object of longing and desire, especially significant. According to Freudian theory, all appetites were expressions of libido or sexual drive. Thus, eating or not eating stood as proxy for basic sexual drives or their absence. Freud believed that the anorectic did not eat because food and sex revolted her; because of prior associations, food had a symbolic significance which made it repugnant. It is important to note that Freud posited a real disgust for food in anorexia nervosa rather than an obsessive control of hunger.

Freud's reading of anorexia nervosa as a neurotic behavior that expressed undeveloped or repressed sexuality was grounded in his important concept of conversion hysteria—that is, that chronic emotional conflicts can be transformed into physical symptoms. In Freudian theory both body and mind were affected by unexpressed emotions. Thus, psychoanalytic treatment emphasized talking and listening to the patient as a way of curing functional nervous disorders. Freud's idea that anorexia nervosa was related to unresolved issues of sexuality was pioneering: no one before him had explicitly put together anorexia and sex.

Although Freud suggested the role of suppressed emotions in anorexia nervosa as early as 1895, it would take nearly a half-century for a full-blown psychosexual interpretation to take hold. In the United States in the first decade of the twentieth century, sophisticated doctors were also exposed to the seeds of a psychodynamic interpretation through the work of Pierre Janet, the distinguished director of the psychology laboratory at Salpêtrière Clinic in Paris and an important practitioner of dynamic psychiatry.[24] Between 1870 and 1900 some French physicians (such as Charles Lasègue) were active in classifying and elaborating nervous disorders and pushing for psychogenic rather than strictly physiological classifications. On the basis of his renown in this area Janet, a former student of Charcot, was invited to Harvard Medical School in 1906 to lecture on the general subject of hysteria. He gave a total of fifteen lectures, one of which centered on anorexia nervosa. Janet declared at the outset that while anorexia nervosa was "difficult to interpret," it definitely was due to a "deep psychological disturbance of which the refusal of food is but the outer expression."[25]

Janet, like Freud, regarded lack of appetite or control of appetite as a representation of underlying emotional difficulty. Janet, however, was unwilling to take literally patient reports of "no appetite." He differed from Freud in emphasizing control of appetite rather than actual revulsion by food. Food refusal, he maintained, could be a voluntary and conscious strategy. As evidence he de-

scribed how some anorexic girls regulated their appetite by submitting to "veritable tortures in order not to yield to the need of
food"; he also described "secret eating," generally at night, of
food garbage or "dirty victuals." According to Janet, the anorectic's chronic refusal of food in the face of real hunger was the
result of a delusion or mental disturbance that became an obsessive idea—what he called an *idée fixe.*

What was the source of the *idée fixe* in anorexia nervosa? In
his lecture at Harvard, Janet was unwilling to specify a single
cause or type of obsession. In fact, he faulted his estranged teacher
and colleague, Charcot, for "seek[ing] everywhere for his rose
colored ribbon" and exaggerating the importance of the "idea of
obesity." Still, Janet did not discredit the power of the aversion
to fat. He enumerated a number of other types of "delirious ideas"
that generated an obsessive concern with appetite control. There
were young women who refused to eat because they were over-
anxious about their stomachs and anticipated pain in digestion;
others who had "scruples" (a commitment to avoiding meat) that
led to finicky eating; some who were preoccupied with "coquetries," feared obesity, and cultivated wan complexions; and
some who deliberately sought to starve themselves to death because of a painful life event ("thwarted marriage, a reproach, a
quarrel . . .").[26]

In his discussion of the emotional sources of anorexia nervosa,
Janet made a brief but important reference to "delirious ideas
relating . . . to pudicity." "Pudicity" (from the Latin *pudic*, having
a keen sense of shame) designated emotional feelings about modesty and chastity, that is, the body and sexuality.[27] In 1903 Janet
wrote a major text on the nature of obsessions that included the
subject of body shame. In that work he provided powerful case
histories and verbatim conversations with anorexic patients who
were preoccupied with anxiety and embarrassment about their
body and its functioning. These young women were ashamed of
the body, obsessed by the idea of its size, and committed to the
maintenance of a "crowd of little specific delusions" relative to
food and eating. The most difficult cases of anorexia nervosa,
Janet implied, involved this unhappy relationship between the girl
and her body.[28]

Body shame was the underlying motif in Janet's 1903 analysis of the case of Nadia, a bourgeois anorectic in her twenties, who regarded eating as immoral and fat as a degraded state. (Janet said that Nadia's case was too extreme to be classified simply as anorexia nervosa, but that her history illustrated a general theme in anorexic cases. Janet, like other sophisticated doctors and psychologists of his time, was familiar with fantasies of altered body image, a symptom associated with the disease we know as schizophrenia.) In conversations with Janet, Nadia said time and again: "I don't insist on being pretty, but it would shame me too much if I became puffy, that would be a horror to me. If by bad luck I were to get fat, I wouldn't dare show myself to anyone, not at home or out on the street; I'd be too ashamed." According to Janet, Nadia refused to eat in the presence of other people; she could not stand the sound of her own chewing; and after tasting some chocolates at Christmas time, she wrote nearly a dozen letters to her doctor confessing each candy as though it were a crime. For Nadia, Janet explained, being asked to eat was tantamount to asking her "to urinate in public." "Being heavy isn't seen only from the point of view of attractiveness," Janet wrote, "it contains something immoral in [her] eyes."

Janet pushed the fear of obesity further than Charcot and postulated, in the manner of Freud, that appetite and eating had symbolic meaning in the psyche of the individual. Janet's text provided a profile of Nadia's personality and the full range of her body-related "torments." From early childhood Nadia had thought of herself as too big; during puberty she became intensely self-conscious about her legs, hips, feet, and arms, which she regarded either as oversized or too muscular. Although she had a clear complexion, Nadia also began to imagine vast numbers of pimples erupting beneath her skin.

Sexual development brought on a complete refusal of food. "The appearance of her period drove her half crazy," Janet reported. Until the age of twenty, Nadia pulled out her pubic hair because she considered it the "ornament of a savage." As her breasts and figure developed, she tried to conceal her sexual maturity by wearing large, ill-fitting clothing; she also cropped her hair. Janet was quick to point out that this behavior was not "inversion," the nineteenth century's term for homosexuality, but the desire to eradicate sex, that is, to have no body at all. Nadia told Janet, "I didn't want to gain weight or grow or look like a woman because I would have liked to stay always a little girl."

Within a decade, then, between 1895 and 1905, two of the major theorists of dynamic psychiatry—Sigmund Freud and Pierre Janet—suggestively linked anorexia nervosa to the issue of psychosexual development.[29] Taken together, Freud and Janet gave birth to the modern psychogenetic idea that anorexic girls refused food in order to keep their bodies small, thin, and childlike, thereby retarding normal sexual development and forestalling adult sexuality. Although they disagreed over the question of control versus lack of appetite, both Freud and Janet promoted the idea that food refusal in anorexia nervosa constituted a form of symbolic behavior that served its predominantly adolescent female clientele as a statement about sexuality. Despite the power and originality of these ideas, dynamic psychiatry did not have a demonstrable effect on the clinical treatment of anorexic patients for nearly thirty years. Because of the consistent popularity of endocrinological explanations, the idea of anorexia nervosa as a psychosexual disturbance lay dormant until the 1930s, when it was integrated into clinical practice through the influence of American psychiatry.

The Pregnancy Fantasy

During the 1930s anorexia nervosa was established as a female psychological or "neurotic" disorder. Although biomedical treatment continued, psychoanalytically informed psychotherapy became an increasingly popular stratagem. Ironically, beginning in the late 1930s, in the wake of the nation's most serious economic crisis, psychiatric interest in "the starving disease" underwent something of a renaissance. But renewed attention to the disease resulted from theoretical developments within medicine rather than from an increase in the number of anorexic patients.

The transformation of treatment and thinking about the disease was generated by at least two factors: the failure of the endocrinologic model to establish either a predictable cure or a definitive cause, and the growing reputation and influence of the Freudian psychoanalytic movement and its emphasis on the unconscious. A third element was the new psychological orientation among physicians that was accompanied by increasing attention to the role of emotions in disease. By the 1930s the scientific study of emotion and of the bodily changes that accompany different emotional states was the focus of a new field called psychosomatic medicine.

Psychosomatic medicine involved practitioners from many different specialty areas, not just psychiatry. Followers of the psychosomatic movement shared a common interest in a more integrated approach to etiology and therapy. Body (soma) and mind (psyche) were considered as one. In 1935 Helen Flanders Dunbar, a psychoanalytically trained psychiatrist and an important theoretician of the relationship between psychic and somatic processes, published an influential text. *Emotions and Bodily Changes* provided a major theoretical concordance for the new movement. Dunbar discussed anorexia nervosa in the context of nutritional disorders, but was quick to point out that "nutritional changes of a very serious nature . . . develop from emotional upsets."[30] And in 1939 a new journal, *Psychosomatic Medicine* (PM), was born. In its first two years, *PM* published two lengthy articles on anorexia nervosa, a disease that was particularly suited to psychosomatic research because of the manner in which bodily changes accompanied neurotic mechanisms.[31] In the medical world of the late 1930s and 1940s, anorexia nervosa presented a fascinating problem and an opportunity for psychiatry to demonstrate its explanatory and curative skills. In the treatment of anorexia nervosa, in particular, psychosomatic medicine was a potential bridge between those who treated only the emaciated body and those who treated only the disturbed mind.

In the 1930s, for the first time, physicians routinely asserted the value and importance of psychotherapy in the treatment of anorexia nervosa. In 1932 Fred Ellsworth Clow (1881–1941), a general practitioner and visiting physician at Huggins Hospital in Wolfeboro, New Hampshire, published a report on two cases of anorexia nervosa in the *New England Journal of Medicine*. Clow, who was eclectic in his approach, declared that there were three essential techniques in the management of the anorexic patient: change of environment, forced feeding, and psychotherapy. Physicians of many different orientations and levels of understanding by now were recommending psychological treatment; yet many, such as Clow, had only a naive faith in the efficacy of the "talking and listening cure" and were unable to describe how the process actually worked.[32] Some claimed that anorexia nervosa could be cured by "a few straightforward conversations."[33] Some were obviously uninformed about the duration of psychotherapy and the tenacity of the condition. Nevertheless, most doctors agreed that in anorexia nervosa permanent recovery, as opposed to simple weight gain, depended on uncovering the "psychologic basis."

What most psychiatrists attempted was something we today call insight-oriented psychotherapy, a regular program of interviews with the physician that would lead the patient to understand rationally that her attitude toward food and the body was abnormal and related to other problems in her life. Repeatedly, doctors stressed the need to expose the "dynamic factors in the personality" or to identify "dynamic material" that would then "impart insight" so that adjustments could be worked out.[34] By "dynamic," the physician meant intimate personal experiences or ideas, both conscious and unconscious, that fueled the patient's neurotic behavior. In most cases, the critical dynamic material was obtained in the interview process, through questioning by the psychotherapist. Only occasionally did psychotherapists resort to sodium amytal, a truth serum, in order to get to the unconscious associations that generated the anorectic's rigid ideas about food and eating. The ultimate goal in the process was to bring the patient to "understanding," that is, to explain the sources of her symptom, refusal of food.

Few published reports detailed how psychotherapy generated dynamic material or how patients were brought to an understanding that changed behavior. Still, many physicians began to suggest that there was a classic anorexic personality. On the basis of psychotherapeutic interviews with anorexic women, doctors began to collate their experiences and assert a personality profile: "Most of them [anorectics] are intelligent, some to a marked degree; all are highly sensitive. Usually they are impulsive, willful, introspective and emotionally unstable . . . Associated with a sense of inferiority, they have a strong desire for prominence and dominance."[35]

In published clinical cases of the 1930s, the clientele for anorexia nervosa was a mix of privileged college girls and young middle-class working women. The disorder was not perceived as a problem with any special affinity for the collegiate setting. Psychotherapeutic interviews did reveal, however, that anorexic girls were often superior but driven students. Although anorectics were classified by psychiatrists in many different ways (as psychoneurotic with anxiety, compulsive, depressive, or schizophrenic features), by the 1940s they were most commonly associated with obsessive-compulsive personality features: perfectionism, stubbornness, overconscientiousness, neatness, meticulousness, and parsimony.[36] This interpretation, while suggesting that the anorectic suffered from a serious personality disorder, did little to explain the primary and most troubling behavioral symptom, the refusal to eat.

Predictably, psychiatrists following Freud and Janet postulated that refusal to eat had something to do with sexual appetite. A 1939 report by George H. Alexander from Butler Hospital, a psychiatric facility in Providence, Rhode Island, stands as one of the first and most complete discussions of the discovery of a psychosexual mechanism in anorexia nervosa. Alexander, reputed to be Rhode Island's first practicing psychoanalyst, described a single case of a 5-foot-4-inch fifteen-year-old girl confined to the hospital after her weight plummeted from 130 to 73 pounds in the course of less than a year. The daughter of a respectable Italian-American family and an honor-roll student in her second year of high school, the patient refused to consume more than a cup of coffee and a few hard crackers each day.[37]

Although the patient said that she began to diet because she considered herself too fat, Alexander did not take her at her word. "It was obvious at the outset that the patient's attitude toward her body and toward food was not that of an average obese individual who starts to diet." The psychiatrist was particularly attentive to the girl's emotional life and relations with her family. He noted that she was "increasingly resentful towards her parents, her mother in particular," because she considered her mother "excessively concerned about her welfare and happiness." At home the patient was very unpleasant; she would become irritable and sullen when urged to eat; she threw food out the window; and she went through stormy periods of "self-blame and weeping" over the worry she caused her parents. Alexander concluded from the case history: "It could be logically assumed that body fat and food had some obscure but powerful emotional significance for her. In other words, fat had come to symbolize something to her unconscious mind which she wished to be rid of, and food represented something dangerous which would prevent the fulfillment of that wish."

Despite Alexander's commitment to a psychiatric understanding of his patient, he initially directed treatment toward the twin goals of weight gain and energy conservation. Confined to bed, the girl took small amounts of milk and cream at two-hour intervals. This nineteenth-century style rest cure was supplemented by small amounts of insulin (given three times daily) in order to stimulate the appetite and was followed by several ounces of fruit juice fortified with lactose. This liquid food was presented to the suspicious girl as a "solvent" for the medicines that would increase her appetite. Consequently, she had to be given placebo capsules with each feeding. To some extent the charade worked. Within a month the emaciated patient gained 7 pounds but she became increasingly restless in her confinement and angry about the constant supervision of nurses who did not trust her to eat her food. After persuading her mother to take her home, the patient was returned to the hospital within twenty-four hours because she continued to refuse food.

In the second month of hospitalization Alexander mobilized an arsenal of endocrine preparations, which he deployed in gradually increasing amounts: thyroid, theelin, antuitrin S, suprarenal substance, and whole-gland pituitary extract. In addition to a diet of 2,000 to 3,000 calories a day, the patient received amino acetic acid, cod-liver oil, fruit juices with lactose, and supplementary vitamins. At the end of four months, despite the endocrine therapy and increased food intake, the girl weighed 78 pounds—a gain of only 5 pounds over her admission weight.

At this point Alexander became convinced that it was time to stop all endocrine therapy and treat the patient as a case of anorexia nervosa with strictly psychogenic origins. The girl was to take only vitamins and a high-calorie diet, combined with regular psychotherapy. Alexander wrote later, "The response to this change was immediate and almost dramatic . . . her appetite immediately improved." By the end of the sixth month, the girl weighed 89 pounds; by the end of the seventh month, 106. At the end of the eighth month, when her weight reached 115, Alexander observed happily, "The greatly altered physical appearance and pleasant personality of the patient at this time, stood in sharp contrast to the emaciated, sullen, irritable, and hypercritical patient of but three months before." He concluded, "It is probably fair to say that, in general, psychotherapy is of more importance in treatment than endocrine-gland preparations."

How did psychotherapy effect this profound mental and physical change? Unlike many doctors of his era, Alexander reported something of the actual process of treatment. His patient was brought to recovery by sixty-eight one-hour sessions conducted by a "psychoanalytically trained physician." Alexander was quick to point out that this did not constitute an endorsement of any one kind of analysis: "No school of psychotherapeutic thought [is] favored." In therapy the anorectic should be exposed to a variety of standard techniques aimed at uncovering dynamic material: "suggestion, persuasion, reeducation, free association and so-called simple 'unloading'."[38] (The last meant allowing the patient to ramble and say whatever came to mind without feeling pressured to justify her emotions or ideas.)

Alexander recommended that the physician administering psychotherapy keep entirely separate from "all matters relative to treatment of the organic aspects of the illness." This was best, he argued, in order to aid transference, the process by which the patient identified with her analyst. In addition, it kept the interview process free from quibbling over food and eating, and separate from any system of reward or punishment employed in the biomedical regimen. First and foremost the therapist wanted to encourage trust and facilitate the free flow of feelings, since his essential task was "to ascertain . . . and then make . . . understandable to the patient the symbolic meaning [to her] of body fat and food."

Within the course of four months Alexander's anorectic patient progressed through three different stages that eventually led to understanding and a return to eating. In stage one, the patient "talked mainly of food in relationship to her feelings of anger" toward her parents and hospital personnel. She felt it unfair, even cruel, to be made to eat. In therapy she tried to enlist the doctor's help in changing or subverting the hospital's food regimen; when she was unable to do so, she became hostile, sullen, and uncooperative.

As the patient began to talk about her own life history, particularly her "sensitivity" to bodily changes at puberty, the psychotherapeutic process entered a critical second stage. At this point the psychotherapist began to uncover the dynamic material that was a key to the patient's neurosis. The emaciated girl now cried easily and openly; she became angry with the therapist and occasionally spent the entire session sitting mute. She also revealed a great deal about herself, including the fact that she was fixated on her stomach. She confessed that fat on her abdomen caused her enormous anxiety, far greater than that associated with the development of her hips or breasts.

From the physician's perspective, this intimate revelation constituted the psychological denouement in the history of the case. In therapy the patient allegedly suggested that her food refusal began after she heard that two of her classmates had become pregnant and had to leave high school. Although she was intellectually aware that she could not be pregnant because she had never had sexual intercourse, she "began to fear in some unknown way [that] she might have become pregnant." What Alexander called an irrational pregnancy fantasy was fueled both by a casual suggestion by her mother that she wear a girdle and by the disappearance of her menses (a result of weight loss). "With the working through of this material," Alexander wrote, "she finally revealed the underlying reason for starting to diet." Alexander ultimately attributed the onset of anorexia nervosa to a fear of pregnancy and not to family dynamics or an obsession with being slim. "It is obvious," he wrote, "that the patient's lower abdominal fat deposits consciously symbolized a pregnant abdomen to her." In turn, "food became symbolic of the dangerous impregnating agent and therefore had to be avoided." Once the patient articulated and understood this fear, she entered the final stage of treatment. In very short order she became congenial, relaxed, and willing to acknowledge her hunger. Almost immediately after conceding her fear, she began voluntarily to eat a regular diet.[39]

George Alexander's 1939 report from Butler Hospital was the first in a series of increasingly complex psychiatric elaborations of psychosexual dysfunction in anorexia nervosa. Throughout the 1940s and 1950s, and well into the 1960s, psychotherapists reported that anorexic women feared eating as impregnation and regarded obesity as pregnancy.[40] Once this essentially Freudian equation of food and sexuality was established, it influenced what psychiatrists chose to ask in the therapeutic interview and what they chose as a strategy for treatment. The anorectic's sexuality (or lack of it) took center stage. In the period 1940 to 1960 anorectics were cast as sexually repressed or puritanical figures: reportedly, they were embarrassed by vulgar stories; preferred reading to going out with boys; claimed never to masturbate; and were easily traumatized by unsolicited overtures or touches by the opposite sex. One adolescent anorectic so loathed her developing body that she appeared on the beach "encased in a huge rain coat that reached from her throat to her ankles." In a 1940 summary of a dozen anorexic cases from New York Hospital and the Payne-Whitney Psychiatric Clinic, the authors observed: "The patients' own statements indicated a strong repudiation of sexuality . . . All our cases had made a poor heterosexual adjustment."[41]

In their early readings of the anorectic as a sexually repressed young woman, Freud and Janet had anticipated a deluge of medical and psychological studies that would make decorous heterosexuality the centerpiece of successful adolescent female adjustment in the twentieth century. A new view of the adolescent girl mandated some "romantic" interest in the opposite sex; a healthy girl did not appear "mannish," and she avoided strong emotional attachments to any particular female friend.[42] The importance of heterosexuality received substantial reinforcement in the work of G. Stanley Hall (1844–1924), the influential Clark University psychologist who popularized the notion that emotional turmoil in adolescence was inevitable because it was biologically based in the process of sexual maturation.[43] According to Hall's theory, adolescent girls were particularly susceptible to environmental influences that could redirect or subvert the "natural" course of heterosexual interest and physical development. Hall and other mental health professionals, physicians, and sexologists were concerned that adolescent girls reach their full reproductive potential, a physiological state marked by the appearance of breasts, hips, and the accumulation of body fat. The anorectic, of course, did not achieve or maintain this desired state; her body was certainly not fecund and until she was cured, her potential for life as a wife or mother was virtually nil. Although the anorectic was not cast as a lesbian, her childlike body was taken as a repudiation of heterosexuality, an issue of enormous concern in the interwar years.

Because the perimeters of the anorexia diagnosis were being extended to include some schizophrenics, the range of pathology associated with anorexia nervosa became wider and more severe. Some patients defined as anorexic by psychotherapists in the 1940s were delusional: allegedly, they feared that they could become pregnant from sperm left by boys on chairs, or they refused slimy foods because they associated them with semen.[44] Psychiatric projections of coitus fear were not, however, the entire story. Anorectics were also portrayed as hysterically exhibitionistic and seductive, and at least one clinical report suggested that the anorectic was a potential prostitute whose inappetence was a subconscious defense against promiscuity.[45] Some psychiatrists claimed that anorectics wanted to be force-fed because of fellatio fantasies.[46]

Freudian suggestions of unresolved oedipal desire came to bear too on the clinical reading of anorexia nervosa. The analyst of a patient who refused food and vomited whenever she ate with men concluded:

The organic dysfunctions are shown to be somatic manifestations of a highly complex personality disorder arising from severe early emotional conflicts, especially in the oral sphere. The most important specific psychodynamism of the vomiting appears to be a symbolic rejection and restitution of the father's phallus, orally incorporated in an attempt to render exclusive her passive dependence on her mother.[47]

Another report described a 52-pound fourteen-year-old who had been tube-fed at home by her father, seven times a day, for over a year. In the hospital she was fed by different doctors, a situation that displeased her. Her psychiatrist observed, "She said that 'only daddy can put it down without hurting' and took it with passive disgust, meanwhile making obvious pelvic movements."[48]

For orthodox psychoanalysts, anorexia nervosa was clearly a painful reenactment of the infantile relationship with mother and father. Clinical reporting in the 1940s demonstrates that when the diagnosis was used to encompass schizophrenic patients, the case histories provided raw material for virtuoso displays of psychoanalytic orthodoxy replete with symbolic interpretations of chocolate (feces), sausages (phallus), and almonds (testicles). Although Freud himself discouraged simplistic one-to-one interpretations of object and meaning, the emphasis on the connection between food and sexuality, particularly phallic fantasies, was heavy-handed. In a paper read before the Chicago Psychoanalytic Society in April 1940, Jules H. Masserman claimed a major analytic breakthrough when his anorexic analysand finally admitted her "fantasy of eating the analyst's penis."[49] It was a rare psychiatrist indeed who admitted that "material explicitly relevant to this complex [the pregnancy fantasy] did not appear in the analysis." Hilde Bruch, the best-known authority on anorexia nervosa, observed that the search for oral impregnation fantasies "dominated" clinical treatment in this era.[50]

A final alteration in pre-1960 treatment strategies is understandable in light of medical developments. In the 1930s and 1940s doctors were more likely than ever before to test and experiment with the reproductive or sexual organs of the anorectic. This resulted from the combined impact of the Freudian view of anorexia nervosa as a form of sexual dysfunction and developments in the field of sex endocrinology. By the late 1930s there was also a range of new diagnostic and therapeutic techniques that made it possible to hone in on the anorectic's sexual functioning: vaginal smears that measured follicular activity, biopsies of the endometrium, and synthetic estrogens that could stimulate ovulation and the development of secondary sex characteristics.

Using these diagnostic techniques, doctors in the 1930s and 1940s found a reflection of the anorectic's alleged sexual maladjustment in both her external and internal sexual organs. In addition to amenorrhea, physicians reported other physical signs that were taken as confirmation of psychosexual dysfunction rather than as a consequence of nutritional deprivation: "underdeveloped" or small genitalia, and "atrophic" breasts and sex organs.[51] Atrophic sex organs implied decline from nonuse; in effect, the anorectic's vagina lacked evidence of vitality. A group report from New York Hospital in 1940 confirmed a diagnosis of atrophic in all anorexia cases where smears were done, and a clinical report in *PM* noted that, on admission, the adolescent anorectic's vaginal smear was of the "atrophic type" found in "menopausal women and castrates."[52]

The reproductive system superseded the gastrointestinal system in this mode of treatment. Physicians did daily vaginal smears in order to monitor the course of the menstrual cycle and its potential for reactivation. When the vaginal smear indicated a lag in ovarian activity, synthetic estrogens, such as estradiol, were administered in order to kick start the girl's system. Estrogens were expected to compensate for the ovarian deficiencies that were linked to the anorectic's psychic state.[53] At least one clinician pointed out, however, that anorexic patients became increasingly unhappy and volatile in this form of treatment, precisely because the hormone stimulated sexual feelings and provoked extremely vivid pregnancy fantasies. The anorectic is more comfortable, argued a New York City psychiatrist, when her "genital tract [is] in a quiescent, more infantile, less differentiated state of sexuality, to correspond with her infantile state of mind."[54]

In the 1930s and 1940s the Freudian conception of the disorder as a psychosexual dysfunction was underscored by psychosomatic medicine and its emphasis on the relationship between mind and body. A 1939 clinical report claimed that anorexia nervosa was "an example of the simplest possible mechanism connecting personality disorders with somatic functions."[55] The interest in more holistic treatment generated by psychosomatic medicine led physicians to the body of the anorectic, where they believed they could see physical confirmation of Freud's notion of repressed or infantile sexuality. In a medical world revolutionized by endocrinology, dynamic psychiatry, and psychosomatic medicine, it was almost inevitable that the treatment of anorexia nervosa would proceed in this way.

The attempt to explain anorexia nervosa with a single psychodynamic formulation was ultimately doomed by the complexity of the disorder and the fact that it is not a static condition. For some, anorexia was chronic; for others, merely episodic. In the course of the illness, individual anorectics experience marked psychological changes in relation to the state of starvation itself and to patterns of interaction within the family.[56] Because the fantasy of pregnancy was not fully articulated in all anorexia cases, many psychoanalysts backed off from a single causal model. Moreover, it was apparent that while the classic form of anorexia nervosa was still confined largely to adolescent females, chronic food refusal could also develop in children, in sexually active or married women, and in males. The recognition of these new anorectics, combined with more sophisticated psychiatric understandings, reduced the explanatory power of the orality interpretation.

After World War II a new psychiatric view of eating disorders, shaped largely by the work of Hilde Bruch, encouraged a broader and more complex view of the significance of food behavior and its relation to the developmental history of the individual. In the introduction to *Eating Disorders* (1973), a book that represented three decades of work with appetite problems, Bruch began with these words:

> This book will concern itself with individuals who misuse the eating function in their efforts to solve or camouflage problems of living that to them appear otherwise insoluble. Food lends itself readily to such usage because eating, from birth on, is always closely intermingled with interpersonal experiences, and its physiological and psychological aspects cannot be strictly differentiated. For normal people, too, food is never restricted to the biological aspects alone. There is no human society that deals rationally with food in its environment, that eats according to the availability, edibility, and

nutritional value alone. Food is endowed with complex values and elaborate ideologies, religious beliefs, and prestige systems.[57]

Throughout her work Bruch stressed the formation of individual personality and factors within the family that preconditioned the patient to respond to his or her problems by means of undereating or overeating. The clinical emphasis on assessing how particular families managed food and eating meant that, for the first time, individuals who ate excessively and those who restricted their intake to the point of dangerous emaciation were linked together as part of a therapeutic puzzle. Although anorexia nervosa and obesity were at opposite ends of the spectrum of eating disorders, according to the new psychiatric gospel both required professional treatment.[58]

Patient statements about food and the body also moved psychiatric thinking in the postwar years in a significant new direction. Bruch's clinical reports indicated a shift in the external articulation of the disease: fears about sexuality were apparently exchanged for endlessly repeated and nearly formulaic statements about being "too fat" and wanting to become ever thinner. Although the dieting litany was always regarded as a rationalization for deep emotional needs, by the 1960s psychiatry began to pay closer attention to the anorectic's day-to-day thinking about food and eating. Physicians now noted that the desire to be thin was coupled with an ardent preoccupation with food, a preoccupation expressed in cooking for others, ritualistic consumption of tiny amounts, compulsive reading of menus, and daydreaming about extravagant dishes. In other words, food was as important to the anorectic as it was to the obese.

Psychiatry came to understand that anorexia nervosa was a misnomer. The condition involved control of appetite rather than loss of it, as the name suggests. The classic anorectic only acted as if she had no appetite; in fact, her life was a constant struggle to deny natural hunger and constantly reduce body weight. Modern psychiatric literature finally put denial at the core of the disorder and concluded that the combination of "conscious and stubborn determination to emaciate herself despite the presence of an intense interest in food" distinguishes anorexia nervosa from other forms of psychological malnutrition and weight loss.[59] For a complicated set of psychological and cultural reasons, the contemporary anorectic adopted a credo of extreme renunciation and self-denial that was expressed through the familiar activity of dieting.

9 · Modern Dieting

In contemporary society young women easily attach themselves to dieting precisely because it is a widely practiced and admired form of cultural expression. A pathology such as anorexia nervosa is not caused by dieting alone, but the centrality of dieting and appetite control in the lives of women is a critical context for explaining the disproportionate number of female anorectics in late-twentieth-century America. Which cultural forces in the twentieth century have contributed to the increasing incidence of anorexia nervosa?

Personal aesthetics have played an obvious role. In the twentieth century the body—not the face—became the special focus of female beauty. As a consequence, dieting moved from the periphery to the center of women's lives and culture. In the modern world dieting involves a self-conscious effort to reduce the body for the purpose of attaining an ideal of outward physical, as opposed to spiritual, beauty.[1] Dieting was already a fact of life for some American women by the 1920s, when the basic institutions of American beauty culture were formalized: the fashion and cosmetics industries; beauty contests; the modeling profession; and the movies.[2] As the rules of physical beauty were elaborated in American popular culture, more and more women, from a variety of class backgrounds and at different stages in their lives, strove to meet the new and increasingly slender ideal.

Not surprisingly, the clinical literature produced by twentieth-century doctors provides only a limited perspective on the birth of this major cultural imperative. When women's dieting was noticed in the early twentieth century, it was most often dismissed as silly, faddish, or a danger to reproductive potential. "Do not blindly follow beauty ideals that endanger your health and even your chances for motherhood," advised Wendell C. Phillips, a former president of the American Medical Association.[3]

By the mid-1920s physicians regarded warnings about feminine weight control as an important part of the Progressive Era's preventive medicine program, for they were beginning to see so many American women pursuing "unwise and fanatical" diets in order to achieve "barber-pole" figures.[4] Because the "mania for thinness" seemed to be accelerating in the 1920s, physicians took potshots at popular quasi-scientific diet programs that promised weight reduction. These were dietary regimens based on lemon juice, milk and bananas, special breads and seaweed; patent medicines or "fat reducers" advertised as Citrophan, Figureoids, Berledets, Allan's Antifat, Rengo, Kellogg's Obesity Food, and Marmola; and treatments with special baths, pastes, and thinning salts.[5]

For medicine, dieting was a problem in the science of metabolism and not a test of salesmanship or psychology. Naturally enough, doctors advised that a diet without professional medical supervision was a serious health risk.[6] What they failed to realize was that for many women appetite control was now a way of life. Modern dieters initiated and discontinued efforts to reduce in response to reigning aesthetic standards and private emotional needs even more than the dictates of scientific medicine. Women dieters were caught up in a process of continual evaluation of their own bodies, and early-twentieth-century science only legitimated their concern.

Mortality and Health

The traditional association of fatness with prosperity and good health all but disappeared in the twentieth century. Between 1900 and 1920 both the medical establishment and the insurance industry began to promote an ideal body type that was decidedly thinner than fifty years before. At the turn of the century most people considered moderate amounts of fat an advantage that improved resistance when disease struck. But if thinness was a sign of ill health associated with feared diseases such as tuberculosis, real obesity—as distinct from plumpness or what the Victorians called embonpoint—was also pathological. Late-nineteenth-century health guides commonly discussed the demerits of both extremes. Between 1900 and 1920 the first medicoactuarial standards of weight and health emerged, and doctors, on the basis of this evidence, suggested that overweight was a serious health liability.[7]

Medicine's interest in the subject of body weight was heightened by new information provided by the insurance industry. Insurance companies characteristically looked for criteria by which to judge the desirability of applicants. Beginning in the middle of the nineteenth century, they used body weight as one indicator of risk. Although companies certainly preferred to insure men of "normal weight," before 1900 they lacked a statistical basis for their opinion that overweight individuals experienced a higher rate of mortality than those of average weight.

After the turn of the century the hypothesis that obesity shortened human life was substantiated by data analyzed by doctors and statisticians. In 1901 Oscar H. Rogers, a physician with the New York Life Insurance Company, reported that the mortality rate of fat policyholders was higher than average. In 1908 Louis I. Dublin, a zoologist who had studied statistics at Columbia University with anthropologist Franz Boas, calculated the average weights of men and women based on information collected from a comprehensive retrospective survey of New York Life policyholders. Dublin's Standard Table of Heights and Weights became the authoritative reference on the issue of what constituted average weight. In 1912 *The Medico-Actuarial Mortality Investigation of 1889–91* provided additional information on over seven hundred thousand insured lives drawn from the records of forty-three insurance companies. The report concluded that before the age of thirty-five, overweight was slightly advantageous; over thirty-five, overweight was a distinct disadvantage.[8]

The idea that excess poundage was a burden rather than a reserve was widely promoted by Dublin in a forty-year career at the Metropolitan Life Insurance Company, where he served as the "house intellectual" and as a publicist for public health and preventive medicine. In the mid-teens Dublin replaced his Standard Table of average weights with a table of "desirable weights," which suggested that both men and women should weigh somewhat less than average for their heights after early adulthood. His charts were published in popular magazines such as *McClure's* and were widely disseminated to physicians in clinical practice.[9]

Dublin's dicta were embraced by the medical community. Doctors writing popular materials on health began to cite his statistical evidence as proof of the general axiom that obesity was an important precipitating agent in a wide variety of diseases including organic heart disease and angina pectoris, arteriosclerosis, diabetes, hypertension, cerebral hemorrhage, apoplexy, gout, nephritis, and female sterility.[10] In the home health guides of the 1920s, medical warnings against overweight and strategies for weight control went hand in hand. Because of the dangers associated with overweight, Morris Fishbein, a physician and editor of the *Journal of the American Medical Association*, recommended that individuals consume only enough food to provide energy for the day's work. Clarence Lieb, a physician at Boston's Peter Bent Brigham Hospital, felt that "obesity should be treated as a disease." Consequently, he felt a responsibility to "engender fear of fat" in his patients.[11]

Medical recognition of the importance of body weight to individual health was formalized in the structure of the modern medical examination. Although doctors had been weighing their patients for some time, they were now trained to make routine notations of "current" and "usual" weight and to inform the patient about his or her supposedly desirable weight, selected from Dublin's table. Between 1900 and 1910 a growing number of Americans wanted to know their exact weight, as determined by a weighing in the doctor's office or on one of the home scales now available for purchase.[12]

In the early-twentieth-century examination room, patients first experienced the direct impact of standardization on the human body. Weight charts, keyed only to height, did not take into account individual and ethnic differences. Instead, the new charts created an abstract ideal that was only indirectly relevant to individual bodies. Yet the influence of Dublin's numbers was pervasive and longstanding. As recently as the 1980s, a doctor wrote critically about the hegemony of Dublin's figures, saying that they "have been accepted as the absolute standard of human normality."[13] Many took the desirable weight to heart and sought to change their body. In 1927 Fishbein observed, "The public has in some way conceived the idea that the human figure can be standardized."[14]

Pediatrics contributed further to the power of standardized weights. As a field, pediatrics built its early reputation on its expertise in feeding and nutrition. At a time when infant mortality was high and a majority of deaths were attributed to gastric and digestive disorders, this was an important asset. Books of information by pediatricians such as Thomas Morgan Rotch (1849–1914) and Luther Emmett Holt (1855–1924) presented middle-class mothers with an elaborate system for how to feed their infants.[15]

But early-twentieth-century pediatricians were also concerned with the eating problems and weight of older children. By the 1930s there was a rich literature on how to deal with children who did not eat enough.[16] According to Joseph Brennemann, a Chicago pediatrician, the emphasis on standardized weights for children in the period after 1910 created enormous anxiety in middle-class parents, which led to a pattern of eating problems in childhood. Brennemann, who was most interested in the psychological aspects of nutrition in childhood, said that educated middle-class mothers were the most likely to attempt to make their children conform to the "tables of weights and measures . . . that [were] found in all the baby books, most nurseries, and on the walls of the offices of nearly all physicians who care for children." He portrayed the middle-class family as preoccupied with the scale and the issue of how to feed its children. In fact, he claimed that children who did not eat constituted as much as 85 percent of a suburban practice. Brennemann implicitly blamed the mothers, who, he said, were liable to "[lay] awake nights planning a Gospel diet."[17]

A heightened sensitivity to the meaning of body weight was the result of other factors as well as the dissemination of medicoactuarial tables and the influence of pediatricians. Large numbers of educated middle-class women were finding meaningful work and careers in the home economics movement, specifically in the burgeoning professional fields of nutrition and dietetics, which had their roots in the nineteenth century.[18] In these new careers women adopted and transformed the canon of nineteenth-century domesticity, turning household management into domestic science. A preoccupation with efficiency in the home was accompanied by an equal concern for efficiency in the body.

Home economists and nutritionists of this period told middle-class homemakers that both underweight and overweight were the result of failing to cook, feed, and eat correctly. "Lack of knowledge of foods is the foundation for both overweight and underweight."[19] Overweight was distressing because it was a clear sign of physiological inefficiency. A person became fat from overeating, which was wasteful, or from consuming foods that were not directly useful in the production of energy; a fat body had to labor longer and harder to accomplish its work. While the home economics literature attached no special stigma to overweight in women, it did assign clear responsibility to the wife and mother for fat or thin family members. Inasmuch as she managed the family kitchen on her own, generally without benefit of domestic help, the Progressive Era homemaker had a special relation to the bodies of those she fed.[20]

The home economics professions worked aggressively to promote a better society through study of the so-called science of feeding. In thousands of books and pamphlets, as well as in urban and rural study groups under the sponsorship of the Department of Agriculture and state-funded cooperative extension programs, American women were taught the basics of food chemistry and metabolism. Central to this curriculum was knowledge of the basic food groups and their components, first provided on a mass scale in 1895 by Department of Agriculture booklet #142 authored by Wilbur O. Atwater, a professor of chemistry at Wesleyan University.[21] Atwater's famous pamphlet contained not only a standard diet but also food composition tables that introduced American housewives to a new food vocabulary: protein, carbohydrate, and fat. Atwater's tables became the building blocks for the spread of scientific nutrition. Atwater also popularized the concept of the calorie, a new unit for measuring heat and food.[22] Classifying foods and nutrients and counting calories became central methodological techniques in the professional fields of nutrition and dietetics. Middle-class homemakers had a whole new quantitative system to learn, to master, and to incorporate into their ideal of domesticity and motherhood. Popular magazines—the *Ladies' Home Journal* for one—hired nutritionists to write regular columns devoted to the needs of middle-class women who wanted to provide their families with the benefits of scientific feeding and eating.[23]

Outside their own homes, many of the same middle-class women participated in the Progressive Era public health movement and its programs to combat child mortality through improved nutrition and preventive medicine. A major public component of the child health movement of the teens and the twenties was the milk station, where children not only received free glasses of "nature's most perfect food" but were also weighed and screened for underweight, a characteristic that in childhood implied poor health. Public schools also participated in massive weighing programs.[24] Having a child of normative weight became important to middle-class parents, because underweight in children conveyed lower-class status and suggested malnourishment and disease. Although the central concern with children continued until the 1940s to be underweight, body size was becoming subject to rationality, control, and interventions associated with social class, age, and gender.

In the Progressive Era, American women embraced scientific feeding as a particularly female contribution to the health of their families and the nation. The frontispiece of Mary Swartz Rose's influential 1916 text, *Feeding the Family*, showed a family of four (parents with a son and a daughter) seated around the dining room table. The caption read, "The welfare of the family is largely in the hands of the one who provides the 'three meals a day.'"[25] Pediatricians, often referred to as baby feeders, were generally women's allies in the cause. As mothers and homemakers, and also as professional dieticians, women viewed their own bodies and those of which they were in charge as an indication of their competence: bodies that were too large or too small spoke badly of their food management skills. In the world of scientific nutrition, the selection and consumption of food was no longer an informal process responsive to the seasons, to the vagaries of individual taste or whim, or to the pocketbook. Now, in the name of science and health, the rules of feeding and eating were codified and women had a moral responsibility to learn the catechism. In this way the feminization of scientific nutrition contributed to women's heightened sensitivity to the body.

Beauty and Guilt

Within the first two decades of the twentieth century, even before the advent of the flapper, the voice of American women revealed that the female struggle with weight was under way and was becoming intensely personal. As early as 1907 an *Atlantic Monthly* article described the reaction of a woman trying on a dress she had not worn for over a year: "The gown was neither more [n]or less than anticipated. But I . . . *the fault was on me* . . . I was more! Gasping I hooked it together. The gown was hopeless, and I . . . I am fat." (Italics added.)[26] While Progressive Era ideology fostered an expectation of personal responsibility for the body in both sexes, women began to internalize the responsibility for weight maintenance in ways that men did not. Although some people in the Victorian era subscribed to the doctrine that "satiety was a conviction of sin," a nineteenth-century woman whose body was large was generally not indicted for lack of self-control.[27] By the twentieth century, however, overweight in women was not only a physical liability, it was a character flaw and a social impediment.[28]

Early in the century elite American women began to take body weight seriously as fat became an aesthetic liability for those who followed the world of haute couture. Since the mid-nineteenth century wealthy Americans—the wives of J. P. Morgan, Cornelius Vanderbilt, and Harry Harkness Flagler, for instance—had traveled to Paris to purchase the latest creations from couturier collections such as those on view at Maison Worth on the famed rue de la Paix. The couturier was not just a dressmaker who made clothes for an individual woman; rather, the couturier fashioned "a look" or a collection of dresses for an abstraction—the stylish woman. In order to be stylish and wear couturier clothes, a woman's body had to conform to the dress rather than the dress to the body, as had been the case when the traditional dressmaker fitted each garment.[29]

In 1908 the world of women's fashion was revolutionized by Paul Poiret, whose new silhouette was slim and straight. Poiret's style, dubbed *le vague* because of its looseness, eliminated the wasp waist, the hips, and the derriere in favor of a high-waisted, small-breasted Empire line. Poiret's "restructuring" of the female body continued into the teens, when his collections featured long, narrow sheaths covered by tunics of different lengths. Almost immediately women of style began to purchase new kinds of undergarments that would make Poiret's look possible; for example, the traditional hourglass corset was cast aside for a rubber girdle to retract the hips.

After World War I the French continued to set the fashion standard for style-conscious American women. In 1922 Jeanne Lanvin's chemise, a straight frock with a simple bateau neckline, was transformed by Gabrielle Chanel into the uniform of the flapper. Chanel dropped the waistline to the hips and began to expose more of the leg: in 1922 she moved her hemlines to midcalf, and in 1926–27 the ideal hem was raised to just below the knee. In order to look good in Chanel's fashionable little dress, its wearer had to think not only about the appearance of her legs but about the smoothness of her form.[30] Women who wore the flapper uniform turned to flattening brassieres constructed of shoulder straps and a single band of material that encased the body from chest to waist. In 1914 a French physician commented on the revised dimensions of women's bodies: "Nowadays it is not the fashion to be corpulent; the proper thing is to have a slight, graceful figure far removed from embonpoint, and *a fortiori* from obesity. For once, the physician is called upon to interest himself in the question of feminine aesthetics."[31]

The slenderized fashion image of the French was picked up and promoted by America's burgeoning ready-to-wear garment industry.[32] Stimulated by the popularity of the Gibson girl and the shirtwaist craze of the 1890s, ready-to-wear production in the United States accelerated in the first two decades of the twentieth century. Chanel's chemise dress was a further boon to the garment industry. Because of its simple cut, the chemise was easy to copy and produce, realities that explain its quick adoption as the uniform of the 1920s. According to a 1923 *Vogue*, the American ready-to-wear industry successfully democratized French fashion: "Today, the mode which originates in Paris is a factor in the lives of women of every rank, from the highest to the lowest."[33]

In order to market ready-to-wear clothing, the industry turned in the 1920s to standard sizing, an innovation that put increased emphasis on personal body size and gave legitimacy to the idea of a normative size range. For women, shopping for ready-to-wear clothes in the bustling department stores of the early twentieth century fostered heightened concern about body size.[34] With a dressmaker, every style was theoretically available to every body; with standard sizing, items of clothing could be identified as desirable, only to be rejected on the grounds of fit. (For women the cost of altering a ready-made garment was an "add-on"; for men it was not.) Female figure flaws became a source of frustration and embarrassment, not easily hidden from those who accompanied the shopper or from salesclerks. Experiences in department-store dressing rooms created a host of new anxieties for women and girls who could not fit into stylish clothing. In a 1924 testimonial for an obesity cure, a formerly overweight woman articulated the power of dress size in her thinking about dieting and about herself: "My heart seemed to beat with joy at the prospect of getting into one of the chic ready-made dresses at a store."[35]

Ironically, standard sizing created an unexpected experience of frustration in a marketplace that otherwise was offering a continually expansive opportunity for gratification via purchasable goods. Because many manufacturers of stylish women's garments did not make clothing in large sizes, heavy women were at the greatest disadvantage. In addition to the moral cachet of overweight, the standardization of garment production precluded fat women's participation in the mainstream of fashion. This situation became worse as the century progressed. Fashion photography was professionalized, a development that paralleled the growth of modern advertising, and models became slimmer both to compensate for the distortions of the camera and to accommodate the new merchandising canon—modern fashion was best displayed on a lean body.[36]

The appearance in 1918 of America's first best-selling weight-control book confirmed that weight was a source of anxiety among women and that fat was out of fashion. *Diet and Health with a Key to the Calories* by Lulu Hunt Peters was directed at a female audience and based on the assumption that most readers wanted to lose rather than gain weight. "How anyone can want to be anything but thin is beyond my intelligence," wrote Peters, a Los Angeles physician and former chair of the Public Health Committee of the California Federation of Women's Clubs.[37] A devotee of scientific nutrition, Peters attempted to "stimulate . . . an interest in dietetics" and recommended books by nutritionists Mary Swartz Rose and Belle Wood-Comstock, as well as Wilbur Atwater's famous Department of Agriculture bulletin #142.

Peters was also a spokesperson for the new quantitative vocabulary. "You should know and also use the word calorie as frequently, or more frequently, than you use the words foot, yard, quart, gallon and so forth . . . Hereafter you are going to eat calories of food. Instead of saying one slice of bread, or a piece of pie, you will say 100 calories of bread, 350 calories of pie."[38]

Peters' book was popular because it was personal and timely. Her 1918 appeal was related to food shortages caused by the exigencies of the war in Europe. Peters told her readers that it was "more important than ever to reduce" and recommended the formation of local Watch Your Weight Anti-Kaiser Classes. "There are hundreds of thousands of individuals all over America who are hoarding food," she wrote. "They have vast amounts of this valuable commodity stored away in their own anatomy." In good-humored fashion Peters portrayed her own calorie counting as both an act of patriotism and humanitarianism:

> I am reducing and the money that I can save will help keep a child from starving . . . [I am explaining to my friends] that for every pang of hunger we feel we can have a double joy, that of knowing we are saving worse pangs in some little children, and that of

knowing that for every pang we feel we lose a pound. A pang's a pound the world around we'll say.[39]

But Peters showed herself to be more than simply an informative and patriotic physician. Confessing that she once weighed as much as 200 pounds, the author also understood that heavy women were ashamed of their bulk and unlikely to reveal their actual weight. Peters observed that it was not a happy situation for fat women. "You are viewed with distrust, suspicion, and even aversion," she told her overweight readers.

Although she tried to make light of the hunger pains suffered by dieters and adorned her book with playful illustrations, Peters' point was clear: dieting was a lonely struggle that involved renunciation and psychological pain. For some women, such as herself, the struggle was for a lifetime. Although she was able to control her weight at 150 pounds, the author confessed it was not easy. "No matter how hard I work—no matter how much I exercise, no matter what I suffer," lamented Peters, "I will always have to watch my weight, I will always have to count my calories."[40]

Peters' book was among the first to articulate the new secular credo of physical denial: modern women suffered to be beautiful (thin) rather than pious. Peters' language and thinking reverberated with references to religious ideas of temptation and sin. For the modern female dieter, sweets, particularly chocolate, were the ultimate temptation. Eating chocolate violated the morality of the dieter and her dedication to her ideal, a slim body. Peters joked about her cravings ("My idea of heaven is a place with me and mine on a cloud of whipped cream") but she was adamant about the fact that indulgence must ultimately be paid for. "If you think you will die unless you have some chocolate creams [go on a] *debauch*," she advised. "'Eat 10 or so' but then *repent* with a 50-calorie dinner of bouillon and crackers." (Italics added.)[41]

Although the damage done by chocolate creams could be mediated by either fasting or more rigid dieting, Peters explained that there was a psychological cost in yielding to the temptation of candy or rich desserts. Like so many modern dieters, Peters wrote about the issue of guilt followed by redemption through parsimonious eating: "Every supposed pleasure in sin [eating] will furnish more than its equivalent of pain [dieting]." But appetite control was not only a question of learning to delay gratification, it was also an issue of self-esteem. "You will be tempted quite frequently, and you will have to choose whether you will enjoy yourself hugely in the twenty minutes or so that you will be consuming the excess calories, or whether you will dislike yourself cordially for the two or three days you lose by your lack of will power." For Peters dieting had as much to do with the mind as with the body. "There is a great deal of psychology to reducing," she wrote astutely.[42] In fact, with the popularization of the concept of calorie counting, physical features once regarded as natural—such as appetite and body weight—were designated as objects of conscious control. The notion of weight control through restriction of calories implied that overweight resulted solely from lack of control; to be a fat woman constituted a failure of personal morality.[43]

The tendency to talk about female dieting as a moral issue was particularly strong among the popular beauty experts, that is, those in the fashion and cosmetics industry who sold scientific advice on how to become and stay beautiful. Many early-twentieth-century beauty culturists, including Grace Peckham Murray, Helena Rubenstein, and Hazel Bishop, studied chemistry and medical specialties such as dermatology.[44] The creams and lotions they created, as well as the electrical gadgets they promoted, were intended to bring the findings of modern chemistry and physiology to the problem of female beauty. Nevertheless, women could not rely entirely on scientifically achieved results. The beauty experts also preached the credo of self-denial: to be beautiful, most women must suffer.

Because they regarded fat women as an affront to their faith, some were willing to criminalize as well as medicalize obesity. In 1902 *Vogue* speculated, "To judge by the efforts of the majority of women to attain slender and sylph-like proportions, one would fancy it a crime to be fat." By 1918 the message was more distinct: "There is one crime against the modern ethics of beauty which is unpardonable; far better it is to commit any number of petty crimes than to be guilty of the sin of growing fat." By 1930 there was no turning back. Helena Rubenstein, a high priestess of the faith, articulated in *The Art of Feminine Beauty* the moral and aesthetic dictum that would govern the lives of subsequent generations of women: "An abundance of fat is something repulsive and not in accord with the principles that rule our conception of the beautiful."[45]

Success and Security

In the 1920s the imperative to diet intensified not only because of medical advice and the flapper style but because of major social changes in the lives of women. In the wake of World War I, American women experienced something of a revolution in their social and political status, a revolution not at all dissimilar to what we have experienced since the 1960s. In both cases, the 1920s and more recently, affluence accompanied social change. In both cases, cultural messages about reducing the body accelerated. This history confirms the thesis of anthropologist Mary Douglas that rapid social change and disintegrating social boundaries stimulate both greater external and greater internal control of the physical body. In short, disorder in the body politic has implications for the individual body.[46]

For women the 1920s were a time of heady optimism and the perception of many new personal and material choices. Prosperity was in the air. In addition to gaining the franchise in 1920, more women worked outside their homes. More American girls were attending high school, as colleges and universities admitted ever larger numbers of women students (who, as a group, were more ethnically diverse than ever before). Advertising and motion pictures stimulated the development of a new mass culture that set styles and sold goods, especially among youth. And many young women—delighted with the prospect of greater personal freedom and more fun—discarded the sexual baggage of the Victorians and pronounced themselves travelers on a new road to increased sexual pleasure and equality with men.[47]

In the fast-paced environment of the 1920s, most women wanted a slim body because of the positive messages it conveyed. Such a body was not only an instrument of fashion, it was also a statement about the social and sexual orientation of the individual. A woman with a slender body distinguished herself from the plump Victorian matron and her old-fashioned ideals of nurturance, service, and self-sacrifice. The body of the "new woman" was a sign of modernity that marked her for more than traditional motherhood and domesticity.

Ironically, the new slim body, with its small breasts and narrow hips, symbolized increased rather than diminished sexuality. Although doctors worried about the consequences of dieting for women's reproductive potential, the new woman pursued svelteness in the name of her sexuality. A lithe figure was an emblem that also marked a woman as separate from the sex-segregated or homosocial world of the Victorians and from the notion of woman's asexuality, a characteristic associated with prudish married women as well as unmarried feminists.[48] Sexual interest and experimentation were novel luxuries, related in part to the availability of birth control, particularly the diaphragm and the condom.[49] In a world where sexuality and reproduction could be separated, a slender body and the willingness to wear more revealing clothes were taken as signs of increased sexual confidence, freedom, and enjoyment. A svelte female figure became, for the first time, the ultimate sign and symbol of heterosexual interest and success.

In the early twentieth century no individual better expressed this idea than Annette Kellerman, the young Australian swimmer who became a star in American silent films.[50] In the new moving pictures, form and grace of movement were particularly important, making slenderness a considerable asset. (Other early female film stars such as Irene Dunne, Clara Bow, Louise Brooks, Billie Burke, and Lillian and Dorothy Gish were all quite slim.) Kellerman's celebrity status was based not only on her swimming (she won the championship of New South Wales and set the record for women's efforts at the English Channel) but on the perfection of her body and her willingness to display it. In the 1916 film *Daughter of the Gods* she appeared nearly au naturel in a series of scenes in vine-covered pools, on coral reefs, amid powerful rapids, and in the fanciful harem of a sultan's palace. What the *New York Times* called Kellerman's "novelties of nudity and natation" spoke to a variety of different interests and symbolized American women's new freedom in manners and morals.[51]

Kellerman was proud of her 5-foot-3¾-inch, 137-pound body. She alleged that Dudley A. Sargent, director of physical training at Harvard, thought her figure "nearer the correct proportions than any he had ever seen." Although Kellerman's weight and measurements (35-26-37) seem quite ample by today's standards, she was an avid campaigner against fat. In *Physical Beauty*, a statement of her own personal beauty code, Kellerman declared:

> "Fat" is a short and ugly word. But "stoutness," "plumpness," "fleshiness," "obesity" and "embonpoint" are only softpedal euphemisms. It is fat just the same, and just as clumsy, as unhealthy, as ugly and awkward spelled with ten letters as with three.[52]

Just as the scientific beauty experts did, Kellerman subscribed to the credo of self-denial, proclaiming "eternal vigilance . . . the price of health and beauty."[53] In order to keep a careful focus on the body, Kellerman advocated daily exercise in the nude before a full-length mirror.

An advocate of the physical culture movement, Kellerman was always more than willing to tell the women's magazines how she used swimming to reach bodily perfection, and she wrote many detailed articles on why and how girls should learn to swim. In this respect she and the movement she represented were important advocates of a healthy female athleticism.[54] Kellerman's magazine lessons always included some version of the following: "Don't wear any more clothes than you need. They hinder your movements and make the body much heavier." Kellerman's popular advocacy of women's swimming had an unintended but critical consequence: by encouraging women to disrobe for more efficient swimming, Kellerman set the stage for the transformation of the female bathing suit into an icon of sexual attractiveness.[55] Beginning in the 1920s, female beauty pageants made bathing suit competitions a centerpiece of their contests, a procedure that underscored the primacy of the body in the definition of feminine good looks. Kellerman reinforced this priority when she declared the figure "even more essential" than the face.[56]

Intensity of interest in the female body was rooted in social insecurity as well as in the physical culturists' credo of self-affirmation. Heterosexual relationships in the 1920s were in transition, much as they are today. Pursuit of the body beautiful was linked to a major dimension of modern social change, the rising rate of divorce. By the late 1920s marital dissolutions were obviously on the rise, a fact that reflected changing expectations of marriage.[57] Personal happiness and satisfaction had replaced duty and sacrifice as the glue that made marriage work; couples came to expect both romance and sexuality in their experience of conjugal love. These attitudinal developments underwrote Annette Kellerman's claim that a great deal of contemporary divorce was the result of the married woman's inattention to her physique. "We should find that in 7 cases out of 10 [cases] the wife had lost her physical charm for her husband," she wrote.[58]

Firmer control of the female body was Kellerman's answer to increasing family insecurity. Instead of challenging the new marital ethic and the heightened legitimacy it gave to male sexual prerogatives, Kellerman urged women to improve themselves by spending more time in the cultivation of good looks. To charges of self-indulgence, Kellerman adamantly replied: "The old lie that the cultivation of feminine beauty is wicked wrecks more homes than poverty, and kills more loves than downright immorality. The new and true gospel of a woman's right to remain beautiful will save more marriages than all the anti-divorce sermons ever preached."[59] Kellerman was not alone in her emphasis on the physical side of marriage. Films by Cecil B. DeMille, such as *Old Wives for New* (1918) and *Why Change Your Wife?* (1920), presented visual tableaux contrasting the frumpy wife with the one who understood appearance as the key to modern marriage.[60] Women were told, often by other women, that their failure to meet the sexual challenge of modern marriage led to divorce court.

Annette Kellerman articulated a basic precept of twentieth-century femininity: to get and hold a man, women needed to preserve their youth and their physical attractiveness. Married women were no longer exempt from such concerns. Traditional wifely virtues, such as excellence in domesticity and a kind heart, could no longer guarantee the success of a marriage—but a beautiful body could. Kellerman declared, "[Beauty] is a more potent sermon on 'How to Keep Your Husband' than all the issues of The Homely Ladies' Journal which tries to answer that question with a lot of drivel about 'tact' and 'sympathy' and 'warmed slippers' and 'attractive dishes from leftovers.'"[61] In effect, by the 1920s outward appearance was more important than inner character because sexual allure had replaced spirituality as woman's "shining ornament."[62]

For individual women this innovative cultural prescription was a decidedly mixed blessing. Although it held out the promise of sexual liberation, it also generated a psychological dilemma that echoed Calvinist religious struggles: How could salvation (that is, beauty) be achieved? Was beauty a state of being, achievable through self-exertion and denial, or was it a commodity, available to be bought? If beauty could be purchased, then consumption was a form of self-improvement rather than self-indulgence. If beauty could be earned, then a righteous woman could achieve it through her "good works": careful attention to complexion, hair, and clothing as well as healthful exercise and, most important, restrained eating.[63]

Not all women could handle these pressures with equanimity.[64] Many internalized the notion that the size and shape of the body was a measure of self-worth; many believed that the process of losing weight would bring spiritual as well as physical transformation. By the 1920s calorie counting was everywhere on the increase and some women turned to bulimic behavior. At the Adult Weight Conference of 1926, a well-known physician reported, "I discovered that many of our flappers have mastered the art of eating their cake and yet not having it, inducing regurgitation, after a plentiful meal, either by drugs or mechanical means."[65] Apparently many women took frequent "high colonic irrigations" (enemas), cathartics, and iodine in the effort to reduce. It was evident that the new woman faced a complicated problem in how to relate to the beauty imperatives of a modern capitalist society. Because weight control was regarded as so important to beauty, women came to feel increasingly at odds with their appetite.

Younger and Thinner

Because of the exigencies of the Great Depression and World War II, women in the 1930s and 1940s involved themselves with major external, collective issues of survival, protection, and work. The canon of style in these decades continued to project a slim image, yet dieting seemed an inappropriate and silly preoccupation in the midst of scarcity and a compelling national emergency.[66] Popular literature on how to reduce never entirely disappeared during this era, but the growth of the diet industry was slowed by other, more pressing national and local concerns, including problems of food shortage and distribution. During the war women who waited in line for a weekly ration of butter and sugar were more likely to savor than to reject items made from these hard-to-get ingredients.

Despite the political and economic emergency that directed attention away from the individual body, the 1940s saw a subtle but important change in the history of modern dieting. Beginning in that decade adolescent girls, known as subdebs, were targeted as an audience for diet information and literature. The post–World War II popularization of adolescent weight control, a phenomenon that set the stage for our contemporary difficulties with anorexia nervosa, had two sources: parents and physicians newly alert to childhood obesity as a pathology, and commercial interests intent on selling to girls the same beauty concerns (and products) that absorbed the attention of their mothers.

Before 1940 the overweight child was mentioned only occasionally in the clinical literature or in popular medical writing.[67] Since the early part of the century, pediatricians and parents had shared a common concern for problems of childhood nutrition, focusing particularly on the poor eater. Underweight was the central problem because of its association with the wasting diseases. As medicine made significant gains in the treatment of these once-devastating illnesses, however, underweight became less of a liability in children.[68] Parents and physicians began to fear for their children what they feared for themselves—overweight. Yet in the 1920s and 1930s, when the first studies of overweight children appeared, most people still regarded overweight in children as a nonproblem. Overweight was simply "baby fat," destined to disappear as children matured into adolescence.

Medicine and psychology were building a different interpretation. They saw the problem of childhood obesity as more serious, complex, and enduring. In 1924 Bird T. Baldwin, a physician at the Iowa Child Welfare Research Station and codesigner of an influential set of height and weight tables for children, wrote, "The decidedly overweight child should be as much a subject of pathologic study as the underweight child."[69] In "Comparative Psychology of the Overweight Child," a doctoral thesis written at Teacher's College, Columbia University, overweight children were reported to be more fearful and less happy than either underweight or normal-weight youngsters.[70] In the mid-1930s Hilde Bruch also began to study obese children. Trained in psychoanalysis, she emphasized the fat child's early development and emotional life within the family. Bruch first gained prominence in 1939 by eliminating a disease of boys, Fröhlich's syndrome, which consisted of excessive obesity, small genitalia, and sluggish behavior. She rejected the idea of a pituitary disturbance and demonstrated that overeating and underactivity were the cause; moreover, boys with Fröhlich's syndrome could be treated with psychotherapy. In a series of influential articles Bruch asserted that the hunger of fat children was deep, psychic, and rooted in the pathology of individual families. And in the first edition of *The Common Sense Book of Baby and Child Care* (1945), Benjamin Spock told concerned parents that "fatness is a complicated problem" and that overeating in children was often a symptom of loneliness or maladjustment.[71] By the close of World War II these ideas were circulating among the middle-class parents who read child-raising literature. Fat children were now a medical, psychological, and social problem.

In adolescence fat was considered a particular liability because of the social strains associated with that stage of life. In the 1940s articles with titles such as "What to Do about the Fat Child at Puberty," "Reducing the Adolescent," and "Should the Teens Diet?" captured the rising interest in adolescent weight control.[72] Women's magazines, reflecting the concerns of mothers anxious to save their daughters from social ostracism, for the first time promoted diets for young girls. According to the *Ladies' Home Journal*: "Appearance plays too important a part in a girl's life not to have her grow up to be beauty-conscious. Girls should be encouraged to take an interest in their appearance when they are very young." Advice to teenagers warned "Not too many fudge sundaes!" and "Resist the three s's: Sundaes, Sodas, and Second Helpings."[73]

Adolescent weight control was also promoted by popular magazines hoping to sell products to young women. As early as the 1920s American business had turned its attention to the youth market.[74] Sales were stimulated by the existence of a youth subculture fostered by a massive increase in school enrollments at the high school and college levels. Between 1900 and 1930 the high school population grew by 650 percent, and colleges and universities experienced a threefold increase in the number of students.[75] In high school and college, young people were exposed to a peer group that generated its own priorities and rules of conduct. In both settings relations between the sexes became a focal point of both student energies and faculty concern. Heterosexual popularity and sexual allure required a certain level of stylistic conformity. High school and college girls, following the model of adult women, adopted beauty and fashion as the coin of the realm.

Advertisers and merchants were heartened by the American girl's devotion to fashion and her insistence on having the best. They also portrayed a young woman's entrance into the consumer culture as an important rite of passage: "No mere man can understand the revolution that takes place in the life of a girl around the ages of eighteen to twenty. For the first time she is buying things for herself on an extensive scale, and yields herself to new fancies, new impressions, new styles . . . She is on the alert to discover the latest and smartest—as they reveal her personality in fashion's setting." In short, "having money to spend on the self was intimately connected to breaking out of the family circle."[76]

By the close of World War II, younger, middle-class high school girls living at home emerged as a discrete new market.[77] These were girls with their own allowances to spend and full-time mothers to escort them on shopping trips. Entrepreneurs embraced popular theories of adolescent development which suggested that girls like these, on the brink of maturity, needed special help in weathering the trials and tribulations of modern adolescence. Advertisements for soaps and skin creams to prevent adolescent acne and displays of attractive clothing to build social confidence were part of the newest marketing strategy. These ideas about adolescence and the hope of profits spawned *Seventeen* magazine, which made its first appearance at the start of the school year in September 1944. Helen Valentine, the first editor, proclaimed, "*Seventeen* is your magazine, High School Girls of America!"[78] The magazine built its success on its ability to sell fashion and beauty products to teenage girls.

Seventeen's adoption of the cause of weight control confirmed that slimness was a critical dimension of adolescent beauty and that a new constituency, high school girls, was learning how to diet. From 1944 to 1948, *Seventeen* had published a full complement of articles on nutrition but almost nothing on weight control. Following the mode of earlier home economists and scientific nutritionists, the magazine had presented basic information about food groups and the importance of each in the daily diet; balance but not calories had been the initial focus. In 1948, however, *Seventeen* proclaimed overweight a medical problem and began educating its young readers about calories and the psychology of eating. Adolescent girls were warned against using eating as a form of emotional expression (do not "pamper your blues" with food) and were given practical tips on how to avoid food binging. No mention was made of the new "diet pills" (amphetamines) introduced in the 1930s for clinical treatment of obesity. Instead, teenagers were encouraged to go on "sensible" and "well-rounded" diets of between 1,200 and 1,800 calories. By the 1950s advertisements for "diet foods" such as Ry-Krisp were offering assistance as they told the readership "Nobody Loves a Fat Girl."[79] Girls, much as adult women, were expected to tame the natural appetite.

Although adolescent girls were consistently warned against weight reduction without medical supervision, dieting was always cast as a worthwhile endeavor with transforming powers. "Diets can do wonderful things. When dispensed or approved by your physician . . . all you have to do is follow whither the chart leads."[80] The process of metamorphosis from fat to thin always provided a narrative of uplift and interest. "The Fattest Girl in the Class" was the autobiographical account of Jane, an obese girl who, after suffering the social stigma associated with teenage overweight, went on a diet and found happiness.[81] Being thin was tied to attractiveness, popularity with the opposite sex, and self-esteem—all primary ingredients in adolescent culture. Nonfiction accounts of "make-overs" became a popular formula in all the beauty magazines of the postwar period and provided a tantalizing fantasy of psychological and spiritual transformation for mature and adolescent women alike.[82]

The popularization of adolescent female weight control in the postwar era is a prime component of the modern dieting story and a critical factor in explaining anorexia nervosa as we know it today. In the 1980s dieting is a central motif in the lives of women of nearly all ages; at least 50 percent of American women are on a diet at any given time.[83] And across the twentieth century the age of those controlling the appetite in the name of beauty has declined. Sadly, recent studies suggest that close to 80 percent of prepubescent girls—sometimes at ages as young as eight or nine—restrict their eating in the interest of not getting fat.[84] The fact that young girls, but not young boys, have such precocious concerns about attractiveness is compelling evidence for the power of sex-role socialization and the potency of the diet message.

The history of the diet industry in America (as yet unwritten) probably represents one of the most astounding triumphs of twentieth-century capitalist enterprise. In 1985 the American people spent over $5 billion on the effort to lose weight. The diet industry is an enterpreneur's delight because the market is self-generating and intrinsically expansive. Predicated on failure (dieters regain weight and must diet again and again), the interest in diet strategies, techniques, and products seems unlimited.[85] For nearly a decade one "diet book" or another has been a fixture on the list of the nation's best-sellers. Moreover, weight control is now a formal scientific subspecialty in American medicine. The American Society of Bariatric Physicians, an association with over six hundred members, describes itself as a group specializing in the treatment of obesity.[86] The existence of bariatrics confirms the fact that many in our society, not just young women, are in hot pursuit of day-to-day assistance and medical guidance on the issue of appetite and weight control.

Since the 1960s the dieting imperative has intensified in two noticeable and important ways that have consequences for anorexia nervosa. First, the ideal female body size has become considerably slimmer. After a brief flirtation with full-breasted, curvaceous female figures in the politically conservative postwar recovery of the 1950s, our collective taste returned to an ideal of extreme thinness and an androgynous, if not childlike, figure.[87] A series of well-known studies point to the declining weight since the 1950s of fashion models, Miss America contestants, and *Playboy* centerfolds.[88] Neither bosoms, hips, nor buttocks are currently in fashion as young and old alike attempt to meet the new aesthetic standard. A Bloomingdale's ad posits, "Bean lean, slender as the night, narrow as an arrow, pencil thin, get the point?"[89] It is appropriate to recall Annette Kellerman who, at 5 feet 3¾ inches and 137 pounds, epitomized the body beautiful of 1918. Obviously, our cultural tolerance for body fat has diminished over the intervening years.

Second, notably since the middle to late 1970s, a new emphasis on physical fitness and athleticism has intensified cultural pressures on the individual for control and mastery of the body. For women this means that fitness has been added to slimness as a criterion of perfection.[90] Experts on the subject, such as Jane Fonda, encourage women to strive for a lean body with musculature. The incredible popularity among women of aerobics, conditioning programs, and jogging does testify to the satisfactions that come with gaining physical strength through self-discipline, but it also expresses our current urgency about the physical body. Many who are caught up in the exercise cult equate physical fitness and slimness with a higher moral state.

More often than not, those who strive for physical perfection are concerned about what they eat. In the 1960s and 1970s many Americans began to change their diet in the interest of fitness and health. (In 1984 we ate more vegetables, fruits, and cereals and less beef and pork than we did in the 1970s.) This interest in a lighter diet sprang from both the social critique of food processing associated with countercultural dietary practices and the powerful medical suggestion that consumption of fats and sodium is linked to coronary disease and perhaps cancer. Given these relationships, many people chose to eliminate from their diet either a particular ingredient (butter, salt, white sugar) or a category of food (meat). Simultaneously, some became food zealots, exalting certain foods or vitamins (bran, cabbage, lecithin, vitamins C and E) for their special properties and proclaiming their own bodily purity. The anorectic's devotion to the ideal of thinness, her elaborate espousal of food theories, and the narrowing of her food repertoire to only the lightest of food is part and parcel of this *mentalité*.[91] In essence, food once again is central to holiness.

According to psychologist Rita Freedman, the contemporary emphasis on fitness and exercise is a double-edged sword. On the one hand, women are profiting in terms of both psychological and physical health from the new athleticism that has accompanied the contemporary women's movement. On the other hand, a "narcissism based on health" is not essentially different from one based on beauty.[92] In fact, spokespersons for the new credo of female fitness espouse the same principles of vanity, self-sacrifice, and physical and spiritual transformation that characterized the beauty zealots of the early twentieth century. What is different is that compulsive exercising and chronic dieting have been joined as twin obsessions.

The way we experience anorexia nervosa in the 1980s is shaped by these recent and powerful accelerations in the imperative for female bodily control. The cult of strenuous exercise and the popularization of the "lite diet," for example, have had a clear effect on the symptom picture in anorexia nervosa. Although hyperactivity was associated with the disorder in the nineteenth century, it was never, until very recently, a culturally sanctioned behavioral symptom. In the 1980s clinical reports and autobiographical statements show a clear-cut pattern of anorexic patients who exercise with ritualistic intensity. How much one runs and how little one eats is the prevailing moral calculus in present-day anorexia nervosa.

Among contemporary anorectics the body becomes an instrument of competition, a way to demonstrate one's mettle. Anorectics not only push themselves for athletic achievement, they also keep a watchful eye out for what is happening to the bodies of their friends. In a manner characteristic of anorexic patients, a young woman told Hilde Bruch, "I don't like it when other girls are skinny." Being the thinnest of her friends was a paramount concern and a source of her competitive energy. A recovered anorectic described the need to excel in thinness with a story about shopping: "Even now it is very difficult for me to go into a store and say, 'Yes, I want a size 5,' because to me that seems so common. Before, I could go in and say, 'I want a size 1,' and everybody would just look around. It was like the whole store, everybody standing around, would go, 'Golly, you are thin—that must be nice!' . . . All my friends seem to wear size 5 or 7, and I didn't like just being one of the crowd."[93] Obviously, the peer group figures prominently in the competition to be thin. Because being thinner than anyone else is so central to her identity, the anorectic finds a curious security in her perilously cadaverous existence.

Anorexia nervosa is a dangerous disease in the 1980s because of the extraordinarily low weights of its victims. An index of body mass in anorexia nervosa hospital admissions since the 1930s shows a marked decline over time, suggesting that more patients with severe weight loss are being admitted today than fifty years ago. In short, today's anorectic is thinner than ever before.[94] These weights are even more significant when we consider that contemporary young women are taller than their mothers and grandmothers and should logically weigh more.[95] The severity of anorexia nervosa today could be the result of delays in treatment or more extended outpatient therapy before hospitalization, but this scenario is unconvincing given our current sensitivity to the disease. Instead, the severity of current cases probably reflects the patients' zealous commitment to both exercise and diet as well as parental and medical tolerance for thinner bodies.

The modern symptom constellation ultimately confirms that modern dieting has a great deal to do with anorexia nervosa. As in many psychiatric disorders, the behavioral symptoms are an expression of prevailing cultural concerns. Although the psychogenesis of anorexia nervosa is largely individual and familial, our present admiration for extremely thin women has certainly contributed to an acceleration in the number who are dieting, a situation that also increases the number of young women who are at risk for anorexia nervosa. To use a model drawn from the literature on substance abuse, there is a correlation between the level of exposure and the prevalence of dependency in a population. Anorexia nervosa seems to behave similarly. As contemporary studies have shown, in occupations such as fashion modeling and ballet, where a slender figure is a criterion for success and dieting is pervasive, the incidence of anorexia nervosa is significantly increased.[96] Given our longstanding and extravagant collective worship at the shrine of slimness, it is no wonder that so many contemporary young women make dieting an article of faith and that anorexia nervosa has become the characteristic psychopathology of the female adolescent of our day.

Afterword

For nearly a century, from the time of William Gull and Charles Lasègue until the 1970s, anorexia nervosa was relatively unknown outside the medical community. Today the disease is all too familiar: if we have not experienced it within our own family, we know about it secondhand or thirdhand. Although a portion of the current "epidemic" is certainly attributable to the spread of information about the disease among girls themselves and to increased use of the diagnosis by doctors, there has also been a real rise in incidence since the mid-1960s. (Today, an estimated 10 percent of American women experience eating disorders, and among those in college the figure is roughly 20 percent.)[1] This is the historical and epidemiological conundrum that the biological and psychological models of anorexia nervosa leave unexplained.

The number of young women who have fallen prey to this dangerous disease since 1960 confirms the general relationship between acute social change and the intensification of bodily controls. But the rise in numbers prompts a more specific question about the recent past and this particular symptom choice: why is it that in the past twenty-five years food and eating have become the psychological battleground for so many middle-class young women?

The proliferation of diet and exercise regimens in the past decade, although an important context for understanding the increase in anorexia nervosa, is not the whole story. For a more complete explanation we must turn to some other recent social changes, keeping in mind that no one factor has caused the contemporary problem. Rather, it is the nature of our economic and cultural environment, interacting with individual and family characteristics, which exacerbates the social and emotional insecurities that put today's young women at increasing risk for anorexia nervosa. Two very basic social transformations are relevant to the problem: one has to do with food; the other, with new expectations between the sexes.

Since World War II, and especially in the last two decades, middle-class Americans have experienced a veritable revolution in terms of how and what we eat, as well as how we think about eating.[2] The imperatives of an expanding capitalist society have generated extraordinary technological and marketing innovations, which in turn have transformed food itself, expanded our repertoire of foods, and affected the ways in which we consume them. Even though much contemporary food is characterized by elaborate processing and conservation techniques that actually reduce and flatten distinctive textures and flavors, the current array of food choices seems to constitute an endless smorgasbord of new and different tastes. In the 1980s an individual in an urban center looking for a quick lunch is able to choose from tacos with guacamole and salsa, hummus and falafel in pita, sushi, tortellini, quiche, and pad thai—along with more traditional "American" fare such as hamburgers. Thirty years ago this diversified international menu was as unknown to most Americans as were many of the food products used to create it: avocados, coriander, garbanzo beans, pita bread, raw or unprocessed tuna, soy sauce, rice noodles, and yogurt. The so-called Global Village has had consequences for our bodies as well as our minds, it seems.

The expansion of our food repertoire, the adoption of ethnic foods, and the more recent "gourmandizing" of America have created enormous activity in the middle-class kitchen and changed the nature of the products on our supermarket shelves. Today, many in the educated middle class spurn iceberg lettuce—not because they are still committed to Cesar Chavez and the cause of farm laborers, but because iceberg is considered boring or tasteless compared to romaine, red leaf, arugula, raddiccio, mâche, and endive. Ice cream is no longer a simple matter of chocolate or vanilla; the ice-cream section of even an ordinary supermarket includes "gourmet" and low-fat selections, sherbets, sorbets, gelatos, nondairy substitutes, and a host of special snack formats designed essentially for children. This kind of differentiation and segmentation, typical of the capitalist marketplace, is both a cause and a consequence of our changing diet and tastes.

Paradoxically, despite the multiplicity of products from which to choose, the contemporary eater probably has less (rather than more) individual control over food than ever before. As anthropologist Sidney Mintz has demonstrated, capitalism—in the interest of food-industry profits—maintains consumption in predictable channels.[3] Despite advertisements that announce increasing ease, convenience, and freedom with respect to food, we consume more and more homogenized, mass-produced foods permeated by sugars and fats, ingredients which many people now regard as necessary, natural, and good—that is, as a matter of taste. Our tastes appear to be as much the product of our economic and social system as they are the interaction of food with the microscopic taste buds on the surface of the human tongue.

In a capitalist society eating, appetite, and taste are all extremely complicated. As a consequence of overstimulation, we are faced with an abundance of food which, in our obesophobic society, necessitates ever greater self-control. On a daily basis many of us struggle with an essential contradiction in our economic system— that is, that hedonism and discipline must coexist.[4] Middle-class Americans feel this tension most acutely in the realm of personal eating behavior. It is no wonder, then, that we talk so incessantly about food and dieting.

The food revolution is a matter of ideas and manners as much as technology and markets. To repeat Hilde Bruch, "There is no human society that deals rationally with food in its environment, that eats according to the availability, edibility, and nutritional value alone."[5] In our society food is chosen and eaten not merely on the basis of hunger. It is a commonplace to observe that contemporary advertising connects food to sociability, status, and sexuality. In an affluent society, in particular, where eating appears to involve considerable individual choice, food is regarded as an important analogue of the self.

In the 1960s, for example, many young people in the counter-culture gave up foods associated with their bourgeois upbringing and turned instead to a diet of whole grains, unprocessed foods, and no meat. This new diet made a statement about personal and political values and became a way of separating one generation from another; independent food cooperatives provided an alternative way to select and purchase foods and at the same time circumvent huge conglomerates. Food was clearly a trope for politics, morality, and purity.

In the 1980s, concern with food as a source of status and personal identity runs particularly deep among well-to-do urbanites, many of whom cast off traditional American fare, embraced the nouvelle cuisine, and are now infatuated with American regional cooking such as TexMex and Cajun. The extent to which the choice of cuisine dominates and defines the sophisticated lifestyle is reflected in a recent *New Yorker* cartoon, which shows a young professional couple after a dinner party given by friends. In complete seriousness they say to each other, "We could get close with David and Elizabeth if they didn't put béarnaise sauce on everything."[6] The anorectic is obviously not alone in her use of food and eating as a means of self-definition. There are many others who internalize the dictum "You are what you eat"—or, for that matter, what you don't eat.[7]

Along with the expansion of our food repertoire and our extraordinary attention to food selection, the eating context has changed. Eating is being desocialized. In American society today, more and more food is being consumed away from the family table or any other fixed center of sociability. This process began in the postwar period with the introduction of convenience foods and drive-in restaurants, precursors of the fast-food chains that now constitute a $45-billion-a-year industry. More recently, sophisticated eaters—particularly style-setting, affluent city dwellers—have adopted a related and highly mobile style of eating known as grazing. Those who graze sample small bits of different, attractive foods throughout the day, as they move from one eating site to another. (Of course, grazing looks different depending on the social class of the eater. Potato chips, pop-tarts, and soft drinks may be the most common snacks among the working class.

Among the elite, one is apt to see an imported chocolate, a bit of chevre or caviar, a glass of Perrier.) In either case, Americans eat everywhere—in the classroom; in theaters, libraries, and museums; on the street; at their desks; on the phone; in hot tubs; in cars while driving. To put it bluntly, we are indiscriminate about where we eat. Signs saying "no food and drink," infrequent in other parts of the world, adorn our public buildings, a clear sign of our pattern of vagabond eating.[8]

On college and university campuses, where eating disorders are rampant, the situation is exaggerated. By the early 1970s most undergraduate students were no longer required to take any sitdown meals at fixed times in college dormitories. The decline of family-style meals on American college campuses was a consequence of the social revolution of the 1960s and the decrease in the university's controversial in loco parentis power. As the university retreated from its commitment to control student social life and sexuality, it also gave up on the business of trying to stimulate fellowship over common meals. Students had always complained about the quality of institutional food, but more and more students were now demanding special dietary consideration as part of the doctrine of entitlement; some wanted no meat or insisted on unprocessed foods; others required macrobiotic or kosher foods; many simply asked for the freedom to individualize the substance and timing of eating, something they were beginning to do increasingly at home.

Today's undergraduate student is a classic vagabond eater because the college environment encourages it. Typically, students frequent a series of university cafeterias or commercial off-campus restaurants where they can obtain breakfast, lunch, or dinner at any time of the day. Some campus food plans allow unlimited amounts, a policy that fuels the behavior of the bulimic: "I used to go to Contract, eat a whole bunch of stuff, go to the bathroom, throw it up, come back, eat again, throw it up, eat again."[9] In addition, the availability of nearly any kind of food at any time contributes to a pattern of indiscriminate eating. Traditions of food appropriateness—that is, that certain foods are eaten at particular times of the day or in a certain sequence—disappear in this unstructured climate. Thus, an ice-cream cone, a carbonated soft drink, and a bagel constitute an easy popular "meal" that may be eaten at any time of day. Most colleges and the surrounding communities have made provisions to gratify student appetites no matter what the hour. Snack bars and vending machines adorn nearly every free alcove in classroom buildings and residence halls; pizza and Chinese food are delivered hot in the middle of the night.

In a setting where eating is so promiscuous, it is no wonder that food habits become problematic. This is not to say that our universities, on their own, generate eating-disordered students. They do, however, provide fertile ground for those who carry the seeds of disorder with them from home. In the permissive and highly individualized food environment of the post–1970 college or university, overeating and undereating become distinct possibilities.[10]

For those young women with either incipient or pronounced anorexia nervosa, the unstructured college life may at first provide relief from a home environment characterized by day-to-day parental supervision of food intake. In some respects, going away to college constitutes the parentectomy that physicians since the time of William Gull have recommended as a cure. Free of parental surveillance, food and eating should become less complicated. Because she is living a more autonomous life, and the act of eating is not under formal scrutiny, the anorexic girl should now be able to respond normally to her hunger.

Instead, the campus environment often accentuates the anorectic's physical and emotional problems. Meals can be skipped so easily that there is increased opportunity for noneating to become habitual and for narrowing the food repertoire to even a single item: apples, soup, cottage cheese, or dry crackers. With no one overseeing the amount that she eats, the collegiate anorectic may experience a precipitous drop in weight as the behavior becomes increasingly addictive. Apparently, the anorectic at college is often troubled by, rather than liberated by, her autonomy with respect to food:

> I don't know any limits here at all. At home, I have my mom dishing out my food . . . But when I'm here it's a totally different story—I can't tell portion size at all. I always get so afraid afterwards, after

eating. Oh my God did I eat that much or this much? So I just pass things up altogether and don't eat.[11]

The anorectic's preoccupation with appetite control is fueled by incessant talk about dieting and weight even among friends and associates who eat regularly. Diet-conscious female students report that fasting, weight control, and binge eating are a normal part of life on American college campuses.[12] Obviously, the anorectic is not the only woman on campus who is anxious about food and her body. Because they came of age in a fat-phobic society, most college women are concerned about how to become or remain slim in an environment that provides constant stimulation to eat (and not to eat). Weight-control techniques are often adopted without regard to safety. For example, recent studies reveal that adolescent women are the fastest-growing market for cigarettes, having taken up smoking precisely because they regard it as a functional aid to appetite control.[13]

Young women in their teens and twenties not only share a notion of an ideal body type, they also learn from one another how to attain it. Information about dieting, purging, and other "disregulating behaviors" is part of their subculture. Techniques are culled from popular stories about anorexia nervosa, the mass-market weight-control industry, women's magazines, and the experience of friends. *The Beverly Hills Diet*, a longtime best-seller, openly advocated a form of bulimia in which binges are "compensated" for by eating enormous amounts of raw fruit in order to induce diarrhea.[14] And a 1981 study demonstrated that a college woman who purges almost always knows another female student who purges, whereas a woman who does not purge rarely knows anyone who does. According to psychologist Ruth Striegel-Moore and her research associates, "A positive feedback loop is thus established: the more women there are with disordered eating, the more likely there are to be even more women who develop disordered eating."[15]

In the 1980s it is not uncommon for an undergraduate woman to tell a faculty adviser or psychological counselor that a roommate or friend is not eating or is regurgitating her food. Some students, caught up in the "therapeutic mentality," become overly zealous in judging and reporting who is anorexic, or they use the term loosely as a self-description; others understand that eating disorders are hard to determine in an environment where so many students are dieting and many eat in nontraditional ways. Nevertheless, for young women already imbued with the ethic of obligation—a characteristic described by psychologist Carol Gilligan—attention to one another's diet and weight may well be a new component in contemporary female morality.[16] Thus, the undergraduate asks: Should I intervene in the personal behavior of a friend? Are my friend's choices about food and eating different from her choices about academic or sexual behavior? Should I report the symptoms to her parents or college authorities? What is my role and responsibility if my friend or roommate *really* has anorexia nervosa or bulimia? For the current college generation of women, learning how to respond to difficulties in handling food constitutes a serious moral dilemma.

Eating disorders have become so prevalent on American college campuses that the *Chronicle of Higher Education* took up the subject, and in the past few years an impressive number of colleges and universities have developed an institutional response to undergraduate eating problems. Many now offer support groups as well as individualized psychotherapy for students who either have eating disorders themselves or have friends who do. The clientele is, of course, predominantly female. In February 1986, representatives from many of the nation's most prestigious colleges and universities met at Radcliffe College for an Intercollegiate Eating Disorders Conference, a two-day program designed to map strategies for effective peer counseling on the nation's campuses. At Cornell University the Office of the Dean of Students sponsors an ongoing workshop program entitled "Women, Food, and Self-Esteem."

These same concerns exist beyond the college, among adult women. Today, even more than in the Victorian period, appetite is an important voice in female identity. In our obesophobic society women struggle with food because, among other things, food represents fat and loss of control. For a contemporary woman to eat heartily, energetically, and happily is usually problematic (and, at best, occasional). As a result, some come to fear and hate their own appetite; eating becomes a shameful and disgusting act, and denial of hunger becomes a central facet of identity and personality. In effect, in our society most women cannot allow their appetite free expression nor are they capable of enjoying (without guilt) the extraordinary food repertoire that postwar affluence has spawned. There are indications of this uncomfortable female predicament outside the confines of the therapeutic establishment: in television commercials, where the female eater consistently constrains and controls her appetite (whereas the male allows his full reign);[17] in the ordinary conventions of middle-class social life, where women ritualistically disclaim their ability to eat all that is on their plate; and in the current rash of feminist cartoons (such as those of Nicole Hollander) about eating as a form of forbidden pleasure and self-expression. By the 1970s and 1980s the cultural imperative for control of appetite became extraordinarily troublesome precisely because the stimulus to eat (and not eat) was everywhere.

Among adolescents concerned with the transition to adulthood, an intense concern with appetite control and the body operates in tandem with increasing anxiety over sexuality and the implications of changing sex roles. For sex is the second important arena of social change that may contribute to the rising number of anorectics. There are, in fact, some justifiable social reasons why contemporary young women fear adult womanhood. The "anorexic generations," particularly those born since 1960, have been subject to a set of insecurities that make heterosexuality an anxious rather than a pleasant prospect. Family insecurity, reflected in the frequency of divorce, and changing sex and gender roles became facts of life for this group in their childhood. These youngsters have grown up with men and women on different sides of the bargaining table; they have heard angry voices, and they have seen relationships torn asunder and families renegotiated. Although there is no positive correlation between divorced families and anorexia nervosa, family disruption is part of the world view of the anorexic generations. Its members understand implicitly that not all heterosexual relationships have happy endings.

As a consequence of these social changes, some young women are ambivalent about commitments to men and have adopted an ideal of womanhood that reflects the impact of post-1960 feminism. Although they generally draw back from an explicitly feminist vocabulary, most undergraduate women today desire professional careers of their own without forsaking the idea of marriage and a family. A 1985 study of college women by sociologist Mirra Komarovsky reveals that finding one's place in the world of work has become essential for personal dignity in this generation—yet a career without marriage was the choice of only 2 percent of the sample.[18] Convinced that individuality can be accommodated in marriage, these young women are interested in heterosexuality, but admit that "relationships with guys" are difficult even in college. Komarovsky describes conflict over dating rituals (who takes the initiative and who pays), decision making as a couple, intellectual rivalries, and competition for entrance into graduate school. Unlike Mother, who followed Dad to graduate school and supported him along the way, today's undergraduate—whether she is a declared feminist or not—wants her own professional career both as a ticket to the good life and as a protection for herself in case of divorce.

Sexual activity also requires an extraordinary degree of self-protection in the modern world of AIDS. While premarital sex is acceptable (if not desirable), it is an understandable source of worry among female undergraduates. An advertisement in a 1986 issue of *Ms.*, aimed at selling condoms to young women, captured the current ambivalence about the physical side of heterosexuality: "Let's face it, sex these days can be risky business, and you need all the protection you can get. Between the fear of unplanned pregnancy, sexually transmitted diseases, and the potential side effects of many forms of contraception, it may seem like sex is hardly worth the risk anymore."[19] For some students the unprecedented privacy and freedom of modern university life generates as much fear as pleasure. It bears repeating that clinical materials suggest an absence of sexual activity on the part of anorectics.

Even though feminine dependency is no longer in fashion, these same young women combine traditional expectations with a quest for equity and power. To be brainy and beautiful; to have an exciting $75,000-a-year job; to nurture two wonderful children in consort with a supportive but equally high-powered husband—

these are the personal ambitions of many in the present college generation. In order to achieve this level of personal and social perfection, young women must be extremely demanding of themselves: there can be no distracting personal or avocational detours—they must be unrelenting in the pursuit of goals. The kind of personal control required to become the new Superwoman (a term popularized by columnist Ellen Goodman)[20] parallels the single-mindedness that characterizes the anorectic. In sum, the golden ideal of this generation of privileged young women and their most distinctive pathology appear to be flip sides of the same record.

My assertion that the post-1960 epidemic of anorexia nervosa can be related to recent social change in the realm of food and sexuality is not an argument for turning back the clock. As a feminist, I have no particular nostalgia for what is deceptively called a "simpler" past. Moreover, historical investigation demonstrates that anorexia nervosa was latent in the economic and emotional milieu of the bourgeois family as early as the 1850s. It makes little sense to think a cure will be achieved by putting women back in the kitchen, reinstituting sit-down meals on the nation's campuses, or limiting personal and professional choices to what they were in the Victorian era. On the basis of the best current research on anorexia nervosa, we must conclude that the disease develops as a result of the intersection of external and internal forces in the life of an individual. External forces such as those described here do not, by themselves, generate psychopathologies, but they do give them shape and influence their frequency.

In the confusion of this transitional moment, when a new future is being tentatively charted for women but gender roles and sexuality are still constrained by tradition, young women on the brink of adulthood are feeling the pain of social change most acutely.[21] They look about for direction, but find little in the way of useful experiential guides. What parts of women's tradition do they want to carry into the future? What parts should be left behind? These are difficult personal and political decisions, and most young women are being asked to make them without benefit of substantive education in the history and experience of their sex. In effect, our young women are being challenged and their expectations raised without a simultaneous level of support for either their specific aspirations or for female creativity in general.

Sadly, the cult of diet and exercise is the closest thing our secular society offers women in terms of a coherent philosophy of the self.[22] This being the case, anorexia nervosa is not a quirk and the symptom choice is not surprising. When personal and social difficulties arise, a substantial number of our young women become preoccupied with their bodies and control of appetite. Of all the messages they hear, the imperative to be beautiful and good, by being thin, is still the strongest and most familiar. Moreover, they are caught, often at a very early age, in a deceptive cognitive trap that has them believing that body weight is entirely subject to their conscious control. Despite feminist influences on the career aspirations of the present college-age generation, little has transpired to dilute the basic strength of this powerful cultural prescription that plays on both individualism and conformity. The unfortunate truth is that even when she wants more than beauty and understands its limitations as a life goal, the bourgeois woman still expends an enormous amount of psychic energy on appetite control as well as on other aspects of presentation of the physical self.

And what of the future? I believe that we have not yet seen the crest of the late-twentieth-century wave of eating disorders. Although historians need to be cautious about prognostication, a few final observations seem in order.

In affluent societies the human appetite is unequivocally misused in the service of a multitude of nonnutritional needs. As a result, both anorexia nervosa and obesity are characteristic of modern life and will continue to remain so.

We can expect to see the evolution of a more elaborate medical classification scheme for eating disorders, and greater attention to distinguishing one syndrome from another. Modern medicine is built on this kind of refinement. There is also the possibility that, as eating behavior is subjected to closer scrutiny by doctors and other health professionals, more eating disorders will be identified. The new syndromes will probably be described in terms that suggest a biomedical (rather than biosocial) etiology. Some clinics specializing in weight and appetite control already advertise a specific treatment for "carbohydrate addiction."

Although eating disorders certainly deserve medical attention, an exclusive concentration on biomedical etiology obscures the ways in which social and cultural factors were implicated in the emergence of these disorders in the past century and in their proliferation today. As we approach the twenty-first century, it will surely become apparent that the postindustrial societies (the United States, Canada, Western Europe, Australia, and Japan) generate many people, not just adolescents, whose appetites are out of kilter. In effect, capitalism seems to generate a peculiar set of human difficulties that might well be characterized as consumption disorders rather than strictly eating disorders.

As Western values and life-styles are disseminated throughout the world and, in the wake of that process, traditional eating patterns disappear, anorexia nervosa will probably spread. Where food is abundant and certain sociocultural influences predominate, there will be some women whose search for perfection becomes misguided, translating into a self-destructive pathology such as anorexia nervosa. Our historical experience suggests that a society marching in a particular direction generates psychopathologies that are themselves symptomatic of the culture.

Finally, we can expect to see eating disorders continue, if not increase, among young women in those postindustrial societies where adolescents tend to be under stress. For both young men and young women, vast technological and cultural changes have made the transition to adulthood particularly difficult by transforming the nature of the family and community and rendering the future unpredictable. According to psychologist Urie Bronfenbrenner and others, American adolescents are in the worst trouble: we have the highest incidence of alcohol and drug abuse among adolescents of any country in the world; we also have the highest rate of teenage pregnancy of any industrialized nation; and we appear to have the most anorexia nervosa.[23]

Although the sexually active adolescent mother and the sexually inactive adolescent anorectic may seem to be light-years apart, they are linked by a common, though unarticulated, understanding. For adolescent women the body is still the most powerful paradigm regardless of social class. Unfortunately, a sizable number of our young women—poor and privileged alike—regard their body as the best vehicle for making a statement about their identity and personal dreams. This is what unprotected sexual intercourse and prolonged starvation have in common. Taken together, our unenviable preeminence in these two domains suggests the enormous difficulty involved in making the transition to adult womanhood in a society where women are still evaluated primarily in terms of the body rather than the mind.

Although the disorder we have examined here is part of a general pattern of adolescent discomfort in the West, anorexia nervosa ultimately expresses the predicament of a very distinct group, one that suffers from the painful ambiguities of being young and female in an affluent society set adrift by social change. Intelligent, anxious for personal achievement, and determined to maintain control in a world where things as basic as food and sex are increasingly out of control, the contemporary anorectic unrelentingly pursues thinness—a secular form of perfection. In a society where consumption and identity are pervasively linked, she makes nonconsumption the perverse centerpiece of her identity. In a sad and desperate way, today's fasting girls epitomize the curious psychic burdens of the dutiful daughters of a people of plenty.

Postscript

Ithaca, New York
April, 1989

Since the publication of *Fasting Girls*, I have received a variety of written reactions from readers. These letters prolonged my engagement with the subject and stimulated many late-night thoughts about how I might answer. I am delighted that a paperback edition provides me with the opportunity to respond, in the form of this brief postscript.

Much of my correspondence was purely informative: it confirmed and elaborated on points made in *Fasting Girls*. For example, from Europe, readers reported on the increasing incidence of anorexia nervosa. (In 1950, there were only 250 cases in France but there have been over 5,000 since 1981.) Academic colleagues who used *Fasting Girls* in their psychology, history, and women's studies courses sent me copies of student papers about the book so that I could judge the effect of my work on the group most at risk for the disorder. And many others—particularly young women and feminist faculty members—sent me pieces of poetry, fiction, and reportage that spoke to the problem of women's bodies and their relationship to food. These selections, which range from the poetry of Emily Dickinson to the diet techniques of Oprah Winfrey, fill my office files, enliven my lectures, and stand as proof of how interactive the writing process can be.

Some other responses have been disturbing and difficult to handle. I received a number of revealing, intimate letters that laid bare the anguish of eating disorders and body image problems in the lives of contemporary women: "I am 5'4" and, on heavy days, I weigh 78 pounds. I have had this lifestyle for five years ... I feel so helpless ..." and "I buy *Big Beautiful Woman* magzine to help boost my self-esteem when I feel so awful and ugly." Occasionally, there was a letter that constituted a covert plea for help and, in those cases, I did the only responsible thing I could: I answered quickly with words of encouragement and current information about the nearest eating disorders organization or clinical facility. Each of these sad and troubled letters reminded me that I was not a clinician but a historian. Despite my best intentions, my work cannot make an anorectic well. Instead, I needed to confront the tough question asked by most readers at the conclusion of my book: "How can this culture be changed?"

Although I am staggered by the enormity of this question, I persevere in the hope that a feminist intellectual critique of the cultural sources of eating disorders can someday generate new social practices and more effective therapeutics. In the wake of the discovery of eating disorders in the 1970s and 1980s, American women began to articulate their problematic relationship to food and the body. Numerous popular books and articles about "body hatred" and learning to "make peace with food" followed. These popular expressions of distress are now paralleled by psychological studies that point to body image problems as a lifetime source of anxiety and stress for women—from childhood to the grave. A series of scholarly conferences, based on women's studies, are being planned to investigate women's special relationship to the production, consumption, and distribution of food. As we prepare to enter the twenty-first century, it seems more important than ever that we come to grips with the unsettling cultural morass that surrounds the female body in a culture of affluence.

I applaud all of the ongoing efforts by feminist groups to change the ways in which women's bodies are currently depicted in advertising and in the entertainment media. All of us—male and female—need to see a more realistic media image of women, one that allows for adult female development, aging, and ethnic variability. But changing a cultural icon is an enormous undertaking, particularly in a society that has so successfully harnessed female sexuality to the interest of capitalist marketing. Still, it is worth the effort. We must continue to protest the insidious ways in which women's bodies are objectified and brutalized in the interest of either stimulating desire or selling us more and more material goods.

There are other ways to stem the tide of eating disorders in addition to the ongoing struggle to transform representations of the female body. First and foremost, we need to turn our attention to the experience of female adolescence. We must reverse the long-standing tendency to trivialize the experience of girls, whether it involves the religious excitement of young nuns in the convents of the sixteenth and seventeenth centuries, the collective enthusiasm of the "Bobby Soxers" of the 1940s, or the formulaic behaviors of the anorectics of today. Somehow, these phenomena are viewed with suspicion, cast as "frenzies" or dismissed as mere "antics." In addition, the very category—"girl"—has shriveled (if not disappeared) in recent years as a result of a feminist distaste for the term and the increasing precocity of our youngsters (i.e., "the disappearance of childhood"). Both of these factors contribute to a profound inattention to the problems of girlhood.

In the case of eating disorders, age seems to be absolutely critical to understanding the problem of vulnerability. Therefore, we need to find out more about how adolescent girls think and, also, develop new lines of communication to them. In our contemporary cultural environment, learning to accept and embrace an adult body makes girlhood particularly excrutiating: this is a fact that should motivate substantive attention to our young women but, unfortunately, it has not.

The issue of the "communicability" of anorexia nervosa ought to be taken up seriously by clinicians, educators, parents, and adolescents themselves. The imitative (or mimetic) aspects of eating disorders are probably related to the cultural environment of girls, the ways in which they are socialized, and the communities in which they live. Yet, clinicians, educators, and feminists have not yet developed effective means of intervention or any way to halt the contagion. With a few notable exceptions (Carol Gilligan, Jeanne Brooks-Gunn), most contemporary researchers are uninterested in the way girls think and there are few who take up the question of the impact of popular culture on their collective behavior and sense of self. In the 1990s, scholars working in a variety of areas—but particularly biomedicine, psychology, and sociology—need to restore girls to the feminist research agenda.

There are other important things that older women can do to begin to curb the spread of eating disorders among adolescent women. These require some simple changes in our own behavior and some honesty between the generations. At the outset, each of us needs to assess the extent to which we have "bought" the beauty ideal. If a major portion of our time, energy, and conversation is spent on dieting and clothes then we are actually part of the problem. We cannot expect our daughters, students, and adolescent friends to be any better than we are. If women's ideal of perfection in adulthood is wearing a size 6, then our girls are doomed.

My lecturing and speaking about the history of anorexia nervosa leads me to conclude that most thinking women want something better for the next generation. At the same time that we all want to look good and feel attractive, we also want to free ourselves, our daughters, and our granddaughters from the tyranny of these body and food imperatives. Some people propose a solution in the form of absolute control and mastery of the body. In other words, they urge the development of the perfect body through hard work, an exquisitely balanced diet, use of a trainer, and effective "de-stressing" at a luxuriuous spa. The problem is that the new narcissism still keeps the focus on the body, it offers hope to only a privileged few, and it ultimately "ups the ante" by setting even higher standards of physical perfection.

What we must develop for ourselves and for our girls is a self-conscious strategy to shift our attention from our bodies to our brains. It is a rare woman indeed who does not admit to having wasted emotional and creative energy on the issue of her own bodily inadequacies. We need to talk with our daughters and our students about what this "brain drain" means for female intelligence and creativity.

We also need to rethink some of our behavior in a deliberate, self-conscious way. Unthinkingly, most of us greet our women friends with comments about how we look because that is the way we have been trained to evaluate how we are doing. Comments about one another's bodies, hair, and clothing are a natural part of our connection to one another and we probably cannot give them up entirely. Yet, we could assign them a less prominent role in our social interactions. Instead of the instantaneous and reflexive "You *look* wonderful," we could begin by asking each other about our work and activities. This point seems particularly important in dealing with younger women. Although we want to encourage self-confidence and assurance in girls, we should not tie that feeling to the experience of receiving compliments for how one looks. To do so is to fuel the addiction to the beauty ideal.

Ultimately, mature women must tell younger women the truth: reliance on beauty as power is a dangerous form of dependency. Those young women who are single-minded in their pursuit of the beauty ideal should be warned that it will not sustain them over a lifetime. Girls need to understand that if beauty is in the eye of the beholder, those who rely on beauty are ultimately controlled by others. Their sense of satisfaction will always depend on the compliments and approval they win, rather than an authentic sense of personal efficacy and worth. These are hard issues to take up with adolescent girls but there is an urgency to our troubles with eating disorders that demands an attempt. If we do not, we will enter the twenty-first century in the same anguished state, without an effective intergenerational strategy for transforming our present and painful preoccupation.

Notes

Introduction

1. I use "anorectic" (the noun) to designate patients with anorexia nervosa; the analogue is "diabetic," "syphilitic," or "dyspeptic." I use "anorexic" (the adjective) to describe behavior that may or may not derive from anorexia nervosa.

2. On contemporary American women and their special relation to food see Jane Rachel Kaplan, *A Woman's Conflict: The Special Relationship between Women and Food* (Englewood Cliffs, N.J., 1980); Kim Chernin, *The Hungry Self: Women, Eating, and Identity* (New York, 1985); Susie Orbach, *Hunger Strike: The Anorectic's Struggle as a Metaphor for Our Age* (New York, 1986). Appetite control is clearly a problem for contemporary women. Psychological research on this issue is cited in Chapter 1; see esp. note 61. Relevant anthropological discussions may be found in Bridget O'Laughlin, "Mediation of Contradiction: Why Mbum Women Do Not Eat Chicken," in *Women, Culture and Society,* ed. Michelle Zimbalist Rosaldo and Louise Lamphere (Stanford, Calif., 1974); Anna Meigs, *Food, Sex and Pollution* (New Brunswick, N.J., 1984); Donald Pollock, "Food and Sexual Identity among the Culina," *Food and Foodways* 1: 1 (1985), 25–41; David McKnight, "Sexual Symbolism of Food among the Wik Mungkan," *Man* 8: 2 (1973), 194–209.

3. Caroline Walker Bynum, *Jesus as Mother: Studies in the Spirituality of the High Middle Ages* (Berkeley, 1982) and *Holy Feast and Holy Fast: The Religious Significance of Food to Medieval Women* (Berkeley, 1986). See also Bynum's "Women Mystics and Eucharistic Devotion in the Thirteenth Century," *Women's Studies* 2: 1–2 (1984), 179–214; and her "Fast, Feast, and Flesh: The Religious Significance of Food to Medieval Women," *Representations* 11 (1985), 1–25.

4. In *The Use of Pleasure: The History of Sexuality,* vol. 2 (New York, 1985), Michel Foucault postulates that hunger, in the Classical period, was one of the appetites that escaped the endless rules, regulations, and judgments that confined sexual behavior. In Chapter 2 I suggest that this was not always the case.

5. This has been the orientation of my earlier work. See Joan Jacobs Brumberg, *Mission for Life: The Judson Family and American Evangelical Cul-*

ture (New York, 1980), esp. chap. 2; "Zenanas and Girlless Villages: An Ethnology of American Evangelical Women, 1870–1910," *Journal of American History* 69 (September 1982), 347–371; "Chlorotic Girls, 1870–1920: An Historical Perspective on Female Adolescence," *Child Development* 53 (December 1982), 1468–77; "'Ruined' Girls: Family and Community Responses to Illegitimacy in Upstate New York, 1890 to 1920," *Journal of Social History* 18 (December 1984), 247–272. Some of what follows appeared as "'Fasting Girls': Reflections on Writing the History of Anorexia Nervosa," in *History and Research in Child Development: In Celebration of the Fiftieth Anniversary of the Society,* ed. Alice Boardman Smuts and John W. Hagen, Monographs of the Society for Research in Child Development (1985), no. 211, 50: 4–5, 93–104. My interest in the history of adolescence follows that of Joseph Kett, *Rites of Passage* (New York, 1977) and John Gillis, *Youth in History* (New York, 1976). Both of these important works deal with the historical experience of adolescence without asking gender-specific questions. My own work has focused on the meaning and experience of female adolescence.

6. Among the best statements of the multiple meanings of food are those of Claude Lévi-Strauss, "The Culinary Triangle," *New Society* 22 (December 1966), 937–940; Mary Douglas, "Deciphering a Meal," *Daedalus* 101 (1972), 61–68; Roland Barthes, "Toward a Psychosociology of Contemporary Food Consumption," in *European Diets from Preindustrial to Modern Times,* ed. Elborg Forster and Robert Forster (New York, 1975), pp. 47–49; Jack Goody, *Cooking, Cuisine and Class* (New York, 1982); Peter Farb and George Armelagos, *Consuming Passions: The Anthropology of Eating* (New York, 1980).

7. For a discussion of the sociological and historical literature on secularization see Chapter 3, note 106. Books of history that deal with the medicalization process are Michel Foucault, *Madness and Civilization: A History of Insanity in the Age of Reason* (New York, 1965); David Rothman, *The Discovery of the Asylum* (Boston, 1971); Andrew Scull, *Museums of Madness: The Social Origins of Insanity in Nineteenth Century England* (New York, 1979); Michael MacDonald, *Mystical Bedlam: Madness, Anxiety, and Healing in Seventeenth Century England* (New York, 1981).

8. On culture and illness see Arthur Kleinman, *Patients and Healers in the Context of Culture* (Berkeley, 1980); George Devereux, *Basic Problems of Ethnopsychiatry* (Chicago, 1979); Jon Streltzer and Terence C. Wade, "The Influence of Cultural Group on the Undertreatment of Postoperative Pain," *Psychosomatic Medicine* 43 (1981), 397–403; Laurence Kirmayer, "Culture, Affect and Somatization, Part II," *Transcultural Psychiatric Research Review* 21 (1984), 237–260. On "the sick role" see Talcott Parsons, *The Social System* (Glencoe, Ill., 1951), chap. 10.

9. My thinking on changing symptomatology is based on my reading of nineteenth-century cases along with twentieth-century material. Hilde Bruch's posthumous manuscript *Conversations with Anorexics* (New York, forthcoming), for instance, includes consultations, between 1973 and 1983, with more than 350 anorexic patients and their families. Bruch wrote: "Once the discovery of isolated tormented young women, it [anorexia nervosa] has now acquired a fashionable reputation, of being something to be competitive about. It is not

unusual to receive inquiries about young girls who express interest in 'trying it' after they have been exposed to a movie on anorexia or if they have been involved in a science project in biology . . . This is a far cry from the twenty-years-ago anorexic whose goal was to be unique and suggests that social factors may impact the prevalence of the disorder" (chap. 1). I argue that not just prevalence has been affected, but symptomatology as well.

10. The recent academic debate over sociobiology, epitomized by the work of E. O. Wilson, *Sociobiology: The New Synthesis* (Cambridge, Mass., 1975), has been particularly relevant. I have followed the general approach marked out by R. C. Lewontin, Steven Rose, and Leon J. Kamin, *Not in Our Genes: Biology, Ideology and Human Nature* (New York, 1984), and Ann Fausto-Sterling, *Myths of Gender* (New York, 1985). In principle I have tried to avoid what Lewontin and his colleagues call the "reductionist" argument, favoring instead a "dialectical" one.

11. See, for example, Charles E. Rosenberg, *The Cholera Years* (Chicago, 1962); Elizabeth Etheridge, *The Butterfly Caste: A Social History of Pellagra in the South* (Westport, Conn., 1972); Barbara Sicherman, "The Uses of a Diagnosis: Doctors, Patients and Neurasthenia," *Journal of the History of Medicine and Allied Sciences* 32 (1977), 33–54; Allan Brandt, *No Magic Bullet: A Social History of Venereal Disease in the United States since 1880* (New York, 1986); Brumberg, "Chlorotic Girls." Other social histories of particular diseases are Ilza Veith, *Hysteria* (Chicago, 1965); Erwin Ackerknecht, *Malaria in the Upper Mississippi Valley, 1760–1900* (Baltimore, 1945); H. Tristam Engelhardt, Jr., "The Disease of Masturbation: Values and the Concept of Disease," *Bulletin of the History of Medicine* 48 (1974), 234–248. Susan Sontag's *Illness as Metaphor* (New York, 1978) continues to be a major, suggestive text for the social history of medicine.

12. I am sympathetic to the view of Michel Foucault and Erving Goffman that psychiatric classification and treatment is problematic, to be analyzed as a reflection of social history and values. Nonetheless, my thinking about anorexia nervosa as a disease has also been influenced by provocative new critiques of the "mental-illness-as-social-construct" field; see Peter Sedgwick, "Illness—Mental and Otherwise," *Hastings Center Report* 1: 3 (1973), 19–40, and Martin Roth and Jerome Kroll, *The Reality of Mental Illness* (New York, 1986). I share with these authors a more complex view of the problem, including suspicion of the idea that all psychiatric classifications are mystifications and that mental suffering is merely nonillness or, alternatively, social protest. The most forthright advocates of the antipsychiatry school are Foucault, *Madness and Civilization*; Thomas Szasz, *The Myth of Mental Illness* (New York, 1974); and Erving Goffman, *Asylums* (Garden City, N.Y., 1961).

13. Rosenberg, *The Cholera Years*, p. 5, n. 8.

1. Anorexia Nervosa in the 1980s

1. Carol Amen, "Dieting to Death," *Science Digest* 67 (May 1970), 27–31. A shorter version of this article appeared earlier in *Family Weekly*.

2. Sam Blum, "Children Who Starve Themselves," *New York Times Mag-*

azine (November 10, 1974), 63–79; C. Michael Brady, "The Dieting Disease," *Weekly World News* 4 (March 22, 1983), 23. The *Star* of March 23, 1983, proposed that Britain's Diana, Princess of Wales, and her sister, Lady Sarah McCorquodale, are both anorectics. The *National Enquirer* has speculated that Michael Jackson is anorexic.

3. Between March 1974 and February 1984 the *Readers' Guide* lists almost fifty articles on anorexia nervosa. For early examples see Majorie Stein, "Dieting to Disaster," *Mademoiselle* 78 (January 1974), 8–10; "The Self Starvers," *Time* (July 28, 1975), 30–31; Kathryn Lynch, "You Can Overdo Dieting," *Seventeen* 34 (March 1975), 106–107; Beverly Solochek, "Why Some Girls Starve Themselves," ibid. 37 (June 1978), 140–168; Elissa Koff and M. Patricia Boyle, "Thin Is Beautiful Until," *Wellesley Magazine* 67 (Winter 1983), 4–9.

4. Hilde Bruch, *The Golden Cage: The Enigma of Anorexia Nervosa* (Cambridge, Mass., 1978), pp. vii–viii. Bruch received her medical degree from the University of Freiberg (1929); her postgraduate work and psychoanalytic training were at the Baltimore Institute for Psychoanalysis (1941–1945). Bruch practiced first in New York and then (beginning in 1964) in Houston. At the time of her death in 1984, she was Professor Emerita in Psychology, Baylor College of Medicine. Her many articles and books include *The Importance of Overweight* (New York, 1957); *Eating Disorders: Obesity, Anorexia Nervosa and the Person Within* (New York, 1973); and *Learning Psychotherapy: Rationale and Ground Rules* (Cambridge, Mass., 1974). Bruch's interest in eating disorders and appetite was longstanding and based on the Freudian view that the feeding situation is always an important interpersonal experience "charged with the emotional complexities of interaction between mother and child." See her "Food and Emotional Security," *Nervous Child* 3 (1944), 165–173. Bruch did not, however, hold to the strict Freudian notion that abnormal food attitudes or behavior must always be "deviations of psychosexual development." In "Role of Emotions in Hunger and Appetite," *Annals of the New York Academy of Science* 63 (1955), 68–75, Bruch argued that sociocultural factors had significant influence. She also wrote for women's magazines; see for example "The Psychology of Dieting," *Ladies' Home Journal* 82 (January 1965), 66. In the 1940s Bruch figured prominently in the new recognition of the problems of overweight in children. See Theodore Lidz, "In Memoriam: Hilde Bruch, M.D. (1904–1984)," *American Journal of Psychiatry* 142 (July 1985), 869–870, and Chapter 9 of this book.

5. Mara Selvini-Palazzoli, "Anorexia Nervosa: A Syndrome of the Affluent Society," translated from the Italian by V. F. Di Nicola, *Transcultural Psychiatric Research Review* 22: 3 (1985), 199.

6. Hilde Bruch, "Perceptual and Conceptual Disturbances in Anorexia Nervosa," *Psychosomatic Medicine* 24: 2 (1962), 187–194. Bruch said in this article: "I have come to the conclusion . . . that it is essential to delineate differences in the clinical course and psychological manifestations of various forms of eating disorders. Without clearcut distinctions, investigations are meaningless, and appropriate treatment impossible" (p. 188).

7. American Psychiatric Association, *Diagnostic and Statistical Manual of*

Mental Disorders 69 (3rd ed., Washington, D.C., 1980; 3rd ed., rev., Washington, D.C., 1987).

8. On weight criteria see N. Rollins and E. Piazza, "Diagnosis of Anorexia Nervosa: A Critical Reappraisal," *Journal of the American Academy of Child Psychiatry* 17 (1978), 126–137. On amenorrhea see Katherine Halmi and J. R. Falk, "Behavioral and Dietary Discriminators of Menstrual Function in Anorexia Nervosa," in *Anorexia Nervosa: Recent Developments in Research,* ed. P. L. Darby et al. (New York, 1983), 323–329. On hyperactivity see L. Kron et al., "Hyperactivity in Anorexia Nervosa: A Fundamental Clinical Feature," *Comparative Psychiatry* 19 (1978), 433–440.

9. In bulimia (without anorexia nervosa) weight loss may be substantial, but the weight does not fall below a minimal normal weight. An astute analysis of the heterogeneity of the disorder is that of Gordon Harper, "Anorexia Nervosa: What Kind of Disorder? The 'Consensus' Model, Myths, and Clinical Implications," *Pediatric Annals* 13 (November 1984), 812–828. See also David B. Herzog and Paul M. Copeland, "Eating Disorders," *New England Journal of Medicine* 313: 5 (1985), 295–303; M. Strober et al., "Validity of the Bulimia-Restrictor Distinction in Anorexia Nervosa: Parental Personality Characteristics and Family Psychiatric Morbidity," *Journal of Nervous and Mental Disorders* 170 (1982), 345–351; R. C. Casper et al., "Bulimia: Its Incidence and Clinical Importance in Patients with Anorexia Nervosa," *Archives of General Psychiatry* 37 (1980), 1030–35; G. F. M. Russell, "Bulimia Nervosa: An Ominous Variant of Anorexia Nervosa," *Psychological Medicine* 9 (August 1979), 429–448. The bulimic anorectic is reported to be the most difficult to treat and the least likely to recover.

10. William J. Swift, "The Long Term Outcome of Early Onset of Anorexia Nervosa: A Critical Review," *Journal of the American Academy of Child Psychiatry* 21 (January 1982), 38–46; D. J. Jones et al., "Epidemiology of Anorexia Nervosa in Monroe County, New York: 1960–1976," *Psychosomatic Medicine* 42 (1980), 551–558. See also M. Duddle, "An Increase in Anorexia Nervosa in a University Population," *British Journal of Psychiatry* 123 (1973), 711–712; A. H. Crisp, R. L. Palmer, and R. S. Kalucy, "How Common Is Anorexia Nervosa? A Prevalence Study," ibid. 128 (1976), 549–554.

11. R. E. Kendell et al., "The Epidemiology of Anorexia Nervosa," *Psychological Medicine* 3 (1973), 200–203.

12. Herzog and Copeland, "Eating Disorders," p. 295; Jane Y. Yu, "Eating Disorders," *Vital Signs* (September 1986), Cornell University Health Services, p. 2.

13. Paul E. Garfinkel and David M. Garner, *Anorexia Nervosa: A Multidimensional Perspective* (New York, 1982), pp. 103, 190; Gloria R. Leon and Stephen Finn, "Sex Role Stereotypes and the Development of Eating Disorders," in *Sex Roles and Psychopathology,* ed. C. S. Wilson (New York, 1984), pp. 317–337; A. H. Crisp et al., "The Long Term Prognosis in Anorexia Nervosa: Some Factors Predictive of Outcome," in *Anorexia Nervosa,* ed. R. A. Vigersky (New York, 1977), pp. 55–65. The fact that anorexia nervosa only rarely exists in males supports the idea that cultural factors play a role in producing the

disorder. On the differential sex distribution of anorexia nervosa see Garfinkel and Garner, *Anorexia Nervosa,* pp. 103–104; A. H. Crisp, "The Possible Significance of Some Behavioral Correlates of Weight and Carbohydrate Intake," *Journal of Psychosomatic Research* 11 (1967), 117–131; E. L. Falstein, S. C. Feinstein, and I. Judas, "Anorexia Nervosa in the Male Child," *American Journal of Orthopsychiatry* 26 (1956), 751–770; D. B. Herzog et al., "Sexual Conflict and Eating Disorders in 27 Males," *American Journal of Psychiatry* 141 (1984), 989–990; Hilde Bruch, "Anorexia Nervosa in the Male," *Psychosomatic Medicine* 33 (1971), 31–47.

14. There are some reports of anorexia nervosa among blacks: see A. J. Pumariega, P. Edwards, and L. B. Mitchell, "Anorexia Nervosa in Black Adolescents," *Journal of the American Academy of Child Psychiatry* 23 (1984), 111–114; T. Silber, "Anorexia Nervosa in Black Adolescents," *Journal of the National Medical Association* 76 (1984), 29–32; George Hsu, "Are Eating Disorders More Common in Blacks?" *International Journal of Eating Disorders* 6 (January 1987), 113–124. Hsu presents an excellent survey of the literature on black anorectics and suggests that the number of referrals for eating disorders is increasing in the black population. According to his review, there are only eighteen reported cases of anorexia nervosa among blacks in the United States and Western Europe, and only two among African blacks. Of the Africans, one was a young woman from an upper-class family who was sent to school in England. See L. D. Gregory and T. Buchan, "Anorexia Nervosa in a Black Zimbabwean," *British Journal of Psychiatry* 145 (1984), 326–330. No black normal-weight bulimics have ever been reported. According to Hsu, the rarity among blacks of anorexia nervosa and bulimia is the result of cultural differences that protect young black women from the negative self-image and intense pressure for slimness that are part of the white middle-class experience. These data, if correct, are telling evidence of the separateness of black culture and white culture and their differential strengths.

15. See Hiroyuki Suematsu et al., "Statistical Studies on the Prognosis of Anorexia Nervosa," *Japanese Journal of Psychosomatic Medicine* 23 (1983), 23–30. A report from Malaysia links the disease to upper-class status and westernization; see N. Buchrich, "Frequency of Presentations of Anorexia Nervosa in Malaysia," *Australian and New Zealand Journal of Psychiatry* 5 (1981), 153–155. See also Noriaki Mizushima and Yo Ishii, "The Epidemiology of Anorexia Nervosa in Junior and Senior High School Students in Ishikawa Prefecture," ibid. 23 (1983), 311–319. The report by a Russian psychiatrist is that of G. K. Ushakov, "Anorexia Nervosa," in *Modern Perspectives in Adolescent Psychiatry,* ed. John G. Howells (New York, 1971), pp. 274–289. The only Russian-language case I have been able to identify is A. A. Kissyel, "A Case of Severe Hysterical Anorexia in a Girl of Eleven," *Medicinskoie Obozrenie* 42 (1894), 17; but it is not clear that this case involves anorexia nervosa as we know it. In general, physicians have looked unsuccessfully for anorexia nervosa in other cultures. See Raymond Prince, "The Concept of Culture Bound Syndromes: Anorexia Nervosa and Brain-Fag," *Social Science Medicine* 21: 2 (1985), 197–203; Pow Meng Yap, "The Culture Bound Reactive Syndromes," in *Mental Health Research in Asia and the Pacific,* ed. William Caudill and

Tsung-yi Lin (Honolulu, 1969), pp. 33–53; Satish Varma, "Anorexia Nervosa in Developing Countries," *Transcultural Psychiatric Research Review* 16 (April 1979), 114–115; R. Prince, "Is Anorexia Nervosa a Culture Bound Syndrome?" ibid. 20: 1 (1983), 299–300; Eleanor S. Nash, "Letter," ibid. 21: 3 (1984), 227; Leslie Swartz, "Anorexia Nervosa as a Culture Bound Syndrome," ibid. 22: 3 (1985), 205–207; R. Prince, abstract of "Frequency of Presentation of Anorexia Nervosa in Malaysia," plus "Letters," ibid., 208–214; Burton G. Burton Bradley and Shridhar Sharma, "Letters," *American Journal of Social Psychiatry* 2 (Summer 1982), 58.

16. There have been a number of attempts to place anorexia nervosa within other established psychiatric categories. See for example G. Nicolle, "Prepsychotic Anorexia," *Lancet* 2 (1938), 1173–74; D. P. Cantwell et al., "Anorexia Nervosa: An Affective Disorder?" *Archives of General Psychiatry* 34 (1977), 1087–93; H. D. Palmer and M. S. Jones, "Anorexia Nervosa as a Manifestation of Compulsive Neurosis," *Archives of Neurology and Psychiatry* 41 (1939), 856. More recently, the focus has been on the behavioral signs and symptoms, and on biological similarities to depressive disorder. An argument against classifying eating disorders as affective disorder is Katherine A. Halmi, "Relationship of the Eating Disorders to Depression: Biological Similarities and Differences," *International Journal of Eating Disorders* 4: 4 (1985), 667–679. For a review of this question see also Alan B. Levy and Katharine N. Dixon, "The Relationship between Anorexia Nervosa and Depression: A Reevaluation," ibid., 382–405.

17. Katherine A. Halmi, G. Broadland, and C. A. Rigas, "A Follow Up Study of 79 Patients with Anorexia Nervosa: An Evaluation of Prognostic Factors and Diagnostic Criteria," in *Life History Research in Psychopathology*, ed. R. D. Wirt, G. Winokur, and M. Roff, vol. 4 (Minneapolis, 1975). L. K. G. Hsu, "Outcome of Anorexia Nervosa: A Review of the Literature," *Archives of General Psychiatry* 37 (1980), 1041–42, reviews studies that show a mortality rate of 0 to 19 percent. There is a good overview of the literature on outcome in Kelly M. Bemis, "Current Approaches to the Etiology and Treatment of Anorexia Nervosa," *Psychological Bulletin* 85 (1978), 593–617.

18. *New York State Journal of Medicine* 84 (May 1984), 228. On the overdiagnosis of bulimia see George Groh, "You've Come a Long Way, Bulimia," *M.D., Medical Newsmagazine* 28 (February 1984), 48–57.

19. Quote from Steven Levenkron in the newsletter of AA/BA, based on Bruch, *The Golden Cage*, p. xii.

20. See the coverage of Karen Carpenter's death in *People Weekly* (February 21 and November 21, 1983; May 31, 1985). In the earliest accounts, low serum potassium was reported to have caused an irregularity in Carpenter's heartbeat. By 1985, the reports were that Carpenter had died of "cardiotoxicity" brought on by the chemical emetine. The suggestion is that Carpenter was abusing a powerful over-the-counter drug, Ipecac, used to induce vomiting in case of poison.

21. Some examples of novels about anorexia nervosa are Deborah Hautzig, *Second Star to the Right* (New York, 1981); Steven Levenkron, *The Best Little Girl in the World* (New York, 1978); Rebecca Joseph, *Early Disorder* (New York, 1980); Ivy Ruckman, *The Hunger Scream* (New York, 1983); Margaret

Willey, *The Bigger Book of Lydia* (New York, 1983); John Sours, *Starving to Death in a Sea of Objects* (New York, 1980); Emily Hudlow, *Alabaster Chambers* (New York, 1979); Isaacsen-Bright, *Mirrors Never Lie* (Worthington, Ohio, 1982). With the exception of *Alabaster Chambers* all of these focus on adolescence. Novels about eating disorders are also popular among women readers. In her novel *Good Enough to Eat* (Ithaca, N.Y., 1986), Leslea Newman explores the twin themes of lesbian identity and food addiction in the life of a twenty-five-year-old Jewish woman who is trying to control her life through the food she eats (or does not eat). Margaret Atwood's *Lady Oracle* (New York, 1976) also deals with the issue of food and identity.

22. See Andrew W. Brotman, Theodore A. Stern, and David B. Herzog, "Emotional Reactions of House Officers to Patients with Anorexia Nervosa, Diabetes, and Obesity," *International Journal of Eating Disorders* (Summer 1983), 71–77, and, for the comment of John Schowalter, *AA/BA Newsletter* 8 (September–November 1985), 6. Eugene V. Beresin reported these weight avoidance techniques in a lecture, "Inpatient Treatment of Anorexia Nervosa," at the Harvard Medical School–Massachusetts General Hospital postgraduate course on June 25, 1983.

23. For personal testimonials see Sheila MacLeod, *The Art of Starvation: A Story of Anorexia and Survival* (New York, 1983); Cherry Boone O'Neill, *Starving for Attention* (New York, 1983); Aimee Liu, *Solitaire* (New York, 1979); Sandra Heater, *Am I Still Visible? A Woman's Triumph over Anorexia Nervosa* (Whitehall, Va., 1983); Camie Ford and Sunny Hale, *Two Too Thin: Two Women Who Triumphed over Anorexia Nervosa* (Orleans, Mass., 1983). The last-named work shares with O'Neill's book an evangelical Christian emphasis.

24. Fonda's experience with bulimia, although the author never used the clinical term, was described by Thomas Kiernan in *Jane: An Intimate Biography of Jane Fonda* (New York, 1973), p. 67: "Like many other girls at the college, Jane became caught up in obsessive anxieties about her weight. She began to practice the trick of eating a full meal, then hastily retreating to the bathroom to vomit it up before it had a chance to do its deadly work on her system." In the early 1980s, Fonda spoke about her eating disorder in television and film interviews. By 1985, her struggles with bulimia were a standard part of her biography. See "Private Lives," *Ladies' Home Journal* 102 (October 1985), 202.

25. See for example Lisa Messinger, *Biting the Hand that Feeds Me: Days of Binging, Purging and Recovery* (Moonachie, N.J., 1985); Jackie Barrile, *Confessions of a Closet Eater* (Wheaton, Ill., 1983); K. B., "A First Anniversary—A Recovering Bulimic's Story," *AA/BA Newsletter*, 8 (September–November 1985), 8; Greg Foster and Susan Howerin, "The Quest for Perfection: An Interview with a Former Bulimic," *Iris: A Journal about Women* 12 (1986), 18–22. See also Geneen Roth, *Feeding the Hungry Heart: The Experience of Compulsive Eating* (New York, 1982); Paulette Maisner and Jenny Pulling, *Feasting and Fasting* (London, 1985).

26. *AA/BA Newsletter* 8 (November 1985–February 1986), 5; in 1984 the AA/BA, in conjunction with Columbia University Press, published *When Will We Laugh Again?*, edited by Barbara P. Kinnoy in collaboration with Estelle B.

Miller and John A. Atchley. The book begins with a personal testimony by an anorectic, then goes on to describe research on the families of anorectics and bulimics. Some additional self-help titles are Steven Levenkron, *Treating and Overcoming Anorexia Nervosa* (New York, 1982); Elaine Landau, *Why Are They Starving Themselves? Understanding Anorexia and Bulimia* (New York, 1983); Peter Lambley, *How to Survive Anorexia* (London, 1983); Janice M. Cauwels, *Bulimia: The Binge Purge Compulsion* (New York, 1983); Suzanne Abraham and Derek L. Jones, *Eating Disorders: The Facts* (New York, 1984); Roger Slade, *The Anorexia Nervosa Reference Book* (New York, 1984); Ann Erichsen, *Anorexia Nervosa: The Broken Circle* (London, 1985); Marilyn Lawrence, *The Anorexic Experience: From Dieting to Compulsive Eating* (Topsfield, Mass., 1985); Susan Kano, *Making Peace with Food: A Step-by-Step Guide to Freedom from Diet/Weight Conflict* (Allston, Mass., 1985); Geneen Roth, *Breaking Free from Compulsive Eating* (New York, 1985); Lindsay Hall and Leigh Cohn, *Bulimia: A Guide to Recovery* (Santa Barbara, Calif., 1986); Terence J. Sandbek, *The Deadly Diet: Recovery from Anorexia and Bulimia* (Oakland, Calif., 1986); Patricia M. Stein and Barbara Unell, *Anorexia Nervosa: Finding the Life Line* (Minneapolis, 1986); Barbara G. Bauer et al., *Bulimia: A Book for Therapist and Client* (Muncie, Ind., 1986).

27. *AA/BA Newsletter* 8 (June–September 1985), 1.

28. These included: *Journal of the American Medical Association, Journal of Clinical Psychiatry, International Journal of Psychoanalysis, Journal of Adolescent Health Care, American Journal of Clinical Nutrition, Journal of Nervous and Mental Disease, Psychosomatics, International Journal of Neuroscience, Journal of Developmental and Behavioral Pediatrics, Journal of Endocrinological Investigations, Adolescence, Journal of Primatology, Journal of School Health, Journal of College Student Personnel, Hospital Practice, International Journal of Family Therapy, British Journal of Addiction, American Journal of Clinical Hypnosis,* and *Wisconsin Law Review.*

29. There are eating disorder units or clinics in hospitals associated with the following medical schools: Harvard, University of Pennsylvania, UCLA, Johns Hopkins, Cornell, University of Virginia, and University of Rochester. See the *Renfrew Perspective* (Spring 1987) and the *Palm Beach Post,* March 23, 1987.

30. On the diet industry see "Dieting: The Losing Game," *Time* (January 20, 1986), 54–60, and Chapter 9 of this book.

31. This view is challenged by Rebecca Dresser, "Feeding the Hunger Artists: Legal Issues in Treating Anorexia Nervosa," *Wisconsin Law Review* 2 (1984), 297–374. Dresser asserts that renourishment is a violation of the patient's rights. She regards the anorectic as engaged in a conscious, autonomous struggle against parents, physicians, and a hostile environment. For an excellent legal discussion of what is wrong with Dresser's argument that anorexia nervosa is "chosen behavior with adaptive functions," see Norman Fost, "Food for Thought: Dresser on Anorexia," ibid., 375–384. Dr. William Bennett explained to me the intricacies of total parenteral nutrition.

32. Herzog and Copeland, "Eating Disorders," p. 300. On therapy and prognosis see W. Stewart Agras and Helena C. Kramer, "The Treatment of

Anorexia Nervosa: Do Different Treatments Have Different Outcomes?" *Psychiatric Annals* 13 (December 1983), 928–935. See also A. H. Crisp, "Treatment and Outcome in Anorexia Nervosa," in *Eating and Weight Disorders*, ed. R. K. Goodstein (New York, 1983); L. K. G. Hsu, "Outcome of Anorexia Nervosa: A Review of the Literature (1954 to 1978)," *Archives of General Psychiatry* 37 (1980), 1041–43; D. M. Schwartz and M. G. Thompson, "Do Anorectics Get Well? Current Research and Future Needs," *American Journal of Psychiatry* 138 (1981), 319–323.

33. The best statements of this interactive view are Garfinkel and Garner, *Anorexia Nervosa*, and Alexander R. Lucas, "Toward the Understanding of Anorexia Nervosa as a Disease Entity," *Mayo Clinic Proceedings* 56 (1981), 254–264. Biologic vulnerability includes genetic and physiological components; psychological predisposition includes early experiences, family influences, and intrapsychic or personality conflict.

34. See Philip W. Gold et al., "Responses to Corticotropin-Releasing Hormone in the Hyper Cortisolism of Depression and Cushing's Disease: Pathophysiologic and Diagnostic Implications," *New England Journal of Medicine* 314 (May 22, 1986), 1329–34, and idem, "Abnormal Hypothalamic-Pituitary-Adrenal Function in Anorexia Nervosa: Pathophysiologic Mechanisms in Underweight and Weight Corrected Patients," ibid., 1335–42. The best reviews of the biomedical literature are in Bemis, "Current Approaches," pp. 607–611, and Herzog and Copeland, "Eating Disorders," pp. 296–298.

In *The Tangled Wing: Biological Constraints on the Human Spirit* (New York, 1982), pp. 363–364, Melvin Konner confirms that stress in mammals provokes both overeating and noneating: "Stress . . . has been shown in various experiments in laboratory animals to increase food intake to abnormal levels in several different species. This fascinating finding evokes the possibility . . . that mammals have been provided by evolution with a motivational system that is not entirely specific; that is, we do not always know what we want. In particular, various different motivations seem to be handled in part by a generalized arousal system in the lateral portion of the hypothalamus." According to Konner, stress produces arousal, which can then, depending on "context," be expressed as overeating or undereating.

35. Bemis, "Current Approaches," p. 609; Lennart Heimer, *The Human Brain and Spinal Cord* (New York, 1983), p. 306.

36. R. S. Mecklenburg et al., "Hypothalamic Dysfunction in Patients with Anorexia Nervosa," *Medicine* 53 (1974), 155.

37. According to Bemis, "Current Approaches," p. 609, anorexia nervosa does not appear to have a genetic component.

38. J. Mayo Berkman, "Anorexia Nervosa, Anorexia Inanition, and Low Basal Metabolism Rate," *American Journal of Medical Sciences* 180 (1930), 411–424; D. Kylin, cited in S. Theander, "Anorexia Nervosa: A Psychiatric Investigation of 94 Female Patients," *Acta Psychiatrica Scandinavica* (1970), suppl. 214; J. C. Patel, "Loss of Appetite," *Indian Journal of Medical Sciences* 11 (1957), 268–273; B. Gottesfield and A. Novaes, "Narco-analysis and Subshock Insulin in the Treatment of Anorexia Nervosa," *Digest of Neurology and*

Psychiatry 13 (1945), 486–494; G. W. Thorn et al., "The Clinical Usefulness of ACTH and Cortisone," *New England Journal of Medicine* 242 (1950), 783–800; T. M. Chalmers et al., "Treatment of Anorexia Nervosa by Ethyl-nortestosterone," *Proceedings of the Royal Society of Medicine* 52 (1959), 514–515; H. A. Gross et al., "A Double-Blind Controlled Trial of Lithium Carbonate in Primary Anorexia Nervosa," *Journal of Clinical Psychopharmacology* 1 (1981), 376–381; A. J. Johnson and N. J. Knorr, "Treatment of Anorexia Nervosa by Levodopa," *Lancet* (1974), 591; Peter Sifneos, "A Case of Anorexia Nervosa Successfully Treated by Leucotomy," *American Journal of Psychiatry* 109 (1952), 356–360; H. K. Davis, "Anorexia Nervosa: Treatment with Hypnosis and ECT," *Diseases of the Nervous System* 22 (1961), 627–631; M. D. Altschule, "Adrenocortical Function in Anorexia Nervosa before and after Lobotomy," *New England Journal of Medicine* 248 (1953), 808–810.

39. The leading contemporary proponents of the use of antidepressants are Harrison G. Pope and James I. Hudson, *New Hope for Binge Eaters* (New York, 1984). See Herzog and Copeland, "Eating Disorders," p. 303, for citations to literature that evaluates different antidepressants.

40. Herzog and Copeland, "Eating Disorders," p. 300, state that "there is no established pharmacotherapy for eating disorders." The November 1986 report is by Andrew Brotman, Massachusetts General Hospital, quoted in *AA/BA Newsletter* 9 (February–April 1986), 1.

41. Herzog and Copeland, "Eating Disorders," pp. 296–298; Bemis, "Current Approaches," p. 594; DSM-III-R, pp. 65, 68.

42. On body fat and menstruation see Rose Frisch and J. McArthur, "Menstrual Cycles: Fatness as a Determinant of Minimum Weight Necessary for Their Maintenance and Onset," *Science* 185 (1974), 949–951.

43. Simone de Beauvoir, *The Second Sex*, trans. H. M. Parshley (New York, 1971), p. 308.

44. Louise Kaplan, *Adolescence: The Farewell to Childhood* (New York, 1984), p. 261.

45. Quotation from *The Standard Edition of the Complete Psychological Works of Sigmund Freud*, trans. and ed. James Strachey, vol. 17, *An Infantile Neurosis and Other Works* (London, 1966), p. 106. See also vol. 1, *Pre-Psychoanalytic Publications and Unpublished Drafts*, pp. 200–201. Bruch, *The Golden Cage*, p. 88, takes issue with the fear of impregnation idea. The sexual inactivity of anorectics was informally noted in a number of different presentations by clinicians at the Harvard Medical School–Massachusetts General Hospital postgraduate course, "Anorexia Nervosa and Bulima," June 24–26, 1983. Two Jungian interpretations of anorexia nervosa are those of Marion Woodman, *The Owl Was a Baker's Daughter: Obesity, Anorexia Nervosa, and the Repressed Feminine* (Toronto, 1980), and Noelle Caskey, "Interpreting Anorexia Nervosa," in *The Female Body in Western Culture*, ed. Susan Suleiman (Cambridge, Mass., 1985), pp. 175–192.

46. Bruch, *Eating Disorders*, pp. 250–255.

47. See Albert Rothenberg, "Eating Disorder as a Modern Obsessive-Compulsive Syndrome," *Psychiatry* 49 (February 1986), 45–53. Rothenberg's article

is a clear-cut statement of this point of view; his argument is convincing precisely because his explanation of the symptomatology takes account of the culture in which young women live.

48. See R. Liebman, Salvador Minuchin, and Lesley Baker, "The Role of the Family in the Treatment of Anorexia Nervosa," *Journal of the American Academy of Child Psychiatry* 13 (1974), 264–274; Bernice L. Rosman, Salvador Minuchin, and R. Liebman, "Family Lunch Session: An Introduction to Family Therapy in Anorexia Nervosa," *American Journal of Orthopsychiatry* 45 (1975), 846–853; Salvador Minuchin, Bernice L. Rosman, and Lester Baker, *Psychosomatic Families: Anorexia Nervosa in Context* (Cambridge, Mass., 1978).

49. Kim Chernin, *The Hungry Self: Women, Eating and Identity* (New York, 1985); Mara Selvini-Palazzoli, "The Families of Patients with Anorexia Nervosa," in *The Child in His Family*, ed. E. J. Anthony and C. Koupernick (New York, 1970), pp. 319–332; Angelyn Spignesi, *Starving Women: A Psychology of Anorexia* (Dallas, 1983). The latter includes a review of the literature on the mother-daughter bond in eating disorders. The emotional makeup of the mother of the anorectic was also discussed by psychoanalyst Ana-Maria Rizzuto, "Eating and Monsters," and social worker Lois Sims Slovik, "Family Therapy Assessment and Its Implication for Treatment: A Structural and Systems Perspective," lectures given at the Harvard Medical School–Massachusetts General Hospital postgraduate course. Marcia Creighton, "Dear Diane," *Bostonia* 61 (February/March 1987), 54–58, is a statement by the mother of an anorectic who died. Mothers were also a focus in some of the Victorian literature (see Chapter 6).

50. See David M. Garner and Paul E. Garfinkel, "The Eating Attitudes Test: An Index of the Symptoms of Anorexia Nervosa," *Psychological Medicine* 9 (May 1979), 273–279; Paul Williams, David Hand, and Alex Tarnopolsky, "The Problem of Screening for Uncommon Disorders: A Comment on the Eating Attitudes Test," ibid. 12 (May 1982), 431–434; David M. Garner et al., "The Eating Attitudes Test: Psychometric Features and Clinical Correlates," ibid. 12 (November 1982), 871–878; David Garner, Marion Olmstead, and J. Polivy, "Development and Validation of a Multi-dimensional Eating Disorder Inventory of Anorexia Nervosa and Bulimia," *International Journal of Eating Disorders* 2 (1983), 15–34.

51. David Garner et al., "Comparison between Weight-Preoccupied Women and Anorexia Nervosa," *Psychosomatic Medicine* 46 (1984), 255–266. For studies that deal with ineffectiveness, self-esteem, and autonomy see also H. Basseches and S. Karp, "Field Dependence in Young Anorectic and Obese Women," *Psychotherapy and Psychosomatics* 41 (1984), 33–37.

52. The best summary of the literature on perceptual and conceptual disturbances in anorexia nervosa is Garfinkel and Garner, *Anorexia Nervosa*, pp. 123–163.

53. The Bem Sex Role inventory is a well-known self-report questionnaire that asks individuals to describe themselves on a series of gender-specific attributes. See Catherine Steiner-Adair, "The Body Politic: Normal Female Adolescent Development and the Development of Eating Disorders" (Ed.D. thesis, Harvard University, 1984); P. K. Dunn and P. Ondercin, "Personality Variables

Related to Compulsive Eating in College Women," *Journal of Clinical Psychology* 1 (1981), 43–49; Linda D. Lewis and Craig Johnson, "A Comparison of Sex Role Orientation between Women with Bulimia and Normal Controls," *International Journal of Eating Disorders* 4 (August 1985), 247–258. The Dunn-Ondercin and Lewis-Johnson studies both disprove the thesis that women with eating disorders are "hyperfeminine." See Marlene Boskind-Lodahl, "Cinderella's Stepsisters: A Feminist Perspective on Anorexia Nervosa and Bulimia," *Signs* 2: 2 (1976), 342–356.

54. George I. Szmukler and Digby Tatum, "Anorexia Nervosa: Starvation Dependence," *British Journal of Medical Psychology* 57 (1984), 303–310. On anorexia nervosa and abuse disorders see D. Scott, "Alcohol and Food Abuse: Some Comparisons," *British Journal of Addiction* 78 (1983), 339–349, and M. Bachmann and H. Rohr, "A Speculative Illness Model of Over-eating and Anorexia Nervosa," *Psychological Reports* 53 (1983), 831–838. Also relevant to the discussion of anorexia nervosa and habitual behaviors is Margaret MacKenzie, "The Pursuit of Slenderness and Addiction to Self Control: An Anthropological Interpretation of Eating Disorders," *Nutrition Update* 2 (1985), 174–194.

55. Judith Rodin, Lisa Silberstein, and Ruth Striegel-Moore, "Women and Weight: A Normative Discontent," in *1984 Nebraska Symposium on Motivation*, ed. Theodore B. Sonderegger (Lincoln, 1985); April E. Fallon and Paul Rozin, "Sex Differences in Perceptions of Desirable Body Shape," *Journal of Abnormal Psychology* 94 (1985), 102–105; Susan C. Wooley and Orlando Wayne Wooley, "Obesity and Women. I: A Closer Look at the Facts," *Women's Studies International Quarterly* 2 (1979), 69–79, and "Obesity and Women. II: A Neglected Feminist Topic," ibid., 81–92; "Should Obesity Be Treated at All?" in *Eating and Its Disorders*, ed. A. J. Stunkard and E. Stellar (New York, 1984), pp. 185–192; "Women and Weight Obsession: Toward a Redefinition of the Underlying Problem," in *For Alma Mater: Theory and Practice in Feminist Scholarship*, ed. Paula A. Treichler, Cheris Kramerae, and Beth Stafford (Urbana, Ill., 1985).

56. See *Time* (January 20, 1986), 54, and *Los Angeles Times*, February 15 and March 29, 1984, for a report on the work of anthropologist Margaret MacKenzie. For a report of the *Glamour* survey see *Palm Beach Post*, December 26, 1985. The term "obesophobic" was used by many doctors at the Harvard Medical School–MGH postgraduate course in 1983. See Albert J. Stunkard, *The Pain of Obesity* (Palo Alto, Calif., 1976) and A. L. Stewart and R. H. Brooks, "Effects of Being Overweight," *American Journal of Public Health* 73 (February 1983), 171–178. Sixty percent of the women in the Stewart-Brooks sample thought they were overweight despite the fact that their weight was normal by conservative medical criteria. On legal aspects of obesophobia see Jane Baker, "The Rehabilitation Act of 1973: Protection for Victims of Weight Discrimination?" *UCLA Law Review* 29 (April 1984), 947–971; Lynne Reaves, "Fat Folks' Rights: Weight Bias Issues Emerging," *American Bar Association Journal* 69 (1983), 878; Lauren Reskin, "Employers Must Give Obese Job Applicants a Fat Chance," ibid., 71 (1985), 104.

57. These studies are summarized in Ruth Striegel-Moore, Gail McAvay,

and Judith Rodin, "Psychological and Behavioral Correlates of Feeling Fat in Women," *International Journal of Eating Disorders* 5: 5 (1986), 935–947; quoted in Ana-Maria Rizzuto, Ross K. Peterson, and Marilyn Reed, "The Pathological Sense of Self in Anorexia Nervosa," *Psychiatric Clinics of North America* 4 (December 1981), 38.

58. Sanford M. Dornbusch et al., "Sexual Maturation, Social Class, and the Desire to Be Thin among Adolescent Females," *Journal of Developmental and Behavioral Pediatrics* 5 (December 1984), 308–314. See also A. J. Stunkard, "From Explanation to Action in Psychosomatic Medicine: The Case of Obesity," *Psychosomatic Medicine* 37 (1975), 195–236; P. B. Goldblatt, M. E. Moore, and A. J. Stunkard, "Social Factors in Obesity," *Journal of the American Medical Association* 192 (1965), 97–102; April E. Fallon and Paul Rozin, "Sex Differences in Perceptions of Desirable Body Shape," *Journal of Abnormal Psychology* 94 (1985), 102–105.

59. Susie Orbach, *Fat Is a Feminist Issue: The Anti-Diet Guide to Permanent Weight Loss* (New York, 1978); idem, *Hunger Strike: The Anorectic's Struggle as a Metaphor for Our Age* (New York, 1986); Kim Chernin, *The Obsession: Reflections on the Tyranny of Slenderness* (New York, 1981); idem, *The Hungry Self*; Marcia Millman, *Such a Pretty Face: Being Fat in America* (New York, 1980); Marlene Boskin-White and William C. White, *Bulimarexia: The Binge Purge Cycle* (New York, 1983). For a collective review of this literature see Carole M. Counihan, "What Does It Mean to Be Fat, Thin, and Female in the United States?: A Review Essay," *Food and Foodways* 1 (1985), 77–94. See also Marilyn Lawrence, "Anorexia Nervosa—the Control Paradox," *Women's Studies International Quarterly* 2 (1979), 93–101; Marlene Boskin-Lodahl, "Cinderella's Stepsisters: A Feminist Perspective on Anorexia and Bulimia," *Signs* 2 (1976), 342–356; Susan Bordo, "Anorexia Nervosa: Psychopathology as a Crystallization of Culture," *Philosophical Forum* 17 (Winter 1985–86).

60. Orbach, *Hunger Strike*, p. 63.

61. Feminist analysis has begun to suggest that the medical models for understanding obesity are inadequate and that rigid appetite control and body-image preoccupations have negative developmental consequences for many women. See for example Barbara Edelstein, *The Woman Doctor's Diet for Women* (Englewood Cliffs, N.J., 1977); C. P. Herman and J. Polivy, "Anxiety, Restraint, and Eating Behavior," *Journal of Abnormal Psychology* 84 (December 1975), 666–672; Janet L. Surrey, "Eating Patterns as a Reflection of Women's Development," *Work in Progress* no. 83-06, Stone Center (Wellesley, Mass., 1984); Elaine Hatfield and Susan Sprecher, *Mirror, Mirror: The Importance of Looks in Everyday Life* (Albany, N.Y., 1985); Rita Freedman, *Beauty Bound* (Lexington, Mass., 1986); Vicki Druss and Mary Sun Henifin, "Why Are So Many Anorexics Women?" in *Women Look at Biology Looking at Women*, ed. Ruth Hubbard et al. (Boston, 1979).

62. For examples see Sandra Gilbert and Susan Gubar, *The Madwoman in the Attic* (New Haven, 1979); Elaine Showalter, *The Female Malady: Women, Madness and English Culture, 1830–1980* (New York, 1985); Mary Poovey, "Scenes of an Indelicate Character: The Medical Treatment of Victorian

Women," *Representations* 14 (Spring 1986), 137–168. Showalter (pp. 18, 121, 126–129) and Gilbert and Gubar (pp. 53–58) explicitly discuss anorexia nervosa. Jeffrey Masson, in *A Dark Science: Women, Sexuality and Psychiatry in the Nineteenth Century* (New York, 1986), focuses on a few select clinical cases but follows the interpretation laid out by literary critics.

63. See Bryan Turner, *The Body and Society: Explorations in Social Theory* (Oxford, 1984). Turner talks about asceticism, training, and denial as part of the "government of the body" and posits that women's bodies are, historically, a focus of social control. On pp. 183–197 he describes anorexia nervosa as a paradoxical condition that reproduces the contradictions of bourgeois thought. I see my interpretation as essentially congruent with his.

64. Personal communication to the author, April 1987. In *Conversations with Anorexics* (New York, forthcoming) Hilde Bruch described the anorectic as characteristically overcompliant to the wishes of others. As a result, she considered it progress if a patient swore at her, dropped a course, or shouted at a parent.

65. Orbach's *Hunger Strike* (1986) implies in its title that anorexia nervosa is a form of political protest. See the review of this book by Angela Barron McBride, "The Body as Battlefield," *Women's Review of Books* (September 1986), 8. On the early-twentieth-century English suffragists see David Morgan, *Suffragists and Liberals: The Politics of Women Suffrage in England* (Oxford, 1975); David J. Mitchell, *The Fighting Pankhursts: A Study in Tenacity* (New York, 1967); E. Sylvia Pankhurst, *The Suffragette: The History of the Women's Militant Suffrage Movement, 1905–1910* (New York, 1911).

66. Dresser, "Feeding the Hunger Artists," p. 338.

67. Showalter, *The Female Malady*, p. 162, writes of the suffragists in 1912, "The hunger strikes of militant women prisoners brilliantly put the symptomatology of anorexia nervosa to work in the service of a feminist cause." The fact that the British government demeaned the suffragists by labeling them "hysterical" should not obscure the real distinctions between conscious political strategies involving refusal of food until a goal is reached and forms of food refusal that are unrelentingly self-destructive.

68. Bruch, *The Golden Cage*, p. ix.

69. J. Blumenthal, "Is Running an Analogue of Anorexia Nervosa? An Empirical Study of Obligatory Running and Anorexia Nervosa," *Journal of the American Medical Association* 252 (1984), 520–523.

70. I refer here to cartoons by Sylvia (Nicole Hollander), Cathy (Cathy Guisewaite), and Linda Barry.

71. Ruth Striegel-Moore, Lisa R. Silberstein, and Judith Rodin, "Toward an Understanding of Risk Factors in Bulimia," *American Psychologist* 41 (March 1986), 256–258, make a similar argument: "We certainly do not mean to imply that psychopathology is merely learned behavior—but we suggest that the public's heightened awareness of eating disorders and a young woman's likelihood of personal exposure to the behaviors may be a significant factor in the increased emergence of eating disorders in the last several decades."

72. The distinction between recruitment and career evolved in conversa-

tions with Dr. William Bennett, whose command of the medical literature (and sensitivity to historical concerns) improved my understanding of the relationship between etiology and symptoms.

2. From Sainthood to Patienthood

1. This is not to say that medieval men did not engage in ascetic food practices. They did, but their level of involvement and the characteristics of their asceticism are quite different. On gender differences in medieval piety see Donald Weinstein and Rudolph Bell, *Saints and Society: The Worlds of Western Christiandom, 100–1700* (Chicago, 1982), esp. table 18, p. 234. Weinstein and Bell demonstrate that all types of penitential asceticism were significantly more common in female religiosity (pp. 233–235). This thesis is confirmed by Richard Kiechefer, *Unquiet Souls* (Chicago, 1984), a study of religious practices (including penitential asceticism) of fourteenth-century saints. I am indebted to Caroline Walker Bynum for this point and for my general understanding of medieval women and their food habits. Bynum discusses the gender difference in food concerns, drawing on a wide range of sources both quantitative and qualitative; she concludes that food asceticism as well as charitable food distribution and the performance of food-related miracles were particularly female roles in the High Middle Ages. On Saint Veronica see Rudolph Bell, *Holy Anorexia* (Chicago, 1985), pp. 54–81.

2. Caroline Walker Bynum, "Women Mystics and Eucharistic Devotion in the Thirteenth Century," *Women's Studies* 2: 1–2 (1984), 179–214.

3. Use of the word "anorexy" or "anorexia" to denote want of appetite dates, according to the *Oxford English Dictionary,* to the sixteenth century. "Inedia prodigiosa" is associated with Guilhelm Fabricius Hildanus (1560–1634), a German physician, who spent nearly thirty years observing fasting cases and wrote about them in *Opera Quae Extant Omnia* (Frankfurt, 1646). Anorexia mirabilis is associated with François Boisser de Sauvages de la Croix (1706–1767), author of *Nosologie méthodique,* 5 vols. (Lyon, 1772), and Royal Professor of Botany at the University of Montpellier beginning in 1752. Sauvages, noted for his classifications of mental diseases, described many forms of anorexia that accompanied different diseases. Aside from anorexia associated with dyspepsia, these fell into three general categories. The first was anorexia humoralis (caused by humors oppressing the stomach); the second, anorexia atonica (resulting from loss of tone in the fibers of the stomach). A third category contained anorexias of a doubtful nature, including anorexia mirabilis. In "Some Account of the Fasting Women of Tutbury . . . ," *Edinburgh Medical and Surgical Journal* 5 (1809), 322–333, Benjamin Granger briefly discusses the use of the two terms. He suggests that anorexia mirabilis was more inclusive: "The *anorexia mirabilis* of Sauvage[s] has an extensive signification, not only including the disease at present under review [inedia prodigiosa], but also diseases in general in which individuals have fasted long" (p. 323). On Fabricius Hildanus and his observations of prolonged abstinence cases see Petr Skrabanek, "Notes towards the History of Anorexia Nervosa," *Janus* 70: 1–2 (1983), 109–128. See note 5 for my methodological objections to Skrabanek's approach. On Sauvages see Greg-

ory Zilboorg, *A History of Medical Psychology* (New York, 1941), pp. 306–307, and William Cullen, *A Methodological System of Nosology* (Stockbridge, Mass., 1808).

4. Bell, *Holy Anorexia,* p. 20.

5. See J. Hubert Lacey, "Anorexia Nervosa and a Bearded Female Saint," *British Medical Journal* 285 (December 18–25, 1982), 1816–17; Wilma Paterson, "Was Byron Anorexic?" *World Medicine* (May 15, 1982), 35–38. Petr Skrabanek, a physician in the Department of Endocrinology, Mater Misercordiae Hospital, Dublin, Ireland, posits that anorexia nervosa has existed since the fifth century. He argues that "food-avoidance among young girls due to psychological causes (as opposed to religious fasting or anorexia due to somatic disease) has a venerable history." Thus Skrabanek, like Bell, argues for a fairly consistent psychological disorder across time. Although I reject this approach, Skrabanek's article provides a useful catalogue of notable fasting cases. See also John Demos, *Entertaining Satan* (New York, 1982), pp. 152 ff. for a brief discussion of the possibility that seventeenth-century New England witches were actually anorectics. Two additional examples of the current enthusiasm for finding historical cases of anorexia nervosa are Fady Hajal, "Psychological Treatment of Anorexia: A Case from the Ninth Century," *Journal of the History of Medicine* 37 (July 1983), 325–328; Carol R. Lewis, "Elizabeth Barrett Browning's 'Family Disease': Anorexia Nervosa," *Journal of Marital and Family Therapy* (January 1982), 129–134; Tilmann Habermas, "Friderada: A Case of Miraculous Fasting," *International Journal of Eating Diseases* 5 (March 1986), 555–561.

6. Joseph Silverman, "Richard Morton, 1637–1698: Limner of Anorexia Nervosa: His Life and Times," *Journal of the American Medical Association* 250 (November 25, 1983), 2830–32. My objections to Silverman's approach are historical as well as methodological. Silverman, who is actually following the suggestion of Bruch, *Eating Disorders,* p. 211, has overlooked the fact that Fabricius Hildanus reported cases of inedia prodigiosa at least fifty years before Morton. See also Eugene L. Bliss and C. H. Hardin Branch, *Anorexia Nervosa: Its History, Psychology, and Biology* (New York, 1960), p. 1; and W. Langdon Brown, *Anorexia Nervosa,* Individual Psychology Publications, Medical Pamphlets I (1931–32), ed. F. G. Crookshank (London, 1932); C. W. Ross, "Anorexia Nervosa with Special Reference to Carbohydrate Metabolism," *Lancet* 234 (May 7, 1938), 1041; John A. Ryle, "Anorexia Nervosa," *Lancet* 231 (October 17, 1936), 894. It appears that English doctors, beginning in the 1930s, attributed the "first" identification to one of their own.

7. Caroline Walker Bynum, "Fast, Feast, and Flesh: The Religious Significance of Food to Medieval Women," *Representations* 11 (1985), 1–25.

8. In *Holy Anorexia* Rudolph Bell discusses the decline of the "holy anorexic behavior model" and dates it to the sixteenth century. He attributes the decline to closer scrutiny by male clerics and to the general "male domination . . . intrinsic to the Reformation." In the medieval world, he says, men did not control female religiosity; after the seventeenth century, women turned to "good works" rather than "radical holiness."

9. Keith Thomas, *Religion and the Decline of Magic* (New York, 1971). An exceedingly useful ethnographic discussion of another cultural fiction (ab-

sence of defecation) is that of Sally Falk Moore, "The Secret of the Men: A Fiction of Chagga Initiation and Its Relation to the Logic of Chagga Symbolism," *Africa* 46: 4 (1976), 357–370.

10. For the stories of Katerine Cooper (or Binder), Eva Fleigen, Jane Balan, Vietken Johans, and Jane Stretton, see Hyder E. Rollins, "Notes on Some English Accounts of Miraculous Fasts," *Journal of American Folklore* 34 (1921), 357–376. According to E. A. Axon, "The Fasting Girl of Schmidweiller in the Sixteenth Century," *Antiquary* 37 (September and October 1901), 269–272, 305–309, Katerine Cooper was one of seven famous fasting girls in the sixteenth century; in the seventeenth, according to Axon, there were only two or three (including Martha Taylor, whom I shall discuss later), and in the eighteenth, Ann Walsh of Harrogate and Katherine (or Janet) McLeod. On Walsh see *London Magazine* 31 (1762), 340; on McLeod see "Account of a Woman in the Shire of Ross Living without Food or Drink," *Philosophical Transactions of the Royal Society of London* 14 (1776–80), 121–124. Rebecca Smith is cited in Robert Plots, *The Natural History of Oxfordshire* (1677), chaps. 8–9, pp. 196–197. See Skrabanek, "Notes," for a catalogue of names, as well as Herbert Thurston, *The Physical Phenomena of Mysticism* (Chicago, 1952), pp. 363 ff. In *Immodest Acts: The Life of a Lesbian Nun in Renaissance Italy* (New York, 1986), pp. 64–65, Judith C. Brown describes the fasting of Benedetta Carlini who, following an order from Jesus, refused to eat meat, eggs, and milk products in order to maintain her bodily purity. Brown regards Benedetta's rejection of food as a "troubled and negative act" rather than the "positive act of penitence, mystical union, and physical self control" associated with medieval female mystics. See pp. 190–191, n. 49, for her discussion of the differences between Bynum and Bell.

11. Miraculous maidens avoided meat, as did Victorian girls. The anthropological literature demonstrates that food taboos are not uncommon in adolescence. At the time of menarche, girls in a number of different cultures apparently abstain from flesh foods, which are believed to heighten the dangers associated with the critical period of sexual maturation. As I argue in Chapter 7, meat eating stands as a proxy for sexual activity. See Mary Douglas, *Natural Symbols* (New York, 1973) and *Purity and Danger* (London, 1966); Peter Farb and George Armelagos, *Consuming Passions: The Anthropology of Eating* (Boston, 1980); G. Eichinger Ferro-Luzzi, "Food Avoidance at Puberty and Menstruation in Tamilnad," in *Food, Ecology and Culture: Readings in the Anthropology of Dietary Practices,* ed. J. R. K. Robson (New York, 1980), pp. 93–100.

12. See Rollins, "Some English Accounts," pp. 364–371.

13. Skrabanek, "Notes," p. 114. Fabricius Hildanus concluded after thirty years of studying fasting girls that most of the tales were fraudulent (ibid., p. 117). Medieval theologians and natural philosophers were also interested in naturalistic explanations of prolonged abstinence. See Bynum, *Holy Feast,* chap. 3.

14. George Hakewill, *Apologia, or Declaration of the Power and Providence of God,* 3rd ed. (London, 1935), I: 7: 9, p. 441.

15. Rollins, "Some English Accounts," pp. 361–362.

16. Ibid., pp. 363, 367–368.

17. Quoted in Samuel Gee, *Medical Lectures and Aphorisms* (London, 1908), pp. 45–47.

18. Both pamphlets were by T. Robins. See *News from Darby-shire, or The Wonder of all wonders, that ever yet was Printed, being a perfect and true relation of the handy work of Almighty God shown upon the body of one Martha Taylor* (London, 1668) and *The Wonder of the World, being a perfect relation of a young maid, about eighteen years of age, which hath not tasted of any food this two and fifty weeks* (London, 1669).

19. John Reynolds, *A Discourse on Prodigious Abstinence* (London, 1669), reprinted in *Harleian Miscellany* 4 (London, 1809), 43–58. My interpretation of this seventeenth-century case confirms the thesis of Michael McDonald, *Mystical Bedlam: Madness, Anxiety and Healing in Seventeenth Century England* (New York, 1981), in which the author argues that deviant behaviors generated eclectic explanations borrowed from religious, magical, and scientific thought.

20. For an example of this view see Moses Pitt, *An Account of Ann Jeffries Who Was . . . Fed by Fairies* (London, 1696).

21. Cotton Mather, "An Account of the Sufferings of Margaret Rule," pt. 1, in *More Wonders of the Invisible World*, ed. Robert Calef (Salem, Mass., 1823), p. 27. Mather followed the literature on abstinence and fasting. See George Lyman Kittridge, "Cotton Mather's Scientific Communications to the Royal Society," *Proceedings of the American Antiquarian Society* 36 (April 12–October 18, 1916), 32–34.

22. I am indebted to Audrey Davis, Curator of Medical Sciences, Smithsonian Institution, for her explanation of seventeenth-century fermentation theory. See *The Remaining Works of . . . Dr. Thomas Willis I. Fermentation* (London, 1681); Audrey B. Davis, *Circulation Physiology and Medical Chemistry in England, 1650–1680* (Lawrence, Kans., 1973). On seventeenth-century scientific developments see Walter Pagel, *William Harvey's Biological Ideas: Selected Aspects and Historical Background* (New York, 1967).

23. Erasmus Darwin, *Zoonomia, or The Laws of Organic Life* (London, 1796), pp. 308–309, 318–319, 357, 604. Von Haller's text, *First Lines of Physiology* (Edinburgh, 1779) is quoted in Granger, "The Fasting Woman of Tutbury," p. 319.

24. "Odd Phases in Literature: Abstinence," extracted from *Oeuvres complètes de Tabarin* (Paris, 1622) and *L'esprit dans l'histoire de recherches et curiosités* in *Irish Quarterly Review* 9 (January 1860), 1028. See also George M. Gould and Walter L. Pyle, *Anomalies and Curiosities of Medicine* (Philadelphia, 1897), pp. 413–415.

25. Ibid.; Benjamin Granger, "On Unusual Cases of Anorexy," *Edinburgh Medical and Surgical Journal* (April 1813), 157–159; Caleb Green, "Remarkable Case of Abstinence," *Buffalo Medical Journal and Monthly Review* 4 (March 1849), 729; Jonathan Harris, "A Remarkable Case of Abstinence from Food," *Cincinnati Medical Observer* 1 (May 1856), 199–200; "Extraordinary Abstinence," *Leisure Hour Monthly Library* 18 (1869), 806–807; Henry Barber, "Cases of Long-Continued Abstinence from Food," *British Medical Journal* 1 (May 28, 1870), 544–545; "A Fasting Woman in Ipswich," *Medical Press and*

Circular 31 (January 12, 1881), 36–37; L. S. Forbes Winslow, "Fasting and Feeding," *Journal of Psychological Medicine* 6 (1880), 253–299; "Fasting and Feeding," *Spectator* 64 (May 3, 1890), 618–619; "Lessons from the Fasting Mania," *Ascepliad* 7 (1890), 236–239.

26. M. Charles Richet, "Long Fastings and Starvation," *Popular Science Monthly* 36 (February 1890), 543.

27. L. S. Forbes Winslow, "Fasting and Feeding," *Journal of Psychological Medicine* 6 (1880), 253–255, 258, 264–265; Kittridge, "Mather's Scientific Communications," p. 32.

28. The details of the case of Ann Moore as given here are extracted from the following: *A Faithful Relation of Ann Moore of Tutbury, Staffordshire, Who for Nearly Four Years, Has and Still Continues to Live without Any Kind of Food*, Published by Her Request, 4th ed. (Birmingham, 1811); Legh Richmond, *A Statement of Facts Relative to the Supposed Abstinence of Ann Moore of Tutbury, Staffordshire, and Account of the Circumstances Which Led to the Recent Detection of Her Imposture* (London, 1813); *An Account of the Extraordinary Abstinence of Ann Moore, of Tutbury, Staffordshire, England Who has for more than three years, lived entirely without food*, 3rd American ed. (Springfield, Mass., 1811); James Ward, *Some Account of Mary Thomas of Tanyrault . . . and of Ann Moore, commonly called the Fasting Woman of Tutbury* (London, 1813); Granger, "The Fasting Woman of Tutbury," and idem, "On Unusual Cases"; Robert Taylor, "Letter," *London Medical and Physical Journal* 20 (December 1808), 402; C. Bede, "Ann Moore, the Fasting Woman of Tutbury," *Leisure Hour Monthly Library* 19 (1870), 155–156. There are other sources on Ann Moore: see the bibliography in "Ann Moore," *Dictionary of National Biography*, ed. Sir Leslie Stephen and Sir Sidney Lee, vol. 13 (London, 1921), p. 786, and *British Museum General Catalogue of Printed Books*, vol. 163 (London, 1963), pp. 549–550.

29. *A Faithful Relation*, p. 5. Note the similarity to medieval women who ingested fluids from the bodies of the people they nursed.

30. Granger, "The Fasting Woman of Tutbury," pp. 319–320.

31. *A Faithful Relation*, p. 8.

32. Richmond, *Statement of Facts*, p. 7.

33. *A Faithful Relation*, pp. 5–6.

34. Ibid., p. 4; Richmond, *Statement of Facts*, p. 51.

35. *An Account of the Extraordinary Abstinence*, pp. 23–24; Granger, "On Unusual Cases," p. 158, also believed that Ann Moore lived on air: "What the blood loses, in these cases of anorexy, by the organs of excretion, is replaced by absorption from the atmosphere."

36. See Richard Morton, *Phthisiologia, or a Treatise on Consumptions* (London, 1694), chap. 1, pp. 4–9; Darwin, *Zoonomia*, pp. 308–309, 318–319, 357; Granger, "The Fasting Woman of Tutbury," pp. 322–323.

37. On Legh Richmond see *Annals of the Poor. Authentic Narratives Consisting of the Dairyman's Daughter, The African Servant, and the Young Cottager with a Brief Memoir of the Author by Reverend Joel Hawes* (Springfield, Mass., 1856), pp. 7–14.

38. Richmond, *Statement of Facts*, pp. 23–44; *A Faithful Relation*, p. 21.

39. *A Faithful Relation,* p. 21. See also the article in *Dictionary of National Biography* on Ann Moore (p. 787).

40. Richmond, *Statement of Facts,* pp. 23–44.

3. The Debate over Fasting Girls

1. [Charles Dickens, ed.], *All the Year Round* 2 (October 9, 1869): 442.

2. *New York Times,* July 6, 1880.

3. Both the *Lexicon of Medicine* (London, 1879), published by the New Sydenham Society, and Robley Dunglison's widely used *Dictionary of Medical Science* (Philadelphia, 1865), p. 72, offered the diagnostic category "anorexia mirabilis" to denote a form of religiously inspired fasting or lack of appetite.

4. See Sally Falk Moore, "The Secret of the Men: A Fiction of Chagga Initiation and Its Relation to the Logic of Chagga Symbolism," *Africa* 46: 4 (1976), 357–370.

5. Henry Sutherland, "On the Artificial Feeding of the Insane," *Journal of Psychological Medicine and Mental Pathology* 1 (April 1875), 101.

6. *New York Times,* December 15, 1878.

7. On Spiritualism in post–Civil War America see R. Laurence Moore, *In Search of White Crows: Spiritualism, Parapsychology and American Culture* (New York, 1977). On the connections between feminism and Spiritualism see Joan Jacobs Brumberg, *Mission for Life: The Judson Family and American Evangelical Culture* (New York, 1980), pp. 145–179.

8. See Paul Boller, Jr., *American Thought in Transition: The Impact of Evolutionary Naturalism, 1865–1900* (Chicago, 1969); Paul A. Carter, *The Spiritual Crisis of the Gilded Age* (DeKalb, Ill., 1971); Donald H. Meyer, "American Intellectuals and the Victorian Crisis of Faith," in *Victorian America,* ed. Daniel Walker Howe (Philadelphia, 1976). On the rise of scientific medicine in the nineteenth century see Morris Vogel and Charles E. Rosenberg, eds., *The Therapeutic Revolution: Essays in the Social History of American Medicine* (Philadelphia, 1979); Charles E. Rosenberg, *No Other Gods: Science and American Social Thought* (Baltimore, 1976); Donald Fleming, *William H. Welch and the Rise of Modern Medicine* (Boston, 1954); Paul Starr, *The Social Transformation of American Medicine* (New York, 1982).

9. The story of Sarah Jacob has been reconstructed from Robert Fowler, *A Complete History of the Welsh Fasting Girl* (London, 1871), pp. 4–25; *British Medical and Surgical Journal,* beginning April 24, 1869, and continuing through 1870; *Lancet,* beginning February 27, 1869; John Cule, *Wreath on the Crown* (Llandysul, Wales, 1967); H. Gethin Morgan, "Fasting Girls and Our Attitudes to Them," *British Medical Journal* 2 (1977), 1652–55. There was some controversy over Sarah Jacob's age: it is unclear whether she was ten or twelve when the fast began. The medical man who did the postmortem was aware of the age discrepancy, saying, "She had more hair on her pubes than children of twelve often have," and identified her as a fourteen-year-old (Fowler, *Welsh Fasting Girl,* pp. 4, 9, 10, 12–13, 116). On Fowler see *British Biographical Archives* (microfiche), ed. Laureen Baillie and Paul Sieveking (New York, 1986), #308.

10. Fowler, *Welsh Fasting Girl,* p. 1.

11. *British Medical and Surgical Journal* (December 25, 1869), 686.

12. *Lancet* (May 1, 1869), 624; ibid. (May 6, 1869), 663.

13. Fowler, *Welsh Fasting Girl*, p. 100; *Lancet* (March 27, 1869), p. 448. On Fowler see [J. and A. Churchill], *London and Provincial Medical Directory* (London, 1872), p. 79.

14. *British Medical and Surgical Journal* (September 11, 1869), 315.

15. Ibid. (September 7, 1869), 6.

16. *Lancet* (December 25, 1869), 680.

17. Both Evan and Hannah Jacob were brought to trial, but only the father was found guilty of criminal negligence. See Fowler, *Welsh Fasting Girl*, pp. 85–93, for a description of the prosecution case against Jacob; see also the *Law Times* for 1870; and *Lancet* (February 5, 1870), 215; (February 19, 1870), 282; (March 5, 1870), 360–361; (March 19, 1870), 430.

18. London *Times,* December 24, 1869.

19. *Lancet* (December 25, 1869), 680–681.

20. Fowler, *Welsh Fasting Girl*, pp. 193, 197.

21. Quoted in ibid., p. 193.

22. Ibid., p. 129.

23. On nineteenth-century medical views of the female adolescent see Joan Jacobs Brumberg, "Chlorotic Girls, 1870–1920: A Historical Perspective on Female Adolescence," *Child Development* 53 (1982), 1468–77. On the general subject of female nervous disorders in the Victorian period see Ann D. Wood, "The Fashionable Diseases: Women's Complaints and Their Treatment in Nineteenth Century America," *Journal of Interdisciplinary History* 4 (1973), 25–52; John S. Haller and Robin M. Haller, *The Physician and Sexuality in Victorian America* (Urbana, Ill., 1974); Charles E. Rosenberg and Carroll Smith-Rosenberg, "The Female Animal: Medical and Biological Views of Woman and Her Role in Nineteenth Century America," *Journal of American History* 60 (September 1973), 332–356; Carroll Smith-Rosenberg, "From Puberty to Menopause: The Cycle of Femininity in Nineteenth Century America," in *Clio's Consciousness Raised: New Perspectives on the History of Women,* ed. Mary Hartman and Louis V. Banner (New York, 1974), pp. 23–37, and "The Hysterical Woman: Sex Roles and Role Conflict in 19th Century America," *Social Research* 39 (1972), 652–678; Elaine Showalter, *The Female Malady: Women, Madness and English Culture, 1830–1980* (New York, 1985).

24. Sir William W. Gull, "The Address in Medicine," *Lancet* (August 8, 1868), 171.

25. In London, nearly two decades later, a doctor who heard the first clinical discussion of anorexia nervosa remarked that in past time anorectics "were sent to Dr. [Morrell] MacKenzie." MacKenzie, a well-known specialist in diseases of the throat, did write about "neuroses of sensation" in the throat and related this to "hysterical girls and women." See Morrell MacKenzie, *Diseases of the Pharynx, Larynx, and Trachea* (New York, 1880), pp. 83–85, 308. Note that in the 1890s MacKenzie's son, Stephen, treated a patient with anorexia nervosa at London Hospital (see Chapter 6).

26. Fowler, *Welsh Fasting Girl*, pp. 23, 32, 98, 142.

27. Ibid., pp. 32, 100. Asitia is defined in the New Sydenham Society's

Lexicon of Medicine, ed. Henry Power and Leonard W. Sedgwick (London, 1879) as a "loathing for food; but more probably and more correctly a want of food." The term "anorexia" was much more commonly used than "asitia."

28. Fowler, *Welsh Fasting Girl,* p. 203.

29. Ibid., p. 114.

30. Samuel Fenwick, *On Atrophy of the Stomach and on the Nervous Affections of the Digestive Organs* (London, 1880), p. 99. A similar commentary about "fasting girls" can be found in early-twentieth-century discussions of anorexia nervosa. In *Medical Lectures and Aphorisms* (London, 1908) Samuel Gee wrote: "Should such a case as this become the topic of gossip in a neighborhood of ignorant and silly people, the patient may attain to the notoriety of a fasting girl" (p. 44). In *A System of Medicine by Many Writers* 8 (London, 1910), p. 710, the authors (Clifford Albutt and Humphry Davy Rolleston) stated: "This state is fraught with danger to life, unless judicious and energetic treatment be adopted. Out of such material, where the friends and surrounds supply the elements of fraud or credulity, are made the fasting girls, who from time to time become notorious, and whose exploits have been known to terminate in death."

31. *New York Times,* March 13, 1876, and May 2, 1881; London *Times,* August 26 and September 15, 1871; "Another Fasting Girl," *British Medical Journal* (February 9, 1878), 200; Frederick Grant, "The Market Harborough Fasting Girl," ibid. (February 2, 1878), 152; D. McNeill, "An Extraordinary Fasting Case," ibid. (June 24, 1882), 938.

32. J. A. Campbell, "Fasting and Feeding," *British Medical Journal* 1 (February 23, 1878), 255.

33. Nathan G. Hale, *Freud and the Americans, The Beginning of Psychoanalysis in the U.S., 1876–1917* (New York, 1971), pp. 47–51, 58. Between 1870 and 1910 the "somatic style" predominated; by explaining many mental conditions as somatic in origin, the neurologists brought them increasingly within the medical model of involuntary illness.

34. George Beard, *Eating and Drinking. A Popular Manual of Food and Diet in Health and Disease* (New York: G. P. Putnam, 1871), p. 8. On Beard, see Charles E. Rosenberg, "The Place of George M. Beard in Nineteenth-Century Psychiatry," *Bulletin of the History of Medicine* 36 (1962), 245–259.

35. In particular, the neurologists were familiar with studies by Chossat that documented a 40-percent weight loss in healthy animals between the onset of starvation and death. Charles Chossat, *Recherches expérimentales sur l'inanition* (Paris, 1843).

36. William Hammond, *Fasting Girls: Their Physiology and Their Pathology* (New York, 1879), p. 71.

37. William Hammond, *Spiritualism and Allied Causes and Conditions of Nervous Derangement* (New York, 1876), p. vi.

38. The best studies of late-nineteenth-century Spiritualism and Seventh-Day Adventism are Moore, *In Search of White Crows*; Ronald Numbers, *Prophetess of Health: A Study of Helen Gould White* (New York, 1976). On Christian Science see Robert Peel, *Mary Baker Eddy,* vol. 1: *The Years of Decision*; vol. 2: *The Years of Trial*; vol. 3: *The Years of Authority* (New York, 1966, 1971, 1977).

In his book on Spiritualism, William Hammond took special aim at women who claimed miraculous powers relating to health care. For example, Hammond chose to retell in graphic detail the story of Charlotte La Porte, the "Sucker," a woman who cured ulcers, cancers, and open sores by sucking them while in a state of ecstasy. According to Hammond, La Porte had "her imitators—women all. They applied their tongues and lips to the most disgusting ulcers, full of pus and horrible to see, and sucked them till they were perfectly clean. They even swallowed the foetid exudations with impunity and even relish. They washed the dressing which had been applied to such sores, and then drank the water." The model for La Porte was clearly Saint Catherine of Siena. Hammond wrote, "We see, therefore, that four hundred years before Charlotte La Porte began her horrible operations, there was a proto-sucker in the person of one of the most worthy saints of the calendar." The message here was obvious: women driven by ecstatic religious experiences did not observe principles of scientific hygiene nor did they maintain a normal distance from decaying flesh (Hammond, *Spiritualism,* p. 302).

39. On Hammond see James M. Phalen, "William Hammond," in *Dictionary of American Biography,* ed. Allen Johnson and Dumas Malone, vol. 4 (New York, 1957), pp. 210–211, and Bonnie Blustein, "A New York Medical Man: William Alexander Hammond, M.D. (1828–1900)" (Ph.D. diss., University of Pennsylvania, 1979). Blustein does not discuss Hammond's involvement with the food abstinence issue in any detail. However, she proposes that "neurological antifeminism" was a basic component of Hammond's medical thought and career.

40. Hammond, *Fasting Girls,* p. 6.

41. Hammond, *Spiritualism,* p. vi.

42. William Hammond, *A Treatise on the Diseases of the Nervous System* (New York, 1892), pp. 741, 764.

43. Hammond, *Spiritualism,* p. vi.

44. The story of the Fancher case is taken from the following: Abram Dailey, *Mollie Fancher: The Brooklyn Enigma* (Brooklyn, 1894); *Brooklyn Daily Eagle,* June 7, 1866; *New York Times* and *New York Sun,* between 1878 and 1881; George M. Beard, "The Scientific Lessons of the Mollie Fancher Case," *Medical Record,* 14 (November 30, 1878), 446–448; Clark Bell, "The Case of Mollie Fancher," *Medico-Legal Journal* 11: 3 (1893), 335–336; "The Case of Mollie Fancher," *Medico-Legal Journal,* 12: 1 (1894), 73–74; Hammond, *Fasting Girls*; T. E. Allen, "The Clairvoyance of Mollie Fancher," *Arena* 12 (1895), 329–336.

45. *Brooklyn Daily Eagle,* June 7, 1866.

46. Dailey, *Mollie Fancher,* p. 11.

47. Ibid., p. 12.

48. The author is referring here to a larger syndrome, designated neurasthenia.

49. The *Brooklyn Daily Eagle* article called her desire for education a "mistaken enthusiasm growing out of class-emulation," by which I assume the author meant to convey Fancher's desire to better herself through schooling. Neither the nature nor the timing of these accidents is terribly clear. The *Eagle,*

for example, never mentioned the streetcar accident, which according to Abram Dailey was extremely serious.

50. *Brooklyn Daily Eagle,* June 7, 1866; Dailey, *Mollie Fancher,* p. 144.

51. *New York Sun,* November 24, 1878. In addition to claiming to communicate with the spirit of her mother, Mollie Fancher claimed to have a "sextuple consciousness" and identified five other "personalities": Sunbeam, Idol, Rosebud, Pearl, and Ruby. These names, of course, reflected the sentimental culture of Victorian women. See the *Brooklyn Daily Eagle* article for a discussion of the spiritual views of Fancher.

52. On the problematic relationship between medicine and Spiritualism see Edward M. Brown, "Neurology and Spiritualism in the 1870s," *Bulletin of the History of Medicine* 57 (Winter 1983), 562–577.

53. Hammond did not explicitly record his objections to the fact that in the Spiritualist community women were also allowed to preach from the pulpit and serve as association presidents.

54. *New York Sun,* November 24, 1878.

55. Dailey, *Mollie Fancher,* p. 112. On female hunger artists, see note 103 below.

56. Ibid., p. 249.

57. Ibid., p. 224.

58. *New York Sun,* November 25, 1878.

59. *New York Times,* January 19, 1880.

60. Hammond, *Spiritualism,* pp. 287–288.

61. Hammond, *Fasting Girls,* p. 69. Although he did not publicly call Mollie Fancher an anorectic, Hammond did reveal his familiarity with the clinical literature on anorexia nervosa. Of her alleged total abstinence Hammond said, "M. Lasègue, in a very interesting memoir, has discussed this part of the subject with great precision, and has shown that though such patients take very little food they do take some."

62. See Walter Riese and Ebbe C. Hoff, "A History of the Doctrine of Cerebral Localization," *Journal of the History of Medicine* 5 (1950), 50–71, and ibid., 6 (1951), 439–470.

63. Hammond, *Fasting Girls,* pp. 58–59.

64. Ibid., p. 71.

65. *New York Times,* January 26, February 12, and February 15, 1916.

66. Ibid., December 15, 1878.

67. Hammond, *Treatise,* p. 762; *New York Times,* December 15, 1878.

68. *New York Sun,* November 25 and November 26, 1878.

69. Ibid., November 17, 1878.

70. Ibid., November 24, 1878.

71. For biographies of these men see, for John Tyndall (1820–1893), *Dictionary of National Biography,* ed. Sir Leslie Stephen and Sir Sidney Lee, vol. 19 (London, 1921–22), pp. 1358–63; for Thomas Henry Huxley (1825–1895), ibid., vol. 22 (London, 1909), pp. 894–903; for Louis Agassiz (1807–1873), *Dictionary of American Biography,* ed. Dumas Malone, vol. 1 (New York, 1964), pp. 114–122.

72. *New York Sun,* November 26, 1878.

73. Ibid. Two vocal supporters of Mollie Fancher who were known beyond Brooklyn were Epes Sargent (1813–1880) and Henry Martyn Parkhurst (1825–1908). Sargent, a Boston writer and author of a well-known rhetoric text, wrote three books between 1869 and 1881 arguing the truths of Spiritualism. In *The Scientific Basis of Spiritualism* (Boston, 1881), he wrote sympathetically about the Fancher case and accused Beard of slander (pp. 225–230). See *Dictionary of American Biography*, vol. 8, pp. 356–357. Parkhurst made his living as a reporter who wrote books on stenophonography and astronomy. He was always referred to in the Fancher debate as a "scientist" who supported her supernatural claims to clairvoyance and abstinence.

74. *New York Sun*, November 26, 1878; George Beard, "Scientific Lessons of the Mollie Fancher Case," *Medical Record* 14 (1878), 446.

75. *New York Sun*, November 27, 1878.

76. "Regulars" is the term used to denote nineteenth-century practitioners who adopted and prescribed standardized therapies; "irregulars" refers to homeopaths, eclectics, and other sectarian practitioners. For a discussion of sectarian medicine in the nineteenth century see Martin Kaufman, *Homeopathy in America: Rise and Fall of a Medical Heresy* (Baltimore, 1971), and William G. Rothstein, *American Physicians in the Nineteenth Century: From Sects to Science* (Baltimore, 1976). On therapeutics among the regulars see John Harley Warner, *The Therapeutic Perspective: Medical Practice, Knowledge, and Identity in America, 1820–1885* (Cambridge, Mass., 1986).

77. *New York Sun*, November 24, 1878.

78. Ibid., December 8, 1878.

79. Ibid.

80. For a classic description of intraprofessional rivalries in nineteenth-century medicine see Charles E. Rosenberg, *The Trial of the Assassin Guiteau: Psychiatry and Law in the Gilded Age* (Chicago, 1968). For a discussion of the neurologist–asylum superintendent feud see Barbara Sicherman, *The Quest for Mental Health in America, 1880–1917* (New York, 1979), and on a specific medical community, Bonnie Ellen Blustein, "New York Neurologists and the Specialization of American Medicine," *Bulletin of the History of Medicine* 53 (1979), 170–183.

81. *New York Sun*, December 8, 1878. In his well-known 1901 Gifford Lecture, William James also discussed the medical materialism of his day as too simpleminded. See William James, *The Varieties of Religious Experience* (Garden City, N.Y.: Doubleday, n.d.), pp. 23, 27, 33.

82. *New York Sun*, December 8 and December 9, 1878.

83. *New York Times*, November 25, 1878.

84. Ibid., January 18, August 9, August 20, and November 2, 1880. As late as 1908 Tanner's record was cited by individuals wishing to demonstrate their own superior abstemiousness (*New York Times*, March 22, 1908). Tanner's accomplishment was widely known, provoking what *Ascepliad* 7 (1890), 1, called a fasting mania. Tanner was widely discussed, and in some cases imitated. A report about a "Fasting Woman in Ipswich" captured the measure and impact of Tanner's fame: "It is not long since that the good people of Ipswich were excited over the exploits of the notorious Dr. Tanner, three thousand miles away little dreaming that in their own town, close to their own homes, was a person

whose fast puts the American starver entirely in the shade." *Medical Press and Circular* 31 (January 12, 1881), 36. See also L. S. Forbes Winslow, "Fasting and Feeding," *Journal of Psychological Medicine* 6 (1880), 299; J. C. Noyes, "Prolonged Abstinence from Food," *Boston Medical and Surgical Journal* 103 (August 5, 1880), 140; C. H. Webber, *The Strange Case of Josephine Marie Bedard* (Boston, c. 1889), p. 3; M. Charles Richet, "Long Fasting and Starvation," *Popular Science Monthly* 36 (February 1890), 541–542; "Fasting and Feeding," *Spectator* 64 (May 1890), 618–619. The best-known of the scientific fasters who worked in laboratory settings was Giovanni Succi, who fasted in the United States and in Italy. See the *New York Times* for August and September 1886, October 1888, November and December 1890; also *Lancet* (April 28, 1888), 845. Even in 1891 Tanner and Succi were competing for an abstinence record (*New York Times*, January 12, 1891).

85. *New York Times*, August 9, 1880.

86. I am indebted to Martin Pernick for this point.

87. The following female fasting cases have been identified through the *New York Times* or other contemporary newspapers:

1876 Ellen Sudworth, age eleven or twelve (Culcheth, Scotland), *New York Times*, March 13, 1876

1881 Hattie Duell, age fifty-two (Iowa City, Iowa), *New York Times*, April 13, 1881

Christina Marshall, age thirteen (Glasgow, Scotland), *New York Times*, May 21, 1881

Lenora Eaton, age twenty-one (Bremerville, N.J.), *New York Times*, August 11, 1881

Maggie Campbell, age fifteen (San Francisco, Calif.), *New York Times*, August 29, 1881

1884 Kate Smulsey, age twenty (Fort Plain, N.Y.), *New York Times*, August 22, 1884; April 17 and April 25, 1885; *Amsterdam* (N.Y.) *Daily Democrat* sporadic articles, August 20, 1884–April 13, 1885

1886 Lina Finch, age twenty-one (Covert, N.Y.), *Homer Republican*, March 25, 1886

Anna Belle Langan, age nine (La Crosse, Wis.), *New York Times*, April 18, 1886

1889 Paulina King, age thirty-two (Springfield, Ill.), *New York Times*, April 18, 1886

1890 Mrs. Adam Wuchter, age thirty-eight (Whitehall, Pa.), *New York Times*, July 20, 1890

1904 Victoria Kopwicz, age twenty-six (Newark, N.J.), *New York Times*, October 7, 1904

1910 Cora Esek, age twenty-two (Cleveland, Ohio), *New York Times*, March 31, 1910

88. T. Jackson Lears, *No Place of Grace: Antimodernism and the Transformation of American Culture, 1880–1920* (New York, 1981), p. 161. According to Lears, "By the turn of the [twentieth] century, religious practices which had seemed barbarous or bizarre were winning renewed attention and respect" from those who shared the antimodernist sentiment.

89. *New York Times*, August 11, 1881.

90. *Homer Republican*, March 25, 1886. Lina Finch was the granddaughter of Elisha and Adeline Vining, a farm couple in their sixties whose worth in land and personal property, according to the 1870 census, was close to $7,000. Adeline Vining, for whom Lina was named, was a member of the Methodist Church. Apparently, Lina Finch grew up, along with her three siblings, her own widowed mother, and a hired hand and his wife and child, in a house immediately adjacent to her maternal grandparents. Then, in the late 1870s, for reasons not revealed by local or census materials, Lina and her elder brother, William, went to live with their grandparents. Lina appears to have attended local schools until about the age of sixteen, probably in 1881 or 1882 (9th Census [1870] of the United States, Town of Covert, New York State, p. 27; 10th Census [1880], p. 2). I am grateful to Faye Dudden for finding this report.

91. Information on the Smulsey case is drawn from the *New York Times*, August 22, 1884, and April 17 and April 25, 1885. The case also received consistent local coverage in the *Amsterdam Daily Democrat* throughout 1884 and 1885. Examples from 1884 include: "A Living Skeleton," August 20; "Kate Smulsey's Fast," August 25; "Is She a Fraud? Who Shall Decide When Doctors Disagree?" August 26; "Watching the Faster," September 19; "The Smulsey Case Again," September 20; "The Fate of the Faster," November 28; "The Faster Sinks Slowly," November 29.

92. *Amsterdam Daily Democrat*, September 16, 1884.

93. Both William Zoller and Douglas Ayer, local physicians involved in the Smulsey case, are listed in Washington Frothingham, *History of Montgomery County* (Syracuse, N.Y., 1892), p. 167.

94. *New York Times*, August 22, 1884.

95. *Amsterdam Daily Democrat*, August 25, 1884.

96. Quoted in ibid., August 27, 1884.

97. Ibid., September 4, 1884.

98. Ibid., September 9 and November 28, 1884.

99. Dr. William Bennett kindly provided me with information on locomotor ataxia and polydipsia (see note 102 below).

100. *Amsterdam Daily Democrat*, August 25, August 26, and September 20, 1884; *New York Times*, August 22, 1884, and April 10, 1885.

101. *Amsterdam Daily Democrat*, April 13, 1885.

102. Polydipsia, drinking excessive amounts of water, is not atypical of animals or people who are fasting or deprived of food.

103. C. H. Webber, *The Strange Case of Josephine Marie Bedard* (Boston, 1889), pp. 1, 17, 19. Bostonians eventually paid fifty cents to see the curious Marie Bedard. A decade later New Yorkers paid ten cents to watch an explicitly commercial variant of the fasting girl. "Hunger artist" Helen Coppague fasted for sixty days and $8,000 on the stage of Huber's Museum on 14th Street. Coppague, a woman in her early twenties, had performed a similar public feat in Pittsburgh the year before. The New York advertisement heralded her as the "only woman faster," one who "lives on water only, and challenges the world." See the *New York Times*, December 7, 1897, and January 2, 1898. An interesting perspective on the commercial faster can be found in Franz Kafka's "Hunger

Artist" in *Franz Kafka: The Complete Stories*, ed. Nahum Glatzer (New York, 1971), pp. 268–277.

104. George Milbry Gould and Walter Pyle, *Anomalies and Curiosities of Medicine* (Philadelphia, 1897), p. 413. Gould was an ophthalmologist widely known as a medical writer and lexicographer. This comment is included in a discussion of anorexia nervosa.

105. See for example J. Dejerine and E. Gauckler, *The Psychoneuroses and Their Treatment by Psychotherapy* (Philadelphia, 1913). These authors list only two groups of mental anorexias: (a) "emotionally disturbed females who spontaneously or voluntarily begin diets only to persist beyond any reasonable limits," and (b) "gastropaths and enteropaths of both sexes who reject foods they feel are indigestible." Religious explanations thus were replaced by a different set of cultural imperatives.

106. In historical studies of the United States secularization is an imprecise and debatable formulation, used all too often to convey a simplistic notion of a predictable process by which American society moved in linear, orderly fashion from otherworldliness to worldliness. On the sociological debate over whether secularization even occurred and if it is a useful concept, see David Martin, "Towards Eliminating the Concept of Secularization," in *Penguin Survey of the Social Sciences*, ed. J. Gould (London, 1965), pp. 169–182; Andrew Greeley, *Unsecular Man: The Persistence of Religion* (New York, 1972); Thomas Luckmann, *The Invisible Religion: The Problem of Religion in Modern Society* (New York, 1967). In contemporary anthropology the issue emerges somewhat differently in terms of the relationship between the sacred and the profane. Works by E. Evans-Pritchard, *Theories of Primitive Religion* (London, 1965) and Mary Douglas, *Purity and Danger* (London, 1966) underscore, first, that there is no absolute distinction between religious and nonreligious phenomena, and second, that contemporary society is not, by definition, secular. Analysis and description of secularization in late-nineteenth-century America is one part of the work of Lears, *No Place of Grace*; Paul A. Carter, *The Spiritual Crisis of the Gilded Age* (De Kalb, Ill., 1971); Gregory H. Singleton, "Protestant Voluntary Organization and the Shaping of Victorian America," in *Victorian America*, ed. Daniel Walker Howe (Philadelphia, 1976), pp. 47–58; D. H. Meyer, "American Intellectuals and the Victorian Crisis of Faith," in Howe, *Victorian America*, pp. 59–77.

Secularization is usually linked to two other equally complex processes, urbanization and industrialization, and is generally measured in terms of structural or institutional indexes that demonstrate the shrinking reach of formal religious organizations, especially churches. By institutional indexes I mean the following: the decrease in congregational size and number of churches and the restriction of the church's sphere of influence; the decline in the role and function of religious personnel and their subsequent replacement by specialists (professionals); and the retreat of ecclesiastical authority in confrontations between church and state. My interpretation of fasting girls certainly incorporates this institutional perspective, especially with regard to the issue of how physicians gradually challenged and replaced the clergy as the primary interpreters of human behavior.

To talk about secularization without reference to the parish or denomination and without a religious head count is, by and large, unusual, yet it is critically important. As David Martin suggested so perceptively in *A Sociology of English Religion* (London, 1967), "Far from being secular our culture wobbles between a partially absorbed Christianity, biased toward comfort and the need for confidence, and beliefs in fate, luck, and moral governance incongruously joined together" (p. 76). Today, and in the late nineteenth century, religious modes of feeling and questioning survive in our culture—outside formal sanctuaries—at widely different levels. Fasting girls should be viewed as one manifestation of that amorphous process.

4. Emergence of the Modern Disease

1. On the process of establishing nosologies see Charles E. Rosenberg, "The Therapeutic Revolution: Medicine, Meaning and Social Change in Nineteenth Century America," in *The Therapeutic Revolution: Essays in the Social History of American Medicine*, ed. Morris J. Vogel and Charles E. Rosenberg (Philadelphia, 1979), pp. 3–26; Bruce Haley, *The Healthy Body and Victorian Culture* (Cambridge, Mass., 1978), p. 5.

2. Robley Dunglison, *A Dictionary of Medical Sciences* (Philadelphia, 1865), p. 72.

3. Among the wasting diseases, phthisis—a pulmonary condition which incorporated what we now call tuberculosis—attracted much attention. Lack of appetite was unambiguously associated with the disorder, and the relationship of phthisis to insanity was also an issue. Some physicians of stature argued, on the basis of their experience within the asylum, that "phthisis is much commoner among the insane than among the sane" (J. P. Miller, "Phthisis—Its Successful Treatment," *Journal of the American Medical Association* 2 [April 1884], 658). See also W. J. Mickle, "Insanity in Relation to Phthisis," *Lancet* (May 12, 1888), 913–914; Thomas Smith Clouston, *Lectures on Mental Disease* (Edinburgh, 1898), n.p.; Joseph Workman, "Starvation and Insanity," *American Journal of Insanity* 24 (April 1868), 482–488. The problem with phthisis in the asylums was that cause and consequence were not entirely clear, an issue that troubled the British as well as the Americans. See for example S. W. D. Williams, "Remarks on the Refusal of Food in the Insane," *Journal of Mental Science* 5 (October 1864), 378; Mickle, "Insanity in Relation to Phthisis," pp. 913–914; Luther Bell, "On the Coercive Administration of Food to the Insane," *American Journal of Insanity* 6 (January 1850), 226.

4. On intraprofessional competition and social-class considerations in Anglo-American medicine see Nancy Tomes, *A Generous Confidence: Thomas Story Kirkbride and the Art of Asylum Keeping, 1840–1883* (New York, 1984), pp. 107–108, 290–294; and M. Jeanne Peterson, *The Medical Profession in Mid-Victorian London* (Berkeley, 1978), chap. 4. On the distinctiveness of French medicine see Jan Goldstein, "'Moral Contagion': A Professional Ideology of Medicine and Psychiatry in Eighteenth and Nineteenth Century France," pp. 181–221; and Matthew Ramsey, "The Politics of Professional Monopoly in Nineteenth Century Medicine: The French Model and Its Rivals," pp. 225–305, both in *Professions and the French State, 1700–1900*, ed. Gerald L. Geison

(Philadelphia, 1984).

5. On the history of the American asylums see Gerald Grob, *The State and the Mentally Ill: A History of the Worcester State Hospital in Massachusetts, 1830–1920* (Chapel Hill, N.C., 1966); idem, *Mental Institutions in America: Social Policy to 1875* (New York, 1973); idem, "Rediscovering Asylums: The Unhistorical History of the Mental Hospital," *Hastings Center Report* (August 1977), 33–41; David Rothman, *The Discovery of the Asylum* (Boston, 1971); Ellen Dwyer, *Homes for the Mad* (New Brunswick, N.J., 1987); Tomes, *A Generous Confidence.* Both asylum doctors (or "superintendents") and neurologists treated nervous and mental diseases. Asylum superintendents were distinguished from neurologists by their placement within institutions, by the nature of their medical clientele, and by the severity of their patients' illness. In general, neurologists saw in private practice or clinics what we consider neurotic patients, whereas doctors in the asylum handled psychotics whose behavior was so problematic they could not remain in a family or be on their own. See Constance M. McGovern, *Masters of Madness: Social Origins of the American Psychiatric Profession* (Hanover, N.H., 1985).

6. See *New York Medical Journal* 45 (February 5, 1887), 34, for a listing of medical disorders with anorexia; and see Eustace Smith, *On the Wasting Diseases of Infants and Children* (New York, 1884), p. 1. Death by starvation was not an uncommon occurrence, according to contemporary Anglo-American medical reports. At a meeting of the Medical Society of the County of New York in January 1868, Dr. Austin Flint cautioned his colleagues against inattention to the importance of feeding in the treatment of all illness. "Starvation is a cause of death," he warned, "marching silently in front with every disease in which alimentation falls below the natural standard. Starvation reaches its natural termination sometimes sooner and sometimes later than the disease which it covertly accompanies; and it may supersede the disease of which, at first, it was merely an incidental element." Flint, who rejected any therapy that included withholding of food, proposed that it is "always desirable" to feed "to the fullest extent of the capacity of the organism for appropriation" (Austin Flint, "Alimentation in Disease," *American Journal of Insanity* 24 [April 1868], 482–483). Before 1860 some medical men regarded depletion of the body as a positive procedure when a patient fell ill. Many recommended "heroic" treatment such as bloodletting and prolonged abstinence as cures for disease. By the late nineteenth century the "depletionists" had lost ground. For their point of view see Henry Ancell, "Diet and Abstinence," *Lancet* (September 19, 1840), 919–920; J. L. Pierce, "Case of Abstinence," *American Journal of Medical Science* 24 (October 1852), 571–572. See also John Harley Warner, *The Therapeutic Perspective: Medical Practice, Knowledge, and Identity in America, 1820–1885* (Cambridge, Mass., 1986), pp. 5, 95–100, 127 on the decline of heroic depletive therapy.

7. In the published writings of nineteenth-century doctors there is unilateral agreement that anorexia and abstinence both had a special connection to insanity. In fact, in *Commentaries on the Causes, Forms, Symptoms and Treatment, Moral and Medical of Insanity* (London, 1828) George Man Burrows felt called upon to disavow the idea that the insane could "sustain fasting with less

injury to the system." He called that theory "erroneous" because, he argued, "the vital powers . . . are never augmented by insanity" (pp. 295–296, 664). It was not entirely clear, even later in the century, whether anorexia was a symptom of insanity or its cause. Poor diet was widely regarded as a possible predisposing factor in the development of insanity; see Philadelphia Neurological Society, "Forcible Feeding of the Insane," *Journal of Nervous and Mental Disease* 13 (May 1888), 338. Some late-nineteenth-century doctors considered a period of anorexia and wasting to be a predictable first stage in insanity; see L. S. Forbes Winslow, "Fasting and Feeding," *Journal of Psychological Medicine* 6 (1880), 274.

8. Bell, "Coercive Administration," p. 226.

9. "Morbid appetite" meant eating outside the normative food categories (ingesting leaves of trees, seeds, roots, chalk, unripe fruits, and feces or urine) or eating in a bizarre style (without reference to rules of deportment at table). See for example W. A. F. Browne, "Morbid Appetite of the Insane," *Journal of Psychological Medicine* 2 (October 1875), 236–247; Henry Sutherland, "On the Artificial Feeding of the Insane," *Journal of Psychological Medicine and Mental Pathology* 2 (April 1875), 100; Clouston, *Lectures*; Archives of the Institute for Living (formerly the Hartford Retreat), Hartford, Conn., MSS 7132, 7411. On the handling of delusions of poison see William Stout Chipley, "Sitomania: Its Causes and Treatment," *American Journal of Insanity* 16 (July 1859), 4, 41; Bell, "Coercive Administration," p. 225. Forbes Winslow, "Fasting and Feeding," p. 286, used the term "religious monomania"; other descriptions of food refusers motivated by religion are Burrows, *Commentaries*, pp. 294–296; Bell, "Coercive Administration," p. 224; Williams, "Refusal of Food," p. 367; Chipley, "Sitomania," pp. 3, 5; Sutherland, "Artificial Feeding," pp. 98–99. On "religious insanity" as a diagnostic category see Ronald L. Numbers and Janet S. Numbers, "Millerism and Madness: A Study of 'Religious Insanity' in Nineteenth Century America," *Bulletin of the Menninger Clinic* 49: 4 (1985), 289–320.

10. Clouston, *Lectures*.

11. Ibid. See also A. Brierre de Boismont, "On the Treatment of Melancholia," *Journal of Psychological Medicine and Mental Pathology* 2 (April 1875), 22; Landon Carter Gray, "Three Diagnostic Signs of Melancholia," *Journal of Nervous and Mental Disorders* 17 (1890), 1–9; J. Adam, "A Case of Melancholia Presenting Some Exceptional Features: Prolonged Refusal of Food and Forced Alimentation," *British Medical Journal* 1 (1888), 348; D. A. Gorton, "Observations on Melancholia," *New York Medical Times* 15 (1887–88), 353–357.

12. T. S. Clouston, "Forcible Feeding," *Lancet* (November 30, 1872), 797. When a certain doctor who was not an asylum superintendent wrote on this issue, he felt compelled to add, "I suppose, some of these gentlemen [alienists] are rather intolerant of my presuming to bring forth a subject which they conceive belongs essentially to their specialty" (D. Anderson Moxey, "Enforced Alimentation of the Insane," *Lancet* [March 31, 1873], 763).

13. "Forcible Feeding of the Insane," *American Journal of Insanity* 39 (January 1883), 349; Bell, "Coercive Administration," p. 224; John Chapin, "The Forcible Feeding of the Insane," *Medical and Surgical Reporter (Philadel-*

phia) 58 (April 21, 1888), 501; Williams, "Refusal of Food," p. 366; H. I. Manning, Letter on "Forcible Feeding," *Lancet* (January 11, 1873), 73.

14. Samuel Fenwick, *On Atrophy of the Stomach and on the Nervous Affections of the Digestive Organs* (London, 1880), p. 121. Clinical records in general confirm the physician's claim. In 1897 the asylum at Hartford admitted a young woman who stopped eating at home because she believed her food to be poisoned. The delusion of poisoning was only one component of a larger psychological disorder: according to reports, she suffered also from "vague apprehensions and lack of coherence in ideation." Upon admission the girl was tube fed, a procedure that apparently made an impression even in her disordered state. The nurse reported on her third day in the asylum: "[She] took some milk and crackers voluntarily when arrangements for feeding her with the tube had begun." For a food-refusing male melancholic in the same institution, forced feeding had a similar effect. The nasal tubes were "so distasteful to him that he soon consented to take nourishment in a proper manner" (Institute for Living, MSS 7730, 7796).

15. This is not to suggest that forced feeding was never done at home or in the doctor's office.

16. Institute for Living, MS 7158.

17. Dunglison, *Dictionary*, p. 887. Other clinical reports on sitophobia are in Williams, "Refusal of Food," p. 378; Max Einhorn, "Sitophobia of Enteric Origin," *Journal of American Medical Association* 36 (June 15, 1901), 1688–90; idem, "Sitophobia, Inanition and Their Treatment," *American Journal of Medical Sciences*, 126 (August 1903), 228–234. Einhorn's work focused on fear of food related to somatic causes.

18. Chipley came to the asylum in Lexington after earning a medical degree from Transylvania University in 1832; establishment of a private practice in Columbus, Georgia, until 1844; and election to the Chair of Theory and Practice of Medicine, at his alma mater, in 1855. See the memorial to Chipley by O. Everts in *American Journal of Insanity* 38 (October 1881), 177–178, and his biography in Howard A. Kelly, ed., *A Cyclopedia of American Medical Biography*, vol. 1 (Philadelphia, 1912), p. 177; McGovern, *Masters of Madness*, pp. 14, 45, 93–94, 138, 174.

19. Chipley, "Sitomania," p. 2.

20. Adolescents were generally not institutionalized in nineteenth-century mental hospitals. Before World War I one finds few patients, male or female, in the age category thirteen to twenty-one years. Between 1873 and 1906 at the McLean asylum, patients under twenty were a rarity; those between twenty and twenty-five constituted less than 8 percent of the total population in those years. My examination of the records of the Institute for Living and of three British asylums (Camberwell, Chiswick, and Holloway) confirms this pattern. In effect, there was a reluctance to classify as insane individuals in the bloom of youth, although there were specific behaviors—such as excessive masturbation, obscenity, histrionics, precocious sexuality, and food refusal—that were an obvious source of family and community concern and that in some cases led to institutionalization. English superintendents such as Clouston confirmed that the number of adolescent insane in the asylums was small and that insanity, when it

occurred in adolescence, was acute but short-lived. See T. S. Clouston, "The Study of Mental Disease," *Edinburgh Medical Journal* 25 (July 1879), 15–20, and "Puberty and Adolescence Medico-Psychologically Considered," ibid. 26 (July 1880), 5–17.

21. Chipley, "Sitomania," pp. 3, 8.

22. J. A. Campbell, "Feeding and Fasting," *British Medical Journal* 1 (February 23, 1878), 255.

23. Chipley, "Sitomania," pp. 8–9.

24. Ibid., p. 9.

25. Another "vicious habit," masturbation, was regarded as a legitimate reason for institutionalizing adolescent males. For nineteenth-century views of this practice see H. Tristam Engelhardt, "The Disease of Masturbation: Values and the Concept of Disease," *Bulletin of the History of Medicine* 48 (1974), 234–248.

26. Chipley, "Sitomania," pp. 8–9.

27. Ibid.

28. From 1873 until the twentieth century, the British dominated medical writing about anorexia nervosa; between 1900 and 1910, French writing on the subject increased; in the United States, clinical reports on anorexia nervosa began to appear in quantity only in the 1920s and 1930s, as a function of the interest in psychiatry, endocrinology, and pediatrics. Between 1873 and 1900, American writing on anorexia nervosa was very sparse. Any reference to the disease usually involved neurologists reporting on French medicine and using the neurological or French terminology. For example, in *Fasting Girls* (1879) William Hammond wrote of Mollie Fancher's alleged abstinence: "M. Lasègue, in a very interesting memoir, has discussed this part of the subject with great precision, and has shown that though such patients take very little food they do take some" (p. 69). In 1896 [Silas Weir?] Mitchell reported on the work of P. Sollier, a French physician, in "Mental Anorexia," *Journal of Nervous and Mental Disease* 21 (August 1896), 573–574.

29. My understanding and interpretation of the consulting physician and the London medical world is based largely on Peterson, *The Medical Profession.* Another useful contribution to the literature on intraprofessional rivalries is Ivan Waddington, "General Practitioners and Consultants in Early Nineteenth-Century England: The Sociology of an Intra-Professional Conflict" in *Health Care and Popular Medicine in Nineteenth Century England*, ed. John Woodward and David Richards (New York, 1977).

30. Anorexia nervosa was repeatedly described this way. See Thomas Stretch Dowse, "Anorexia Nervosa," *Medical Press and Circular* 32 (August 3, 1881), 95–97, and ibid. (August 17, 1881), 147–148; "A Case of Anorexia Nervosa," *West London Medical Journal* 9 (January 1904), 112, and ibid. (April 1904), 204–206. See Elaine Showalter, *The Female Malady* (New York, 1986), pp. 105–106, 118, for a discussion of the "borderline" (or "borderland") concept.

31. Benjamin Brodie, *Lectures Illustrative of Certain Local Nervous Affections* (London, 1837), p. 37.

32. Samuel Fenwick, *On Atrophy of the Stomach and on the Nervous Affections of the Digestive Organs* (London, 1880), p. 107.

33. Anorexia nervosa tended not to be reported among girls who worked in support of the family economy. I allude here to the model described by Joan W. Scott and Louise Tilly, *Women, Work and Family* (New York, 1978) and Thomas Dublin, *Women at Work: The Transformation of Work and Community in Lowell, Massachusetts, 1826–1860* (New York, 1979). In France medical reports confirm a similar social pattern: the first anorectics were the daughters of the bourgeoisie, not the aristocracy or the working class.

34. These particular enticements are mentioned by British doctors: Sutherland, "Artificial Feeding," p. 100, and D. McNeill, "An Extraordinary Fasting Case," *British Medical Journal* 1 (June 24, 1882), 938.

35. Chiswick Asylum, MS 6651, p. 300, Wellcome Institute.

36. Specialists developed their own institutions (for instance, Royal London Eye Hospital, Maida Vale Hospital for Nervous Diseases, St. John's Hospital for Skin Diseases, St. Peter's Hospital for Stone) but they never achieved the status of the teaching hospitals where the consultants, the crème de la crème of London medicine, built an important network of professional and social associations (Peterson, *The Medical Profession*, pp. 247–248, 272–277).

37. For a report on the first meeting see *Transactions of the Clinical Society of London* 1 (London, 1868), xxv, 2–4 ff. In his inaugural address to the society Sir Thomas Watson, the first president, extolled the group's purposes and told the membership that the "greatest gap in the science of medicine is to be found in its final and supreme stage—the stage of therapeutics." By sharing their clinical experiences with one another, Watson believed that doctors might see an improvement "in the divine art of healing," even within their own time. "Contributions of this order, multiplied in number, contrasted, sifted, and discussed by a variety of keen and instructed minds—of minds sceptical in the best and truest sense of the word—must lead at length to the discovery even of laws, by which our practice shall be guided."

38. Although he was regarded as a fashionable physician and a gentleman, Gull was actually a self-made man. He was raised, from the age of ten, by a widowed mother who worked diligently to bring him into contact with the "best" people she could. She brought her son to the attention of the local clergy; through the Reverend Mr. Brownell, rector of the neighboring village of Beaumont, William made the acquaintance of Benjamin Harrison, treasurer of Guy's Hospital, who became his patron. In 1837, at the age of twenty-one, Gull entered Guy's as a regular medical student but supported himself working as a clerk in the "counting house" of the hospital. After capturing prizes in ophthalmic surgery, midwifery, and other areas, Gull went on to receive a Bachelor of Medicine from the University of London in 1841 and a Doctor of Medicine in 1846. The biographical material on Gull is culled from entries under his name in John H. Talbott, ed., *A Biographical History of Medicine* (New York, 1970); *Dictionary of National Biography*, ed. Sir Leslie Stephen and Sir Sidney Lee (London, 1921); [J. and A. Churchill], *The Medical Directory for 1888* (London, 1888); Samuel Wilks and G. T. Bettany, *A Biographical History of Guy's Hos-*

pital (London, 1892). See also Theodore Dyke Acland, ed., *A Collection of the Published Writing of William Withey Gull* (London, 1896). There are some useful obituaries: *British Medical Journal* 1 (January–June 1890), 256–262; *Guy's Hospital Reports* 47 (1890), xxv–xliii; "Death of Sir William Gull," London *Times*, January 30, 1890; but there is no definitive biography.

39. Sir William W. Gull, "The Address in Medicine," *Lancet* (August 8, 1868), p. 175.

40. William Jenner (1815–1898) received his medical degree from the University of London in 1844 and was elected to the Royal College of Physicians in 1849. In the early 1860s Jenner began to serve the royal family as physician extraordinary to the queen, and he attended Prince Albert in his fatal illness that year. Jenner was created a baronet in 1868. See "Sir William Jenner, 1815–1898," *Journal of the American Medical Association* 214 (November 2, 1970), 907–908; "Sir William Jenner," *Lancet* (December 17, 1898), 1674–76.

41. London *Times*, January 30, 1890. This quote first appeared in the *Times* obituary of December 19, 1871.

42. On Gull's involvement with Edward's illness, see Wilks and Bettany, *Biographical History*, pp. 264–265: "The principal event of Gull's life was attendance on the Prince of Wales during his severe attack of typhoid fever." For a discussion of the national debate over prayer and its efficacy, including information on the national response to Edward's illness, see Frank M. Turner, "Rainfall, Plagues, and the Prince of Wales: A Chapter in the Conflict of Religion and Science," *Journal of British Studies* 13 (May 1974), 46–65.

43. Papers of Sir William Withey Gull, MSS 5873, G/8, Wellcome Institute. Alexandra, wife of the Prince of Wales, also admired Gull and in the period of her husband's recovery wrote Sir William a profuse note of thanks: "Edward is better . . . *how* thankful and happy I am to see him so far recovered . . . I shall *never never* forget what I owe to you dear Dr. Gull who *saved* his life!" (Italics in original.) (Ibid., MSS 5873, F/5/10.) In recognition of Gull's splendid medical performance, the prince, via his secretary, thanked Gull for bringing him "renewed health and strength in the great race of life"; his thanks were accompanied by a check, which the prince described as "inadequate acknowledgement of the professional services which no money can repay." (Ibid., MSS 5873, F/6.)

44. At these functions Gull mixed with civil and religious leaders. Before an 1881 dinner in connection with the International Congress of Medicine, the Prince of Wales' secretary wrote to Gull: "The Prince of Wales thinks that the Crown Prince of Germany had better sit on your right hand and he [the Prince] on your left, and the Archbishop of York should be placed next to the Crown Prince and Cardinal Manning next to him—the Prince of Wales." In this august company Gull, the physician, was not without authority. The note continued: "H.R.H. hopes that you will not object to smoking beginning directly after the toast of the Queen has been given." (Ibid., MSS 5873, H/8; F/16.)

45. Wilks and Bettany, *Biographical History*, pp. 272–273. Gull's correspondence with his son Willie, a student at Eton, was marked by constant religious references and a high degree of concern about avoiding "wickedness" and finding a "calling." (MSS 5873, I/2; I/4; I/10/1; I/13.)

46. *Lancet* (August 15, 1868), 220.

47. William Gull, "Anorexia Nervosa (Apepsia Hysterica, Anorexia Hysterica)," *Transactions of the Clinical Society of London* 7 (1874), 22–28.

48. I have been unable to find this addendum in any of the printed versions of the speech. The only reference to the alleged early marker of Gull's special interest is in the November 1873 summary report of his October 1873 address to the Clinical Society. See "Clinical Society," *Medical Times and Gazette* 2 (November 8, 1873), 534. In 1907, in a lecture at Harvard Medical School, Pierre Janet also observed this curious attempt by Gull to preempt a slightly earlier description of the disease by Charles Lasègue. See Pierre Janet, *The Major Symptoms of Hysteria* (New York, 1907), p. 228. On Lasègue, see Chapter 5.

49. "Dr. Lasègue does not refer to my address at Oxford." Gull, "Anorexia Nervosa," p. 25.

50. Charles Lasègue, "On Hysterical Anorexia," *Medical Times and Gazette* (September 27, 1873), 368. The first portion of Lasègue's translated work appears in the same journal for September 6, 1873, pp. 265–266. The original French report was in *Archives générales de médecine* (April 1873).

51. Gull, "Anorexia Nervosa," p. 22.

52. Ibid., p. 25.

53. Gull's 1873 address gave no recognition of antecedent descriptions that linked anorexia to specific forms of hysteria. In addition to ignoring Lasègue (and Chipley), the eminent practitioner failed to acknowledge a related description of "Temper Disease" published by his colleague John Ogle, a member of the Clinical Society, only three years before. In 1870, in the *British Medical Journal*, Ogle had reported the case of Sarah G, a hysterical twenty-year-old who was hospitalized in a ward for paying patients. Described as "rather delicate and interesting looking," Sarah combined the symptoms of a cough and cold ("catarrh and pulmonary congestion") with a refusal to eat, and sometimes vomited what she was coerced to eat. Ogle cast food refusal as a kind of "Temper Disease" under the larger rubric of hysteria. (John Ogle, "A Case of Hysteria; 'Temper Disease'," *British Medical Journal* [July 16, 1870], pp. 57–60.) Ogle's report is significant because it includes a note written by the patient to another patient, explaining some of her feelings about eating. Ogle, an Oxford graduate and a consultant at St. George's Hospital, coedited the hospital's reports and maintained memberships in English, Scottish, and American neurological societies. On Ogle see [J. and A. Churchill], *London and Provincial Medical Directory* (London, 1870), p. 142.

54. Gull, "Anorexia Nervosa," p. 26.

55. The discussion that follows is drawn from Gull, "Anorexia Nervosa," pp. 22–28.

56. On Kelson Wright see [Churchill], *Medical Directory*, 1870, p. 187.

57. On William Anderson see [Churchill], *Medical Directory*, 1888, p. 442.

58. "Clinical Society," *Medical Times and Gazette* 2 (November 8, 1873), 534–536. Gull, who was obviously acquainted with the Jacob case, corrected his colleague on a technicality. According to his reading of the postmortem, Sarah Jacob died of urinemia (dehydration and lack of fluids) rather than starvation.

59. Ibid., p. 535.

60. "Autointoxication" was often used in nineteenth-century American medicine to describe a condition of excess uric acid, curable through frequent evacuations, drinking water, and "internal cleaning." See Harvey Green, *Fit for America* (New York, 1986), pp. 141, 285, 303. In the instance cited in the text I believe the word is being used differently. Symes Thompson received his medical degree from King's College (1862) and was a Fellow of the Royal College of Physicians (1868). He was a physician to the Consumptive Hospital (Brompton) and held appointments at King's College Hospital. See [Churchill], *Medical Directory*, 1873, pp. 193–194.

61. *Medical Times and Gazette* 2 (November 8, 1873), 535.

62. Ibid.

63. Ibid.

5. Love and Food in the Bourgeois Family

1. Viviana Zellizer makes this argument in *Pricing the Priceless Child: The Changing Value of Children* (New York, 1985). The middle-class female adolescent is an excellent example of Zellizer's formulation but her dating of this transformation in values is debatable. Her work deals primarily with the early twentieth century, although the value revolution she suggests occurred two to three decades before. On the so-called great demographic revolution see J. A. Banks, *Prosperity and Parenthood: A Study of Family Planning among the Victorian Middle Classes* (London, 1954), and Carl Degler, *At Odds: Women and the Family in America from the Revolution to the Present* (New York, 1980). On adolescence in nineteenth-century America see Joseph Kett, *Rites of Passage: Adolescence in America, 1790 to the Present* (New York, 1977); John Modell, Frank Furstenberg, and Theodore Hershberg, "Social Change and Transitions to Adulthood in Historical Perspective," *Journal of Family History* 1 (1976), 7–32. On the Canadian and European experience see Michael Katz, *The People of Hamilton, Canada West: Family and Class in a Mid-Nineteenth-Century City* (Cambridge, Mass., 1976); and John Gillis, *Youth and History: Tradition and Change in European Age Relations, 1770–Present* (New York, 1974).

2. All of the themes described in this paragraph are drawn from Joan Jacobs Brumberg, "'Ruined' Girls: Family and Community Responses to Illegitimacy in Upstate New York, 1890 to 1920," *Journal of Social History* 18 (December 1984), 247–272. On middle-class supervision of girls see also Peter Gay, *The Bourgeois Experience: The Education of the Senses* (New York, 1984), p. 5.

3. On domestic service in the nineteenth-century United States see Faye E. Dudden, *Serving Women: Household Service in Nineteenth Century America* (New York, 1979); David Katzman, *Seven Days a Week: Women and Domestic Service in Industrializing America* (New York, 1978); Leslie Woodcock Tentler, *Wage Earning Women* (New York, 1979). In Britain, some young women were

forced to work outside the home as teachers or governesses. See M. Jeanne Peterson, "The Victorian Governess: Status Incongruence in Family and Society," *Victorian Studies* 14 (September 1970), 7–26.

4. The choice of words here is intentional: Christopher Lasch, *Haven in a Heartless World: The Family Besieged* (New York, 1977).

5. Charles Lasègue, "On Hysterical Anorexia," *Medical Times and Gazette* (September 6, 1873), 265–266, and ibid. (September 27, 1873), 367–369. The original French report was in *Archives générales de Médecine* (April 1873). Although he considered naming the disorder "hysterical inanition" (hysterical starvation), Lasègue ultimately chose "anorexia" because, he said, that term "refers to a phenomenology which is less superficial, more delicate, and also more medical." Still, the physiology of loss of appetite was very confusing, and Lasègue lamented the widespread lack of precision in medical writing on the human appetite. He noted that while anorexia was used to designate a broad pathological condition, there was no way to indicate its range or variety. "We are defective in expressions for the degrees or varieties of inappetence—the poverty of our vocabulary corresponding to the insufficiency of our knowledge" (p. 265). Thus, Lasègue's description of *l'anorexie hystérique* had a twofold purpose: to specify medical knowledge of anorexia and to enrich the medicine of the mind in its search for understanding the manifold forms of hysteria.

6. Lasègue was initially drawn to the study of philosophy and literature, but his friendship with medical students interning at Salpêtrière, the famed public mental hospital for women in Paris, provoked his interest in mental illness. He did a clinical internship with Armand Trousseau at the Faculty of Paris and served for a time as inspector general of French asylums. See the obituaries of Lasègue in *Bulletin de l'Académie de Médecine*, 2nd ser., 12 (March 27, 1883), 385–390; *Archives générales de Médecine* 1 (April 1883), n.p.; *Annales médico-psychologiques*, 7th ser., 12 (April 27, 1885), 88–121. Lasègue first came to public attention in France as a result of his 1848 reporting of the cholera epidemic in Russia; he is best known for his clinical writing on the subject of persecution delirium. American psychiatry is acquainted with Lasègue's paper published in 1877 with J. Falret, "La folie à deux, ou folie communiquée," which was reprinted in translation in October 1964 in the supplement to *American Journal of Psychiatry* 4, 1–23. On his mentor, Armand Trousseau (1801–1867), and on Salpêtrière see *La grande encyclopédie*, vol. 29, p. 377, and vol. 31, p. 431; and Jacques Leonard, *La france Médicale: médecins et malades au XIXe siècle* (Paris, 1978). A summary of Lasègue's work and a bibliography are included in his biography in René Semelaigne, *Les pionniers de la psychiatrie française avant et après Pinel*, vol. 2 (Paris, 1932), pp. 40–49.

7. Lasègue, "On Hysterical Anorexia," p. 265. The discussion that follows is based on Lasègue's reports of September 6 and 27, 1873. See note 5.

8. The use of enticements depended on a family's attitude toward food—and that varied, of course, by social class. In the British upper classes, for example, there was a great deal of austerity with respect to food; the diet of young people at the best private schools was generally repetitive, unstimulating, and spartan. Among the middle classes, however, clinical reports on anorexia

nervosa suggest a willingness to use sweets and other special foods as an entice-
ment to return to eating.

9. Lasègue, "On Hysterical Anorexia," p. 266.

10. Pierre Janet, *The Major Symptoms of Hysteria* (New York, 1907), p. 231.

11. The quotations that follow are from Lasègue, "On Hysterical Anorexia," pp. 367–369.

12. Lasègue did write in the *Annales médico-psychologiques*, as early as
1846, on the general subject of mental therapeutics in "Questions de thérapeu-
tique mentale: La théorie du traitement moral est-elle possible?" He was interested in the moral authority of the doctor, the role of intimidation, and the
concept advanced by Leuret that the physician substituted his personality for
that of the patient. Uneasy with these ideas, Lasègue apparently proposed that
in judicious moral treatment it was incumbent on the doctor to determine if
there were in the patient any traces of the normal state remaining. The goal of
medical intervention, then, was to develop these normal "traces" or "particles"
and to give them strength. See Semelaigne, "Les pionniers," p. 41.

13. Lasègue, "On Hysterical Anorexia," pp. 367–368.

14. Sources that refer to children becoming the objects of increasing expenditure are Kett, *Rites of Passage*, pp. 168–171; and Banks, *Prosperity and
Parenthood*, chap. 2. This literature focuses primarily on the investments parents
made in the professional careers of boys. See W. J. Reader, *Professional Men:
The Rise of the Professional Classes in Nineteenth Century England* (London,
1966). The same general trend was true for girls, although the outcome would
not be the same.

15. Lasègue, "On Hysterical Anorexia," p. 265. In a 1974 analysis of the
internal psychological dynamics of late-nineteenth-century families, one historian
wrote: "The child of the Victorian period was subject to an extraordinary set
of pressures through the social ambitions of the family . . . The pressures brought
to bear on many Victorian children were indeed of explosive intensity." (Stephen
Kern, "The Psychodynamics of the Victorian Family," *History of Childhood
Quarterly* 1 [Winter 1974], 457.) My interpretation of the Victorian middle-
class family is drawn from a variety of secondary sources, including Gay, *The Bourgeois Experience*; Patricia Branca, *Silent Sisterhood: Middle-Class Women in the
Victorian Home* (London, 1975); Lloyd De Mause, ed., *The History of Childhood* (New York, 1975); Deborah Gorham, *The Victorian Girl and the Feminine
Ideal* (Bloomington, Ind., 1982); Lawrence Stone, *The Family, Sex and Marriage
in England, 1500–1800* (New York, 1979); Anthony S. Wohl, ed., *The Victorian
Family: Structure and Stresses* (London, 1978); Steven Mintz, *A Prism of Expectations: The Family in Victorian Culture* (New York, 1983).

16. [Society for Promoting Christian Knowledge], *Talks to Girls by One
of Themselves, on the Difficulties, Duties, and Joys of a Girl's Life* (London,
1894), p. iv. On the idealization of American middle-class girlhood among late-
nineteenth-century evangelical women, see Joan Jacobs Brumberg, "Zenanas
and Girlless Villages," *Journal of American History* 69 (September 1982), 347–
371. Around the turn of the century there developed an elaborate iconography

of girlhood that included visual representations by Charles Dana Gibson and Howard Chandler Christy, poetry by James Whitcomb Riley, serialized novels, popular songs, and college humor. Much of this material venerated the distinctiveness of the American girl and hinged on the idea that in the United States middle-class girls were unencumbered by their sexuality.

17. Karl Krauss (1899–1936), the Viennese satirist and social critic, observed the "business character of bourgeois marriage." See Allan Janik and Stephen Toulmin, *Wittgenstein's Vienna* (London, 1973). Banks, *Prosperity and Parenthood*, pp. 32–47, describes some of the difficulties of the Victorians over the issue of marriage. Many young people were unable to marry because even jointly they did not have enough money; £300 per annum was the commonly given formula for a middle-class marriage that preserved a certain standard of gentility. Much of nineteenth-century British fiction centers on the problems of young women in making love economically viable. Family needs frequently took precedence over personal desires. For example, in George Eliot's *Daniel Deronda* (London, 1876), Gwendolyn Harleth marries the wealthiest man available in order to improve the status of her mother and sisters and save herself from "working-out" as a governess. In Anthony Trollope's *Phineas Finn* (London, 1869) and in *Phineas Redux* (London, 1874) the young Laura Standish elects to wed Robert Kennedy in spite of her affection for Phineas Finn. She chooses to become Lady Laura Kennedy in order to establish a financial position to aid her indebted brother; as Lady Laura she is forever plagued by her decision not to marry the impoverished man she loves. Trollope's *Ralph the Heir* describes the sensible daughter of an ambitious and successful artisan who refuses to succumb to her father's pressure to marry an attractive gentleman who owes him money. Despite the attractions of his gentility, Polly Neefit opts for a man of humbler origins precisely because she knows that the gentleman would ultimately make her parents and herself uncomfortable and self-conscious about their lack of polish. Trollope was a master of the novel that centered on problems of marriage, money, and career.

18. Banks, *Prosperity and Parenthood*, pp. 68–69, makes the point that expansion of standards rather than higher prices accounted for the increased expenditures of the middle class on food and drink. Although there was much discussion of the correct amount to eat and how to distribute food during the day, most authors agreed that two to three meals were commonplace. See Dio Lewis, *Talks about People's Stomachs* (Boston, 1870), pp. 201–204. In *Health Fragments, or Steps towards True Life* (New York, 1875) George Everett and Susan Everett stated the golden rule of eating: "Eat only at regular hours, and never then unless you are hungry, nor oftener than three times a day" (p. 34). For an excellent description of the daily food regimen of a British middle-class family in the 1870s see Banks, *Prosperity and Parenthood*, appendix 2.

For a wide-ranging history of table manners see Norbert Elias, *The Civilizing Process* (Oxford, 1978). Elias traces the transition from communal eating with minimal regulation of individual eating habits to eating that is more individualized but controlled by unarticulated behavioral norms. As manners became more complex and differentiated, each eater had his or her own equipment.

19. Everett and Everett, *Health Fragments*, p. 38.

20. Marion Harland, *Eve's Daughters; or, Common Sense for Maid, Wife, and Mother* (Farmingdale, N.Y., 1885; reprint ed., 1978), p. 152.

21. The troubled relationship between middle-class Victorian mothers and daughters and the grooming of daughters for marriage is discussed in Carol A. Martin, "No Angel in the House: Victorian Mothers and Daughters in George Eliot and Elizabeth Gaskell," *Midwest Quarterly* 24 (1983), 297–314; Lenore Davidoff, *The Best Circles* (Totowa, N.J., 1973), p. 54.

22. See for example Harland, *Eve's Daughters*.

23. Michael Brooks, "Love and Possession in a Victorian Household: The Example of the Ruskins," in Wohl, *The Victorian Family*, pp. 82–100. Another relevant family study is Howard M. Feinstein, *Becoming William James* (Ithaca, N.Y., 1984). In *The Bourgeois Experience*, Peter Gay writes, "The ideology of unreserved love within the family was attractive but exhausting" (p. 444).

24. Gay, *The Bourgeois Experience*, p. 445, notes that "the nineteenth century was an age in which members of the middle classes aspired to rooms of their own." American middle-class attention to the ambience of girls' rooms was pervasive: women's periodicals in the late nineteenth century, the *Ladies' Home Journal* for one, had a regular column on the subject. Advice books in both Britain and the United States assumed that most girls had a room of their own or that they shared it with a same-sex sibling. Reports on nineteenth-century anorectics featured girls doing exercises alone in their own rooms. By contrast, working-class children and adolescents did not have private space. See Anthony S. Wohl, "Sex and the Single Room: Incest among the Victorian Working Class," in Wohl, *The Victorian Family*, pp. 197–216. An undergraduate paper by Amanda Bryans provided me with useful information about the rooms of Victorian girls.

25. On Victorian diary keeping see Gay, *The Bourgeois Experience*, pp. 445–460.

26. Priscilla Robertson, "Home as Nest: Middle-Class Childhood in Nineteenth Century Europe," in De Mause, *History of Childhood*, p. 417.

27. Ibid.

28. Everett and Everett, *Health Fragments*, p. 34.

29. Wet nursing was rapidly disappearing in England by the 1860s; British medicine in the years between 1870 and 1900 strongly disapproved of the practice. But in England domestics did feed children, particularly those of the upper classes, where parents and children often ate separately. See Theresa McBride, "'As the Twig is Bent': The Victorian Nanny," in Wohl, *The Victorian Family*, pp. 46–47. By contrast, in *The Education of American Girls* (New York, 1874), p. 25, Anna Brackett warned mothers against allowing servants to make or even pack lunches for their children. In America, boarding schools were also widely criticized for the food they served girls and for the poor eating habits they encouraged. See W. W. Hall, *Health and Good Living* (New York, 1873), p. 81. In other words, in America no one but Mother would do as cook.

30. Everett and Everett, *Health Fragments*, p. 152.

31. Gay, *The Bourgeois Experience*, p. 451.

32. Ibid., p. 453. We often describe this kind of behavior as passive-aggressive in character.

6. Therapeutic Intervention

1. Samuel Wilks, *Lectures on Diseases of the Nervous System. Delivered at Guy's Hospital* (Philadelphia, 1878), p. 384. On Adams see [J. and A. Churchill], *London and Provincial Medical Directory* (London, 1886), p. 65, and ibid., 1888, p. 72. Adams received an M.D. degree from St. Andrews in 1859 and was a member of the Royal College of Surgeons. He held different municipal positions: medical officer and vaccinator for Barnes district of the Richmond Union, and director of surgery for the Metropolitan Police. W[illiam] S[moult] Playfair, "Note on the So-Called 'Anorexia Nervosa,'" *Lancet* (April 28, 1888), 818. To the best of my knowledge, the scrapbook of anorectics no longer exists. Playfair was the author of *A Handbook on Obstetric Operations* (London, 1865), *A Treatise on the Science and Practice of Midwifery* (London, 1876), *The Puerperal Fever* (London, 1881), and *Systematic Treatment of Nervous Prostration and Hysteria* (London, 1883). In his 1883 work Playfair indicated that he subscribed to the same methods (diet, massage, electricity, seclusion, and rest) that were associated with Silas Weir Mitchell, the famous Philadelphia neurologist who treated many different women with nervous disorders that included anorexia. See note 11 below and pp. 18–39 of *Systematic Treatment*. For biographical details on Playfair see [Churchill], *Medical Directory*, 1888, p. 245. A school for midwives (Playfair School of Midwifery) operated in Chicago in 1898.

2. Clifford Allbutt, *A System of Medicine*, vol. 3 (New York, 1905), p. 474. Clinical reports of anorexic hyperactivity revealed a good deal about the social life of the patients as well as the attitude of doctors toward adolescent girls. The strange unrest that overcame the anorectic was usually expressed in highly individualistic exercise, such as solitary walks, which took the girl away from her family and friends. With rare exceptions, these activities did not interrupt any real work, because these were young women of leisure. In some cases anorectics were so frenzied that they upset the entire household. "Sometimes the girl will think that exercise is very necessary and will take long walks far beyond her strength, or she will try the eccoprotic [purgative] powers of leaping and dancing in her bedroom before daybreak, until the awakened household protests against the continuance of such preposterous therapeutics." Samuel Gee, *Medical Lectures and Aphorisms* (London, 1908), pp. 43–44. On Gee see [Churchill], *Medical Directory*, 1888, p. 159.

The doctor in a different case noted: "The patient is exceedingly fond of long walks. As she is growing thinner with enormous rapidity, they are forbidden to her. She then begins to walk, from morning to night, up and down the little garden of the house, which was likewise forbidden to her. Then she plays all day at shuttlecock. It is prescribed that she stay in her room; there she gives herself up to violent exercises. Even in bed she goes on with her gambols and summersaults." The frantic gymnastics of this seventeen-year-old led her doctor to take away her clothes as a means of controlling her activity. M. Wallet, "Deux cas d'anorexie hystérique," in *Nouvelle iconographie de la Salpêtrière*, ed. J.-M. Charcot (Paris, 1892), pp. 276–277. See also Silas Weir Mitchell, *Lectures on Diseases of the Nervous System, Especially in Women* (Philadelphia, 1885), pp. 229–230, 243–244; John K. Mitchell, *Self-Help for Nervous Women* (Philadelphia, 1909), p. 103; W. J. Collins, "Anorexia Nervosa," *Lancet* (January 27, 1894), 203; Pierre Janet, *The Major Symptoms of Hysteria* (New York, 1907), p. 228.

3. Charles Féré, *Pathology of Emotions: Physiological and Clinical Studies* (London, 1899), p. 79. Lasègue also took this position. See Janet, *The Major Symptoms of Hysteria*, pp. 239–243, and *Les obsessions et la psychasthénie* (Paris, 1903), p. 35, for a somewhat different view. Janet regarded hyperactivity as one of the two primary characteristics of true anorexia nervosa, but he did not think the activity had a conscious motivation.

4. Gee, *Medical Lectures*, p. 42.

5. Thomas Stretch Dowse, "Anorexia Nervosa," *Medical Press and Circular* 32 (August 3, 1881), 96; Playfair, "Note," p. 818; Lockhardt Stephens, "Case of Anorexia Nervosa; Necropsy," *Lancet* (January 5, 1895), 31; Timothy McGillicuddy, *Functional Disorders of the Nervous System in Women* (New York, 1896), p. 178; Féré, *Pathology of Emotions*, p. 78; Gee, *Medical Lectures*, p. 48; Allbutt, *A System of Medicine*, p. 474. See also Wallet, "Deux cas," pp. 277–278, for a description of the "stubbornness" of the patient and the "softness" of her parents, especially the father.

6. Sigmund Freud, of course, is an exception; Freud regarded anorexia nervosa as a depression of sexual appetites.

7. Dowse, "Anorexia Nervosa," pp. 95–96.

8. *AA/BA Newsletter* (November 1985), 7.

9. Gee, *Medical Lectures*, p. 47.

10. J.-M. Charcot, *On Diseases of the Nervous System* (London, 1889), pp. 213–214.

11. Mitchell, *Lectures*, pp. 265–283. See "Silas Weir Mitchell" in *Dictionary of American Biography*, vol. 7, ed. Dumas Malone (New York, 1935), pp. 62–65. In the past two decades Mitchell has been the subject of important new feminist interpretations: see Barbara Sicherman, "The Uses of a Diagnosis: Doctors, Patients, and Neurasthenia," *Journal of the History of Medicine and Allied Sciences* 32 (1977), 33–54; Carroll Smith-Rosenberg, *Disorderly Conduct: Visions of Gender in Victorian America* (New York, 1985), pp. 197–216; G. Barker-Benfield, *The Horrors of a Half-Known Life* (New York, 1976); Jean Strouse, *Alice James* (New York, 1980). Mitchell treated a number of prominent American women: Jane Addams, Winifred Howells (daughter of William Dean Howells), Edith Wharton, and Charlotte Perkins Gilman. Gilman made Mitchell her model for the doctor in "The Yellow Wallpaper," a short story about a woman's struggle with acute depression and with her treatment (the rest cure). See "Why I Wrote 'The Yellow Wallpaper,'" in *The Charlotte Perkins Gilman Reader*, ed. Ann J. Lane (New York, 1980), pp. 19–20.

12. All of the following explicitly recommended removal from home: All-

butt, Charcot, Dowse, Féré, Gee, Gull, Mitchell, Myrtle, Osler, Playfair, and Wallet.

13. H. E. Astles, "Anorexia in Young Girls Unaccompanied with Visceral Disease," *Proceedings of South Australian Branch of the British Medical Association* (1882), 31–32.

14. On the private asylums in Britain see William L. Parry-Jones, *The Trade in Lunacy: A Study of Private Madhouses in England in the Eighteenth and Nineteenth Centuries* (London, 1972). Private asylums were conducted as business propositions for the personal profit of the proprietor(s). "Hysterical homes" were another private-for-profit variation; they serviced a less disturbed clientele but specialized in nervous disorders. The cottage hospital was a medical facility that took paying patients.

In the United States the private "madhouse" trade did not expand until the 1880s and it was never as highly developed as in England. Here, as in Britain, young women with anorexia nervosa usually were not institutionalized. Nevertheless, some anorectics were probably sent to a type of institution known as the private proprietary hospital. For example, in the 1850s Edward Jarvis, a prominent figure in American medicine, provided residential services to eight or nine patients in his home and had five or six in nearby residences. Jarvis and his wife were the primary caretakers, although the families did hire private attendants if the patients required it. According to Gerald Grob, *Edward Jarvis and the Medical World of Nineteenth Century America* (Knoxville, Tenn., 1978), pp. 59–60, the cost of being cared for in this way was three to four times the cost of care in exclusive private hospitals. Still, families were willing to spend larger amounts to avoid institutionalization.

Hydrotherapeutic institutions appear to have been considered appropriate for anorectics in the United States and in France. Charcot, in *On Diseases*, says: "In Paris, during the last fifteen years, establishments of hydrotherapy take patients who are so disposed in hand with much success" (p. 210). By "so disposed," Charcot meant hysterical. For the United States, this was confirmed by McGillicuddy, *Functional Disorders*, p. 178.

Unfortunately, the small, private institutions that treated middle-class patients with anorexia nervosa were notoriously lax in terms of keeping and preserving clinical case records. I have had to rely largely on published materials, along with some unpublished records drawn from institutions where the authors of these articles worked. My review of the records at a number of different mental asylums (public and private) suggests that patients with anorexia nervosa were treated by and large outside institutions, a fact that makes historical investigation of their experience extremely difficult.

15. John Ogle, "A Case of Hysteria: 'Temper Disease,'" *British Medical Journal* (July 16, 1870), 59.

16. William Gull, "Anorexia Nervosa," *Transactions of The Clinical Society of London* 7 (1874), 28.

17. Dowse, "Anorexia Nervosa," pp. 95–97; *Medical Press and Circular* (August 17, 1881), pp. 147–148. Dowse received his medical degree in 1868 from the University of Aberdeen, an institution that did not have enormous

prestige in the London medical world. He held a number of appointments at minor hospitals: North London Hospital for Consumption and the West End Hospital for Diseases of the Nervous System, Central London Sick Asylum, and Charing Cross Hospital. These appointments varied across specialty areas; apparently he dabbled in neurology and dermatology. See [Churchill], *Medical Directory*, 1888, p. 135. On the Hospital for Epilepsy and Paralysis see Sir Henry Burdett, *Hospitals and Charities* (London, 1902), p. 270.

Although Dowse's article is obviously imitative of Gull, he began the report with an overview of the history of the syndrome, mentioning Samuel Fenwick, Samuel Wilks, and Forbes Winslow as contemporary practitioners who published on the subject. Dowse was not an inept reporter; his article is significant in that it notes the presence of hostility between the mother and the daughter and includes engravings of a patient.

18. William Gull, "Anorexia Nervosa," *Lancet* (March 17, 1888), 516–517. On Petersfield in particular see Burdett, *Hospitals and Charities*, p. 450. The doctor who referred the anorexic patient to Gull was Albert Warren Leachman of Fairley, Petersfield, Hants, a settlement of about two thousand persons. Leachman, a member of the Royal College of Surgeons, had received an M.D. degree from St. Andrews in 1860. In 1888 he was head of the six-bed cottage hospital in Petersfield, which charged anywhere between 4 and 8 shillings per week according to the patient's means. Leachman was also the medical officer in charge of public vaccinations for the third district of the Petersfield Union, a position for which he received an annual salary of £65. See [Churchill], *Medical Directory*, 1888, p. 711. In a description of the Petersfield Cottage Hospital (pp. 219–221), Burdett called it "more charming than . . . any other in Hampshire."

19. Gull, "Anorexia Nervosa," p. 516.

20. *Lancet* (March 24, 1888), 583–584.

21. "Death of Sir William Gull," London *Times*, January 30, 1890. Gull's obituary said he was the first to describe the adult cretinoid condition called myxedema, but said nothing about anorexia nervosa.

22. See for example Wilks, *Lectures*, p. 384; Mitchell, *Lectures*, pp. 242–244; William Osler, *The Principles and Practice of Medicine* (New York, 1892), p. 973; Allbutt, *A System of Medicine*, vol. 2, pp. 474–475.

23. Playfair, "Note," p. 817.

24. Because it incorporated so many different symptoms, neurasthenia was a useful catchall diagnosis, quickly becoming the predominant malady of the urban middle classes in the United States. In the 1890s *McClure's Magazine* called it the "national disease of America." American neurasthenics—particularly those with ample resources and time—sought relief in many places: at neurologists' offices, at hydropathic institutes, in Europe, in the hands of masseurs, and in the chairs of doctors who extolled the value of electric shock. On neurasthenia see John S. Haller and Robin M. Haller, *The Physician and Sexuality in Victorian America* (Urbana, Ill., 1974); Sicherman, "The Uses of a Diagnosis"; and Howard M. Feinstein, *Becoming William James* (Ithaca, N.Y., 1984). Edward Wakefield's "Nervousness: The National Disease of America," *McClure's Magazine* (1893–94), 302–307, is only one of many journalistic pieces on the disease. See George M. Beard, *American Nervousness, Its Causes and*

Consequences (New York, 1881) for a complete statement. Beard first used the term "neurasthenia" in the *Boston Medical and Surgical Journal* 3 (1869), 217. On George Beard see Charles E. Rosenberg, *On Science and American Social Thought* (Baltimore, 1978), pp. 98–108.

25. Playfair, "Note," p. 818.

26. Ibid., p. 817.

27. Ibid., p. 818.

28. On women's higher education in the United States and Britain in the nineteenth century see Thomas Woody, *A History of Women's Higher Education in the United States* (New York, 1929); Patricia Albjerg Graham, "Expansion and Exclusion: A History of Women in Higher Education," *Signs* 3 (Summer 1978), 759–773; Helen Horowitz, *Alma Mater: Design and Experience in the Women's Colleges from Their Nineteenth Century Beginnings to 1930* (New York, 1984); Barbara Miller Solomon, *In the Company of Educated Women* (New York, 1985); Mabel Newcomer, *A Century of Higher Education for Women* (New York, 1959). On the coeducational controversy see Rosalind Rosenberg, *Beyond Separate Spheres: Intellectual Roots of Modern Feminism* (New Haven, 1982), pp. 43–44; Woody, *A History*, pp. 295–303. On higher education for women in nineteenth-century Britain see Joan Burstyn, *Victorian Education and the Ideal of Womanhood* (London, 1980) and "Education and Sex: The Medical Case against Higher Education for Women in England, 1870–1900," *Proceedings of the American Philosophical Society* 117 (April 1973), 78–89; Joyce Sender Pedersen, "The Reform of Women's Secondary and Higher Education: Institutional Change and Social Values in Mid and Late Victorian England," *History of Education Quarterly* 19 (1979), 61–91; Martha Vicinus, *Independent Women: Work and Community: For Single Women, 1850–1920* (Chicago, 1985). Vicinus notes that major educational reforms affecting women occurred between 1869 and 1887, the very period in which British medicine became so interested in anorexia nervosa.

29. T. S. Clouston, "Female Education from a Medical Point of View," *Popular Science Monthly* 24 (1884), 322–323.

30. E. H. Clarke, *Sex in Education; or, A Fair Chance for Girls* (Boston, 1873).

31. Ogle, who actually preferred a more sympathetic nursing style in cases of hysteria, called the professional hospital nurse "abrupt, rough, and ready" ("A Case of Hysteria," p. 59). By 1870 British nursing had been affected by the reforms associated with Florence Nightingale. Nightingale's training school at St. Thomas' Hospital, established in 1860, fostered the idea that women of character and intelligence could be attracted into nursing. The "new nursing," as advocated by Nightingale and Margaret Lonsdale at Guy's Hospital, worked to set aside the old conception of nurses as indigent, immoral, and intemperate ex-patients, working only to earn their keep. Women trained in the new nursing were the very best kind of person to place in a private-duty assignment in the home of decent people, but at the same time they were problematic because they provided a constant challenge to medical authority. Recent literature on the history of nursing in the United States and in Britain is rich and instructive, suggesting that there were significant professional tensions between physicians

and nurses as well as among different kinds of nurses. In addition to Lucy Ridgeley Seymer, *A General History of Nursing* (London, 1956) and Lena Dixon Dietz, *History and Modern Nursing* (Philadelphia, 1963), newer work sets out important developments in the Anglo-American world. See for example the essays in Celia Davies, ed., *Rewriting Nursing History* (London, 1980); Ellen Condliffe Lagemann, ed., *Nursing History: New Perspectives, New Possibilities* (New York, 1983); Susan Reverby, *Ordered to Care: The Dilemma of American Nursing, 1850–1945* (New York, 1987).

32. Playfair, "Note," p. 818.

33. Silas Weir Mitchell, *Fat and Blood: And How to Make Them* (Philadelphia, 1878), pp. 36–37. On Mitchell, see note 11 above.

34. Ibid., p. 7.

35. Ibid., p. 42.

36. Astles, "Anorexia in Young Girls," p. 32; Osler, *Practice of Medicine*, p. 973; idem, "A Case of Anorexia Nervosa," *West London Medical Journal* 9 (January 1904), 112, and ibid. (April 1904), 204–206.

37. [A. S. Myrtle], "Anorexia Nervosa," *Lancet* (May 5, 1888), 899. Myrtle received an M.D. degree from the University of Edinburgh in 1844 and served as consulting physician to Harrogate Bath Hospital. He contributed to British medical journals primarily on the subject of chronic diseases and therapies used at the Harrogate spa. See [Churchill], *Medical Directory*, 1888, p. 774.

38. [D. De Berdt Hovell], "Anorexia Nervosa," *Lancet* (May 12, 1888), 949. On De Berdt Hovell see [Churchill], *Medical Directory*, 1888, p. 183. It is not clear where De Berdt Hovell received his medical degree in 1839, but in 1847 he became a fellow of the Royal College of Surgeons.

39. [De Berdt Hovell], "Anorexia Nervosa," p. 949.

40. London Hospital, Physician's Casebooks, MS 107 (1897), n.p. On Stephen MacKenzie see [Churchill], *Medical Directory*, 1888, p. 212. Mac-Kenzie's father, Morrell, was a well-known specialist in diseases of the throat and author of *Diseases of the Pharynx, Larynx, and Trachea* (New York, 1880). Morrell MacKenzie wrote about "neuroses of sensation" in the throat and related this to hysterical women and girls. See *Diseases*, pp. 83–85, 308. At the Clinical Society meeting in 1873 where Gull presented his description of anorexia nervosa, a doctor remarked that in past times such patients (anorectics) were sent to "Dr. (Morrell] MacKenzie" generally for treatment of "globus hystericus." See "Clinical Society," *Medical Times and Gazette* 2 (November 8, 1873), 534–536.

Stephen MacKenzie was the author of "On a Case of Anorexia Nervosa Vel Hysterica," *Lancet* (March 31, 1888), 613–614. In this earlier case, also treated at London Hospital, the patient was a nineteen-year-old who had been a governess for a short period. MacKenzie said of his patient that she was "not of the class usually treated in hospital." The girl was living at home when the malady began, and her mother made the decision to place her in London Hospital when her emaciation became severe.

In "The Victorian Governess: Status Incongruence in Family and Society," *Victorian Studies* 14 (September 1970), 7–26, M. Jeanne Peterson analyzes the contradictory situation of the Victorian governess and suggests that some young women periodically turned to this "ladylike" form of work when their family could not support them. The only other reported case of an anorectic who worked is A. M. Edge, "A Case of Anorexia Nervosa," *Lancet* (April 28, 1888), 818; the patient was a nineteen-year-old who had been employed as a book-folder in or near Manchester.

41. MacKenzie and others continued to use Lasègue's terminology rather than Gull's. In the hospital register, case 107 is classified under the broader headings "Diseases of the Nervous System" and "Hysteria and Hypochon-driasis." The patient's height is not given.

42. Charcot, *On Diseases*, p. 214.

43. Stephens, "A Case of Anorexia Nervosa," p. 31. Stephens' 1895 report was discussed as a landmark in the history of the disease in John A. Ryle, "Anorexia Nervosa," *Lancet* 231 (October 17, 1936), 893–896. Ryle's article was given in London as the Schorstein Memorial Lecture on October 15, 1936. He began by displaying Gull's engravings, then proceeded to show the photo-graph of "the first fully recorded fatal case" of anorexia nervosa—a picture supplied, he said, through "the courtesy of another old Guy's man, Dr. Lockhardt Stephens of Emsworth." Stephens was a reputable provincial practitioner asso-ciated with Emsworth for over forty years; in 1919 he received the C.B.E. for his service in World War I. His obituary in the *British Medical Journal* 1 (June 1, 1940), 915, described him as a "good British Medical Association man . . . the sort . . . who could be depended on to work for the profession and the Association either locally or centrally." On Stephens see [Churchill], *Medical Directory*, 1895, p. 1057.

44. At Emsworth patients were accepted by letter of recommendation from a financial supporter and by payment of 5 to 10 shillings per week. Cottage hospitals took paying patients and were run by country practitioners who sought a convenient "receiving home" for patients who required a professional nursing environment. Individuals with infectious or incurable diseases were not admitted. On the cottage hospital movement see Horace Swete, *Handy Book of Cottage Hospitals* (London, 1870) and Sir Henry Burdett, *Cottage Hospitals* (London, 1896), p. 388.

45. Stephens, "A Case of Anorexia Nervosa," p. 31.

46. Ibid.

47. Ibid. How the mother's presence actually affected the patient is unclear. Did the mother pander to the girl or make her agitated? Did her presence make the girl more resistant to eating? Or did the mother's proximity prevent the doctors from forcibly feeding the girl?

48. As early as 1859 the editors of the *Lancet*, realizing the potential of adapting photographic images to medical purposes, called photography the "Art of Truth." Quoted in Joel Stanley Reiser, *Medicine and the Reign of Technology* (Cambridge, Mass., 1978), pp. 56–57. Reiser briefly discusses still photography in medicine in the context of the evolution of X rays, the ophthalmoscope, and the laryngoscope.

49. Stephen Marcus, *The Other Victorians: A Study of Sexuality and Por-nography in Mid-Nineteenth Century England* (New York, 1966); Ronald Pear-sall, *The Worm in the Bud: The World of Victorian Sexuality* (London, 1969);

Jean Hagstrum, *Sex and Sensibility, Ideal and Erotic Love from Milton to Mozart* (Chicago, 1980); Peter Gay, *The Bourgeois Experience: The Education of the Senses* (New York, 1984); F. Barry Smith, "Sexuality in Britain, 1800–1900. Some Suggested Revisions," in *A Widening Sphere: Changing Roles of Victorian Women*, ed. Martha Vicinus (Bloomington, Ind., 1977), pp. 182–198.

7. The Appetite as Voice

1. The best statement in the extensive literature on the relation of culture to obsessive-compulsive disorder and anorexia nervosa is Albert Rothenberg, "Eating Disorder as a Modern Obsessive-Compulsive Syndrome," *Psychiatry* 49 (February 1986), 45–53. Another historian interested in the changing symptomatology of hysteria is Edward Shorter. See his "The First Great Increase in Anorexia Nervosa," *Journal of Social History* 21 (Fall 1987), 69–96.

2. This point is made by Laurence Kirmayer, "Culture, Affect and Somatization, Part II," *Transcultural Psychiatric Research Review* 21 (1984), 254.

3. London Hospital Physician's Casebooks, MS 107 (1897); quoted in Pierre Janet, *The Major Symptoms of Hysteria* (New York, 1907), p. 234; Max Wallet, "Deux cas d'anorexie hystérique," in *Nouvelle iconographie de la Salpêtrière*, ed. J.-M. Charcot (Paris, 1892), p. 278.

4. See Janet, *Major Symptoms*, p. 234, for these terms. Janet did, however, have a more sophisticated interpretation based on his idea of "body shame."

5. My description of late-nineteenth-century examinations is drawn from clinical case records and from Joel Stanley Reiser, *Medicine and the Reign of Technology* (Cambridge, Mass., 1978), and Charles E. Rosenberg, "The Practice of Medicine in New York a Century Ago," *Bulletin of the History of Medicine* 41 (May–June 1967), 223–253; D. W. Cathell, *The Physician Himself and What He Should Add to His Scientific Acquirements* (Baltimore, 1882).

6. I have tried to incorporate, and move beyond, the perspective on male doctor–female patient relations provided in Barbara Ehrenreich and Deirdre English, *Witches, Midwives and Nurses* (New York, n.d.) and *Complaints and Disorders: The Sexual Politics of Sickness* (Old Westbury, N.Y., 1973). At the outset I asked, Can the absence of a patient voice be attributed solely to misogyny and authoritarianism on the part of doctors? I think not. Without discounting the relevance of both these well-known attributes of nineteenth-century medical men, I posit that the silence stemmed from a complex of medical and social factors that shaped interactions between doctors and patients in such a way that doctors really had no coherent, firsthand information to give. In a system of medicine that emphasized physical diagnosis, somatic complaints were primary. Traditional ideas about hysteria in women and girls prevailed, providing the rationale for medical and moral therapy.

7. J.-M. Charcot, *Clinical Lectures on Diseases of the Nervous System* (London, 1889), p. 214.

8. See for example John Ogle, "A Case of Hysteria: 'Temper Disease,'" *British Medical Journal* (July 16, 1870), 59; William Gull, "Anorexia Nervosa (Apepsia Hysterica, Anorexia Hysterica)," *Transactions of the Clinical Society of London* 7 (1874), 22–28; Thomas Stretch Dowse, "Anorexia Nervosa," *Medical Press and Circular* 32 (August 3, 1881), 95–97, and ibid. (August 17, 1881), 147–148; W. J. Collins, "Anorexia Nervosa," *Lancet* (January 27, 1894), 203.

9. Charles Féré, *The Pathology of Emotions* (London, 1899), pp. 79–80. The home was designated a Maison de Santé.

10. Ogle, "A Case of Hysteria," pp. 57–58.

11. The strongest statement on the separation of male and female spheres is Carroll Smith-Rosenberg, "The Female World of Love and Ritual: Relations between Women in Nineteenth-Century America," *Signs* 1 (1975), 1–29. In addition to this generative article see Nancy Cott, *The Bonds of Womanhood* (New Haven, 1977); Ann Douglas, *The Feminization of American Culture* (New York, 1977); Mary Ryan, *Cradle of the Middle Class* (New York, 1982). Ellen Rothman's *Hands and Hearts: A History of Courtship in America* (New York, 1984) provides some rethinking of the Smith-Rosenberg thesis.

12. John Ryle to Parkes Weber, January 27, 1939, PP/FDW F. Parkes Weber Papers, Wellcome Institute, London.

13. Ann Douglas Wood, "The Fashionable Diseases: Women's Complaints and Their Treatment in Nineteenth Century America," *Journal of Interdisciplinary History* 4 (1973), 25–52; John S. Haller, Jr., and Robin Haller, *The Physician and Sexuality in Victorian America* (Urbana, Ill., 1974). See also Judith Walzer Leavitt, ed., *Women and Health in America: Historical Readings* (Madison, Wis., 1984).

14. Augustus Hoppin, *A Fashionable Sufferer; or, Chapters from Life's Comedy* (Boston, 1883), pp. 16–17, 35, 55, 135.

15. Marion Harland, *Eve's Daughters; or, Common Sense for Maid, Wife, and Mother*, with an introduction by Sheila M. Rothman (Farmingdale, N.Y., 1885; reprint ed., 1978), pp. 135, 153.

16. See for example Elizabeth Stoddard, *The Morgesons* (New York, 1862). Stoddard's novel depended in large part on the contrast between two adolescent sisters in a wealthy New England family. Thirteen-year-old Veronica was in a premature adolescent decline and remained at home, isolated from society; sixteen-year-old Cassandra was vigorous and "about in the world." Cassandra served as narrator of the story and presented many intimate details of the behavior of her ailing and dyspeptic sister.

Stoddard never told the reader what was exactly wrong with the invalid Veronica, but she appeared to combine both dyspepsia and anorexia. Cassandra explained: "Delicacy of constitution the doctor called the disorder. She had no strength, no appetite, and looked more elfish than ever. She would not stay in bed, and could not sit up, so father had a chair made for her, in which she could recline comfortably." Much of the trouble with Veronica revolved around her lack of appetite, complicated by a simultaneous interest in food preparation and in the consumption habits of others. From her chair she directed the family maid to cook elaborate dishes that she would not eat.

For long periods of time Veronica Morgeson ate only a single kind of food. "As we began our meal," Cassandra recounted, "Veronica came in from the kitchen with a plate of toasted crackers. She set the plate down, and gravely shook hands with me, saying she had concluded to live entirely on toast, but supposed I would eat all sorts of food as usual." Although Veronica ate virtually nothing at the family table, she asked many questions about food and cast aspersions on her sister's normal appetite. Whenever Cassandra said she was hungry, Veronica's eyes "sparkled with disdain." Above and beyond her physical problems with digestion, Veronica Morgeson took some strange emotional delight in her denial of hunger. Her reclusive existence, her listless appetite, and her sensitive stomach all implied that her body was subordinated to other, higher, more spiritual concerns.

17. Bernard Hollander, *Nervous Disorders of Women* (London, 1916), p. 77.

18. For the general history of chlorosis see Frank Panettiere, "What Ever Happened to Chlorosis?" *Alaska Medicine* 15 (May 1973), 68–70; Eugene Stransky, "On the History of Chlorosis," *Episteme* 8: 1 (1974), 26–46; and Ronald E. McFarland, "The Rhetoric of Medicine: Lord Herbert's and Thomas Carew's Poems of Green Sickness," *Journal of the History of Medicine* 30 (July 1975), 250–258. For more perceptive in-depth studies of Great Britain see Karl Figlio, "Chlorosis and Chronic Disease in Nineteenth Century Britain: The Social Constitution of Somatic Illness in a Capitalist Society," *Social History* 3 (1978), 167–197; and Irvine Loudon, "Chlorosis, Anemia, and Anorexia Nervosa," *British Medical Journal* 281 (December 20–27, 1980), 1669–75; and idem, "The Diseases Called Chlorosis," *Psychological Medicine* 14 (1984), 27–36. For the United States see R. P. Hudson, "The Biography of Disease: Lessons Learned from Chlorosis," *Bulletin of the History of Medicine* 51 (1977), 448–463; S. R. Huang, "Chlorosis and the Iron Controversy: An Aspect of Nineteenth-Century Medicine," Ph.D. diss., Harvard University, 1978; Joan Jacobs Brumberg, "Chlorotic Girls, 1870–1920: An Historical Perspective on Female Adolescence," *Child Development* 53 (December 1982), pp. 1468–77; A. C. Siddall, "Chlorosis—Etiology Reconsidered," *Bulletin of the History of Medicine* 56 (1982), 254–260.

19. J. H. Montgomery, *Clinical Observations on Cases of Simple Anemia or Chlorosis Occurring in Young Women in the Decade Following Puberty* (Erie, Pa., 1919), n.p.

20. *Elmira Daily Gazette and Free Press*, March 26, 1898. On women and the patent medicine business see Sarah Stage, *Female Complaints: Lydia Pinkham and the Business of Women's Medicine* (New York, 1979).

21. Loudon, "Chlorosis," posits that after 1850 chlorosis incorporated at least three different kinds of disorders common in young women, each involving loss of weight, anemias, and amenorrhea. He argues that chlorosis was a functional disorder closely related to anorexia nervosa: they were two "closely related conditions, each a manifestation of the same type of psychological reaction to the turbulence of puberty and adolescence" (p. 1675). Loudon is correct that the two diseases had much in common, and his observation probably means that there was more anorexia nervosa than heretofore thought. Anorexia nervosa

was usually a class-specific diagnosis, however. Given the family dynamic that was part of the disorder, working-class girls were unlikely to develop anorexia nervosa. Moreover, if a similar pattern of noneating developed in a working-class girl, family reverberations were different and medicine was more likely to call the disorder chlorosis or depression.

22. G. Stanley Hall, *Adolescence*, vol. 1 (New York, 1904), pp. 252–253.

23. Lillie A. Williams, "The Distressing Malady of Being Seventeen Years Old," *Ladies' Home Journal* (May 1909), p. 10.

24. James Henry Bennet, *Nutrition in Health and Disease* (London, 1877), pp. 59–60, 170. Among others who noted that children and women had more easily disturbed digestive systems are Elizabeth Blackwell, *The Laws of Life* (New York, 1852), and Anna Brackett, *The Education of American Girls* (New York, 1874).

25. Edward Smith, *Practical Dietary for Families, Schools, and the Labouring Classes* (London, 1864), p. 141.

26. These descriptions are from Harland, *Eve's Daughters*, pp. 111–113; see also Charles E. Simon, "A Study of Thirty-One Cases of Chlorosis," *American Journal of Medical Sciences* 113 (April 1897), 399–423; Lucien Warner, *A Popular Treatise on the Functions and Diseases of Women* (New York, 1875), p. 70; E. H. Ruddock, *The Lady's Manual of Homeopathic Treatment* (New York, 1869), p. 32.

27. Simon, "Thirty-One Cases," pp. 413–414.

28. Mary Wood-Allen, *What a Young Girl Ought to Know* (Philadelphia, 1905), p. 89.

29. Harland, *Eve's Daughters*, pp. 111–115. The notion of an adolescent decline had some foundation. Among adolescents tuberculosis was a particularly serious threat with a high mortality rate. Most people agreed that once a child passed beyond infancy and early childhood, adolescence stood as the next critical juncture in the life course. Adolescence required caution, whether one was male or female, but physical decline seemed to occur more often among girls. For a summary of a number of different statements about the vulnerability of the female adolescent see Nellie Comins Whitaker, "The Health of American Girls," *Popular Science Monthly* 71 (September 1907), 240.

30. Harvey W. Wiley, *Not By Bread Alone* (New York, 1915), pp. 245, 248–250, 256; Brackett, *Education of American Girls*, pp. 25–26.

31. Warner, *A Popular Treatise*, p. 54.

32. On meat eating and sexual excess see Vern Bullough and Martha Voight, "Women, Menstruation and Nineteenth Century Medicine," *Bulletin of the History of Medicine* 47 (1973), 66–82. According to many physicians, flesh eating contributed to a "neurotic temperament." T. S. Clouston, superintendent of the Edinburgh asylum, espoused a widely held view: "I have found . . . a large proportion of the adolescent insane h[ave] been flesh-eaters, consuming and having a craving for much animal food"; see his "Puberty and Adolescence Medico-Psychologically Considered," *Edinburgh Medical Journal* 26 (July 1880), 17. This article was reprinted in the *American Journal of Insanity* in April 1881.

33. See Albert J. Bellows, *The Philosophy of Eating* (New York, 1869),

for a typical statement about meat by a health reformer. And see Stephen Nissenbaum, *Sex, Diet and Debility in Jacksonian America: Sylvester Graham and Health Reform* (Westport, Conn., 1980) on nineteenth-century vegetarianism.

34. E. L. Jones, *Chlorosis: The Special Anemia of Young Women* (London, 1897), p. 39; Charles Meigs, *Females and Their Diseases* (Philadelphia, 1848), p. 361; Montgomery, *Clinical Observations*. Susan Williams, *Savory Suppers and Fashionable Feasts: Dining in Victorian America* (New York, 1985), notes that rare or "underdone meat" was "out of fashion" and particularly "disgusting" to women and children (p. 239).

35. Nellie Browne to her mother [April 1859?], Sarah Ellen Browne papers, Schlesinger Library. Jane Hunter called this letter to my attention.

36. J. Clifford Allbutt, *A System of Medicine*, vol. 5 (New York, 1905), p. 517.

37. "The Antagonism between Sentiment and Physiology in Diet," *Current Literature* 42 (February 1907), 222. In reporting on anorexia nervosa, Pierre Janet described the phenomenon of *la crainte d'engraisser*—literally, the fear of taking on grease.

38. Quoted in Claude Fischler, "Food Preferences, Nutritional Wisdom, and Sociocultural Evolution," in *Food, Nutrition and Evolution*, ed. Dwain Walcher and Norman Kretchmer (New York, 1981), p. 58.

39. I borrow the term "subtext" from literary criticism, particularly from the semioticians. Food in nineteenth-century fiction and culture serves as a set of signs and symbols with communicative power. See Roland Barthes, "From Work to Text," in *Textual Strategies: Perspectives in Post-Structuralist Criticism*, ed. J. Harari (Ithaca, N.Y., 1979), pp. 73–81.

40. Williams, *Savory Suppers*, chap. 1, describes a pattern of middle-class concern over eating and correct eating behaviors. See also Jocelyne Kolb, "Wine, Women, and Song: Sensory Referents in the Works of Heinrich Heine," Ph.D. diss., Yale University, 1979, p. 8.

41. Janet, *Major Symptoms*, p. 234. Kolb, "Wine, Women, and Song," writes, "In the early 19th century, when Heine was writing, the mere mention of food in a lyrical passage was generally shocking enough to achieve ironic distance" (p. 71). The Romantic conception of food as an emblem of both the positive and negative sides of sensuality continued into the late nineteenth century.

42. Harland, *Eve's Daughters*, p. 81.

43. Although middle-class women were frequently assisted by a household servant, resulting in some reduction of time spent in the kitchen, they spent more and more energy planning meals, purchasing food, and determining ways to make eating an aesthetic experience. See Ruth Schwartz Cowan, *More Work for Mother: The Ironies of Household Technology from the Open Hearth to the Microwave* (New York, 1983).

44. George Everett and Susan Everett, *Health Fragments; or, Steps Toward a True Life* (New York, 1875), p. 35.

45. Fannie Munn Field diary, December 17, 1886, Box 9:18, Munn-Pixley Papers, Department of Rare Books and Special Collections, Rush Rhees Library,

University of Rochester, Rochester, N.Y. Susan Williams kindly brought this example to my attention.

46. Everett and Everett, *Health Fragments*, p. 25; Sarah Josepha Hale, *Receipts for the Million* (Philadelphia, 1857), p. 509.

47. [Society for Promoting Christian Knowledge], *Talks to Girls by One of Themselves* (London, 1894), p. 104.

48. Everett and Everett, *Health Fragments*, pp. 26, 29; Leslie A. Marchand, *Byron: A Portrait* (New York, 1970), p. 386.

49. George Eliot, *Daniel Deronda* (New York, n.d.), p. 104.

50. Jane Austen, *Mansfield Park* (New York, 1963), pp. 311–312; Anthony Trollope, *Ralph the Heir* (London, 1871), p. 195.

51. Mark Twain, *The Prince and the Pauper* (New York, 1881).

52. Elizabeth Gaskell, *Cranford* (New York, 1906), pp. 41, 53. Oranges were problematic for American eaters also; see Williams, *Savory Suppers*, pp. 108–109.

53. Eliot, *Daniel Deronda*, p. 104. The actual text of Byron's statement is, "A woman should never be seen eating or drinking, unless it be lobster salad and champagne, the only truly feminine and becoming viands" (Marchand, *Byron*, p. 133). In William Makepeace Thackeray's *History of Pendennis* (London, 1848–50) the character of Blanche is delineated by her peculiar appetite and secret eating: "When nobody was near, our little sylphide, who scarcely ate at dinner more than six grains of rice . . . was most active with her knife and fork, and consumed a very substantial portion of mutton cutlets: in which piece of hypocrisy it is believed she resembled other young ladies of fashion." (Quoted in Ann Alexandra Carter, "Food, Feasting, and Fasting in the Nineteenth Century British Novel," Ph.D. diss., University of Wisconsin, 1978, p. 3.)

54. Anthony Trollope, *Can You Forgive Her?* (New York, 1983), p. 70.

55. Sanford Bell, "An Introductory Study of the Psychology of Foods," *Pedagogical Seminary* 9 (1904), 88–89. In *Adolescence*, vol. 2 (New York, 1907), pp. 14–15, G. Stanley Hall noted that appetite varied a great deal in adolescence in response to "psychic motives." Hall did not differentiate between male and female adolescents, although Bell certainly did.

56. Kolb, "Wine, Women, and Song," suggests that this idea of higher and lower senses was inherited from the eighteenth century—specifically from Chevalier de Jancourt, who wrote on the subject in the famed *Encyclopédie*.

57. Harland, *Eve's Daughters*, p. 153.

58. On Byron's influence among the Victorians see Donald David Stone, *The Romantic Impulse in Victorian Fiction* (Cambridge, Mass., 1980).

59. Lizzie Eustace in Anthony Trollope's *Eustace Diamonds*, quoted in Stone, *Romantic Impulse*, p. 51.

60. On Byron's life and his struggles with food and eating see Edward John Trelawny, *Records of Shelley, Byron and the Author*, ed. David Wright (London, 1973), pp. 11, 35–36, 86, 97–98, 245. Mary Jacobus pointed out to me that Trelawny, notoriously "pro-Shelley," is a less than totally disinterested source of information on Byron's dieting. It is significant that Shelley too was a picky eater and a vegetarian, contributing further to the romance of undereating.

61. J. Milner Fothergill, *The Maintenance of Health* (London, 1874), pp.

80–81. This report of girls swallowing vinegar is not anomalous. See Brumberg, "Chlorotic Girls."

62. George Beard, *Eating and Drinking* (New York, 1871), p. 104.

63. Harland, *Eve's Daughters*, p. 124.

64. Beard, *Eating and Drinking*, p. v. Beard connected the American propensity for scanty eating to health reformers of an evangelical bent. He spoke of the "vast army of Jeremiahs who have gone up and down the land, predicting that gluttony will be our ruin" (p. iv). The links between parsimonious eating and religiosity are also suggested in Anthony Trollope, *Rachel Ray* (London, 1880). The plot of this novel is interesting because of the contrast between Mrs. Ray, a loving mother who likes tea and buttered toast, and her austere daughter, Mrs. Prime, an asexual, pious, churchgoing widow who likes "her tea to be stringy and bitter" and "her bread stale" (p. 5). The older women who influence Rachel Ray are defined by their appetite and eating behavior.

65. See for example Clouston, "Puberty and Adolescence," p. 14.

66. H. Davenport Adams, *Childlife and Girlhood of Remarkable Women* (New York, 1895), chap. 5; Josephine Butler, *Catherine of Siena* (London, 1878); Vida Scudder, *Letters of St. Catherine of Siena* (New York, 1905).

67. William James, *The Varieties of Religious Experience*, with an introduction by Reinhold Niebuhr (New York, 1961), pp. 79, 221, 238–240. James observed that as a consequence of secularization painful austerities or asceticism were not considered abnormal. "A strange moral transformation has within the past century swept over our Western world. We no longer think we are called on to face physical pain with equanimity. It is not expected of a man that he should either endure it or inflict much of it, and to listen to the recitals of cases of it makes our flesh creep morally as well as physically ... The result of this historical alteration is that even in the Mother Church herself, where ascetic discipline has such a fixed traditional prestige as a factor of merit, it has largely come into desuetude, if not discredit. A believer who flagellates or 'macerates' himself today arouses more wonder and fear than emulation" (p. 238). On asceticism see also Emile Durkheim, *The Elementary Forms of Religious Life*, trans. Robert Nisbet (London, 1976), pp. 299–321.

68. In the twentieth century many ideological followers of G. S. Hall spoke of the idealism of adolescents, that is, their search for moral purity. Asceticism in adolescence is rarely discussed, however. An interesting article that makes this connection and also distinguishes between adaptive and pathological asceticism is S. Louis Mogul, "Asceticism in Adolescence and Anorexia Nervosa," *Psychoanalytic Study of the Child* 35 (1980), 155–175. Mogul is reliant on Anna Freud, *The Ego and the Mechanisms of Defense* (London, 1937).

69. See note 16 above and Stoddard, *The Morgesons*, pp. 30, 57, 61, 140.

70. Trollope, *Ralph the Heir*, p. 29.

71. Thorstein Veblen, *The Theory of the Leisure Class* (New York, 1967).

72. Ibid., pp. 145–149.

73. My argument about the ways in which cultural and class concerns are encoded in the body follows from Michel Foucault, *History of Sexuality*, vol. 1 (New York, 1980), and *Madness and Civilization* (New York, 1965). The dis-

cipline of the body and its relation to social theory is explored by Brian Turner, "The Discourse of Diet," *Theory, Culture and Society* 1: 1 (1982), 23–32.

74. Hester Pendleton, *Husband and Wife; or, The Science of Human Development through Inherited Characteristics* (New York, 1863), p. 66.

75. Ibid., pp. 65–66.

76. Harland, *Eve's Daughters*, p. 134.

77. Trollope, *Can You Forgive Her?* p. 297.

78. Harland, *Eve's Daughters*, p. 111.

79. Allbutt, *A System of Medicine*, vol. 3, p. 485.

80. Harland, *Eve's Daughters*, p. 111.

8. Hormones and Psychotherapy

1. On pediatric anorexia nervosa see Joseph Brennemann, "Psychological Aspects of Nutrition in Childhood," *Journal of Pediatrics* 1 (August 1932), 145–171. Brennemann (pp. 157 ff.) claimed that an "army of anorexia" had descended upon parents and pediatricians and that as much as 85 percent of a private suburban practice was composed of children with anorexia nervosa. Obviously, the range of behaviors so labeled was extremely wide, which suggests that Brennemann's report should be viewed with some skepticism. A more cautious approach that hypothesized many different forms of "psychological anorexia" in children was John A. Rose, "Eating Inhibitions in Children in Relation to Anorexia Nervosa," *Psychological Medicine* 5: 2 (1943), 117–124.

2. My understanding of the history of endocrinology in the late nineteenth and early twentieth centuries is based on Merriley Borrell, "Organotherapy, British Physiology, and Discovery of Internal Secretions," *Journal of the History of Biology* 9 (Fall 1976), 235–268; idem, "Origins of the Hormone Concept: Internal Secretions and Physiological Research, 1889–1905," Ph.D. diss., Yale University, 1976; and Diana Long Hall, "Biology, Sex Hormones, and Sexism in the 1920s," *Philosophical Forum* 5: 12 (1973–74), 81–97. Additional relevant material is in Edward Allen, ed., *Sex and Internal Secretions: A Survey of Recent Research* (Baltimore, 1932) and Graham Lusk, "A History of Metabolism," in *Endocrinology and Metabolism*, ed. Lewellys F. Barker (New York, 1922), pp. 3–78.

3. For the story of Murray's research see Borell, "Organotherapy," pp. 244–248; for the clinical report see George R. Murray, "Note on the Treatment of Myxoedema by Hypodermic Injections of an Extract of the Thyroid Gland of a Sheep," *British Medical Journal* 2 (October 10, 1891), 796–797. It is interesting that William Gull is credited with the first clinical description of myxedema in 1893.

4. For the important early discussion of internal secretions and glands see Edward A. Schäfer, "Address in Physiology on Internal Secretions," delivered at the annual meeting of the British Medical Association in London, August 2, 1895, *Lancet* (August 10, 1895), 321–324.

5. On Starling see Diana Long Hall, "The Critic and the Advocate: Contrasting British Views on the State of Endocrinology in the Early 1920s," *Journal*

of the History of Biology 9 (Fall 1976), 275–283; Carleton Chapman, "Ernest Henry Starling, Physiologist," *Annals of Internal Medicine* 51 (1962), 1–43; F. G. Young, "The Evolution of Ideas about Animal Hormones," in *The Chemistry of Life*, ed. Joseph Needham (Cambridge, 1970), pp. 125–127.

6. See George Washington Corner, "The Early History of the Oestrogenic Hormones," *Journal of Endocrinology* 31 (January 1965), pp. iii–xvii. This article was given in London as the Sir Henry Dale Lecture for 1964.

7. M. Simmonds, "Ueber Hypophysisschwund mit tödlichem Ausgang," *Deutsche medizinische Wochenschrift* 40 (1914), 322–323; idem, "Über embolische Prozesse in der Hypophysis," *Virchows Archiv [Pathologische Anatomie]* 217 (1914), 226–239. In "Toward the Understanding of Anorexia Nervosa as a Disease Entity," *Mayo Clinic Proceedings* 56 (1981), 254–264, Alexander Lucas calls the period 1914–1942 the Pituitary Era in the history of etiological models of anorexia nervosa.

8. On the confusion between Simmonds' disease and anorexia nervosa, see Henry B. Richardson, "Simmonds' Disease and Anorexia Nervosa," *Transactions of the Association of American Physicians* 52 (May 1935), 141–145; idem, "Simmonds' Disease and Anorexia Nervosa," *Archives of Internal Medicine* 63 (January 1939), 1–28; Lucas, "Anorexia Nervosa as a Disease Entity," pp. 255–256; R. F. Escamilla and H. Lisser, "Simmonds' Disease: A Clinical Study with Review of the Literature: Differentiation from Anorexia Nervosa by Statistical Analysis of 595 Cases, 101 of which were Proved Pathologically," *Journal of Clinical Endocrinology* 2 (1942), 65–96; R. F. Escamilla, "Anorexia Nervosa or Simmonds' Disease? Notes on Clinical Management with Some Points of Differentiation between the Two Conditions," *Journal of Nervous and Mental Disorders* 99 (1944), 583–587.

9. Berkman received his M.D. degree from the University of Iowa; he was appointed to the staff of the Mayo Clinic in 1931 as a consultant in medicine and was a specialist in gastroenterology. John Mayo Berkman, "Anorexia Nervosa, Anorexia, Inanition and Low Basal Metabolism Rate," Master's thesis, University of Minnesota, 1930; idem, "Anorexia Nervosa, Anorexia, Inanition and Low Basal Metabolism Rate," *American Journal of Medical Science* 180 (July 1930), 411–424. My discussion of Mayo Clinic practice is based on Berkman and my own research in the clinic's archives. Berkman's work encompasses 117 cases between 1917 and 1929. The Mayo doctors who treated anorexic patients in that period were Henry S. Plummer (endocrinology), Frederick A. Willius (cardiology), Samuel F. Haines (endocrinology and internal medicine), Leonard Roundtree (endocrinology), Roger L. J. Kennedy (pediatrics), and Charles H. Mayo. Plummer (1874–1936) was influential in the classification of thyroid diseases and treatment of exophthalmic goiter with iodine. See *Dictionary of American Biography*, ed. Dumas Malone, vol. 8 (New York, 1935), pp. 533–534.

10. Mayo Clinic records, ARL–1, ARL–2, ARL–3; all records from this source have a special code designation, on file with Dr. Alexander Lucas.

11. On the general history of work in nutrition and metabolism see the entries for Francis Gano Benedict, Graham Lusk, and Wilbur Olin Atwater in the *Dictionary of Scientific Biography*, ed. Charles Coulston Gillispie (New York,

1970). On Benedict's "closed circuit method" of estimating the basal metabolism rate by oxygen consumption see Francis Gano Benedict, "An Apparatus for Studying the Respiratory Exchange," *American Journal of Physiology* 24 (1909), 345–374; Henry F. Moore, "The Basal Metabolism Rate: Its Determination and Interpretation," *Lancet* 208 (January 31, 1925), 219–224; John R. Murlin, "Normal Processes of Energy Metabolism," in *Endocrinology and Metabolism*, ed. Lewellys F. Barker (New York, 1922), pp. 544–547. Today oxygen consumption tests have given way to serum measurements.

12. Berkman, Master's thesis, pp. 19–20.

13. Thyroxin was isolated in crystalline form in 1915 by E. C. Kendall; desiccated thyroid is a natural extract.

14. Mayo Clinic records, ARL–4.

15. Ibid., ARL–3. At the Mayo Clinic metabolic balancing was the preferred treatment for anorexia nervosa in over 95 percent of the diagnosed cases. In only one case was there surgical intervention: in 1920 Charles Mayo did an exploratory "plastic operation" on a fifty-year-old woman who reportedly had had anorexia nervosa for more than twenty-five years. Mayo wrote: "I operated on her today finding a marked pyloric contraction, evidently chronic gastric neurosis with a hypertrophied muscle ring. I excised the muscle and made a gastroduodenostomy doubling the normal size of the stomach outlet and hope she will receive benefit. However, Miss [X] had had so much trouble with her nervous system for so many years that it is doubtful whether she will make a good recovery." In cases such as these, Henry Plummer recommended something called a "bougie" or "esophageal dilator"—a spindle and whalebone staff (Mayo Clinic records, ARL–5).

16. Mayo Clinic records, ARL–1.

17. Ibid., ARL–6.

18. Ibid.

19. Insulin, given because low fasting blood sugar and flat sugar tolerance curves were reported in anorexia nervosa, was supposed to increase the appetite. See for example R. F. Farquharson and H. H. Hyland, "Anorexia Nervosa: A Metabolic Disorder of Psychogenic Origin," *Journal of the American Medical Association* 3 (September 1938), 1085–92; and Bernard C. Meyer and Leonard A. Weinroth, "Observations on Psychological Aspects of Anorexia Nervosa," *Psychosomatic Medicine* 19 (September–October 1957), 389–398. Both accounts describe insulin therapy. On drug therapies for mental illness in the early twentieth century see Gerald Grob, *Mental Illness and American Society, 1875–1940* (Princeton, 1983), pp. 296–297, and idem, *The Inner World of American Psychiatry* (New Brunswick, N.J., 1985), pp. 105, 126–127. Apparently, insulin shock therapy was used to treat schizophrenics beginning in the 1920s and throughout the 1930s. "Antuitrin" is probably a term for a growth hormone such as somatotropin, STH.

20. John A. Ryle, "Anorexia Nervosa," *Lancet* 231 (October 17, 1936), 893–899.

21. Farquharson and Hyland, "Anorexia Nervosa," p. 1092.

22. The definitive history of dynamic psychiatry at present is Henri F. Ellenberger, *The Discovery of the Unconscious: The History and Evolution of*

Dynamic Psychiatry (New York, 1970). Ellenberger and others use the term to denote a school of psychiatry that made systematic investigations into the unconscious mind and that saw the mind as dynamic (changing) rather than fixed. (See pp. 289–290 of that history, however, for a discussion of the many different uses of the term "dynamic" within psychiatry.) Dynamic psychiatry is associated with the biosocial theories of Adolf Meyer (1866–1950), one of the most influential figures in American psychiatry from the 1890s through the 1940s. His "psychobiology" blended the life experiences of the individual with physiological and biological data. Early in his career Meyer incorporated and disseminated the ideas of Freud and Jung. On Meyer see Grob, *Mental Illness*, pp. 112–118, and John Burnham, *Psychoanalysis and American Medicine: 1894–1918* (New York, 1967), pp. 67–69.

23. *The Standard Edition of the Complete Psychological Works of Sigmund Freud,* trans. and ed. James Strachey, vol. 1, *Pre-Psychoanalytic Publications and Unpublished Drafts* (London, 1966), pp. 200–201.

24. On Janet see Ellenberger, *Discovery of the Unconscious*, pp. 331–417.

25. Pierre Janet, *The Major Symptoms of Hysteria* (New York, 1907), p. 233.

26. Ibid., pp. 233–237.

27. Ibid., p. 237.

28. The material that follows is from Pierre Janet, *Les obsessions et la psychasthénie* (Paris, 1903), pp. 33–40, 50. The term "sexual inversion" is generally associated with Havelock Ellis, the most influential purveyor of sexology in Britain and the United States. See for example his "Sexual Inversion with an Analysis of Thirty-Three New Cases," *Medico-Legal Journal* 13 (1895–96), 255–263.

29. Another psychogenetic interpretation in roughly the same period was that of J. Dejerine and E. Gauckler, *The Psychoneuroses and Their Treatment by Psychotherapy*, translated from the French by Smith Ely Jelliffe (New York, 1913). Dejerine and Gauckler regarded anorexia nervosa as a "psychic affection" caused by "mechanisms of many kinds." In other words, they did not emphasize the psychosexual etiology. Jelliffe, the translator, was part of the psychoanalytic movement: he was a student of A. A. Brill, a New York analyst who had studied with both Freud and Jung.

30. Helen Flanders Dunbar, *Emotions and Bodily Changes: A Survey of Literature on Psychosomatic Interrelationships, 1910–1933* (New York, 1935), p. 323. On Dunbar see Franz Alexander, "In Memoriam," *American Journal of Psychiatry* (August 1960), 189–190; G. Allison Stokes, "Flanders Dunbar," in *Notable American Women, The Modern Period*, ed. Barbara Sicherman and Carol Hurd Green (Cambridge, Mass., 1980), pp. 210–212; Robert C. Powell, "Healing and Wholeness: Helen Flanders Dunbar (1902–1959) and the Extra-Medical Origin of the American Psychosomatic Movement," Ph.D. diss., Duke University, 1974.

31. See masthead and "Introductory Statement," *Psychosomatic Medicine* 1 (January 1939), 3. On anorexia nervosa see Lincoln Rahman, Henry Richardson, and Herbert S. Ripley, "Anorexia Nervosa with Psychiatric Observations," ibid. (July 1939), 335–365; John V. Waller, M. Ralph Kaufmann, and

Felix Deutsch, "Anorexia Nervosa: A Psychosomatic Entity," ibid. 2 (January 1940), 3–16.

32. See Fred Ellsworth Clow, "Anorexia Nervosa," *New England Journal of Medicine* 207 (October 5, 1932), 613–617. Clow graduated from Harvard Medical School in 1904 and thereafter practiced as an internist in New Hampshire. In 1932 he was secretary of the New Hampshire Board of Registry in Medicine. (Information provided by Richard J. Wolfe, Joseph Garland Librarian, Francis A. Countway Library of Medicine, Harvard Medical School.)

33. See comments of Sir Arthur Hurst, "Discussion of Anorexia Nervosa," *Proceedings of the Royal Society of Medicine* 32 (January 24, 1939), 34.

34. Rahman, Richardson, and Ripley, "Anorexia Nervosa," p. 363; Ruth Moulton, "A Psychosomatic Study of Anorexia Nervosa Including the Use of Vaginal Smears," *Psychosomatic Medicine* 4 (January 1942), 65.

35. Farquharson and Hyland, "Anorexia Nervosa," p. 1090.

36. Rahman, Richardson, and Ripley, "Anorexia Nervosa," p. 355. There is a single report from a university health service in this era: Helen P. Davis, "Anorexia Nervosa," *Endocrinology* 25 (December 1939), 991–995. This report is from the University of Wisconsin Department of Student Health.

37. The discussion that follows is based on George H. Alexander, "Anorexia Nervosa," *Rhode Island Medical Journal* 22 (December 1939), 189–195. Alexander graduated from Brown University in 1921 and received his M.D. degree from Yale University College of Medicine in 1931. See "George H. Alexander," in "Rhode Island Medical Society—Necrology 1955," *Rhode Island Medical Journal* 39 (January 1956), 4. The obituary in the *New York Times*, April 30, 1955, mistakenly says that Alexander was a graduate of the University of Rhode Island.

38. Alexander, "Anorexia Nervosa," p. 193. These terms are common to the period around 1910, during the psychotherapy craze, and are not associated with psychoanalysis.

39. Alexander (ibid., p. 195) explained that he had not pursued the "deeper exploration" of the unconscious that was characteristic of orthodox psychoanalysis, even though he suspected that the girl's pregnancy fantasy was related to some infantile experience. Rather, in this particular case he focused the interview process on conscious awareness. "By strengthening the forces of the conscious mind," he said, psychotherapy helped the patient "resubmerge the anxiety-producing factors to deep, unconscious levels of the mind where they were incapable of expression in the form of neurotic illness."

40. See for example J. V. Waller, R. M. Kaufman, and F. Deutsch, "Anorexia Nervosa: A Psychosomatic Entity," *Psychosomatic Medicine* 2 (1940), 3–16; Sandor Lorand, "Anorexia Nervosa: Report of a Case," ibid. 5: 2 (1943), 282–292; Irving I. Sands, *Neuropsychiatry for Nurses* (Philadelphia, 1948), pp. 335–336; J. Masserman, "Psychodynamics in Anorexia Nervosa," *Psychoanalytic Quarterly* 10 (1941), 211–242; Meyer and Weinroth, "Observations," p. 395.

41. Rahman, Richardson, and Ripley, "Anorexia Nervosa," p. 355.

42. Both Mary Ryan, *Womanhood in America*, 3rd ed. (New York, 1983) and Linda Gordon, *Woman's Body, Woman's Right* (New York, 1976), point

to the growing emphasis on heterosexual behavior in the period between 1890 and 1930. See also Christina Simmons, "Companionate Marriage and the Lesbian Threat," *Frontiers* 4 (Fall 1979), 54–59; Carroll Smith-Rosenberg, *Disorderly Conduct: Visions of Gender in Victorian America* (New York, 1985), pp. 266–286; Sheila Jeffreys, *The Spinster and Her Enemies: Feminism and Sexuality, 1880–1930* (London, 1985). Also relevant is Vern Bullough and Bonnie Bullough, "Lesbianism in the 1920s and 1930s: A Newfound Study," *Signs* 2 (Summer 1977), 895–904.

43. Hall's most important statements on adolescence are his two-volume magnum opus, *Adolescence: Its Psychology and Its Relation to Physiology, Anthropology, Sociology, Sex, Crime, Religion and Education* (1904) and *Youth: Its Education, Regimen, and Hygiene* (1906). The latter was widely used in normal schools for training teachers. On Hall's life and work see Dorothy Ross, *G. Stanley Hall: The Psychologist as Prophet* (Chicago, 1972). Freud came to the United States in 1909 at Hall's invitation. For a literary critic's view of the power of the idea of adolescence, see Patricia Meyer Spacks, *The Adolescent Idea* (New York, 1981).

44. Moulton, "Psychosomatic Study," p. 67.

45. P. Lionel Goitein, "The Potential Prostitute: The Role of Anorexia in the Defense against Prostitution Desires," *Journal of Criminal Psychopathology* 2 (January 1942), 359–367.

46. Moulton, "Psychosomatic Study," pp. 70–71, 73.

47. Masserman, "Psychodynamics," p. 240.

48. Ibid.

49. Ibid., p. 224. In *The Interpretation of Dreams* (1900) Freud argued that the psychoanalyst must work to find the linkage between the object and its meaning.

50. Hilde Bruch, *Eating Disorders: Obesity, Anorexia Nervosa, and the Person Within* (New York, 1973), p. 217.

51. Physicians probably interpreted the lanugo associated with nutritional deprivation as a sign of masculinity. Some also used the distribution of pubic hair as evidence of sexual abnormality: anorectics were sometimes described as having a "masculine" as opposed to "feminine" pattern of hair on the pudendum. See Rahman, Richardson, and Ripley, "Anorexia Nervosa," p. 338.

52. Ibid., p. 356; Moulton, "Psychosomatic Study," p. 71.

53. See for example the two references cited in note 52, and see also Bruch, *Eating Disorders*, pp. 216–222, for a summary of this literature.

54. Moulton, "Psychosomatic Study," p. 68.

55. Rahman, Richardson, and Ripley, "Anorexia Nervosa," pp. 357, 360.

56. Bruch, *Eating Disorders*, p. 215.

57. Ibid., p. 3.

58. In 1920 overweight was not regarded as a psychological problem, but by the 1940s it was. Hilde Bruch figured prominently in this changing medical view. In 1939 she eliminated Fröhlich's syndrome, believed to be a pituitary disturbance, by demonstrating that the condition (usually in fat boys with delayed pubertal development) could be treated with dietary restriction and increased activity. Moreover, she related the symptoms to psychological problems

created by the mother-child interaction. See Bruch's own account of this discovery, "The Constructive Use of Ignorance," in E. James Anthony, *Explorations in Child Psychiatry* (New York, 1975), pp. 247–264.

Obese people increasingly were distinguished from others on the basis of personality characteristics. By 1951 a U.S. Public Health Service study of obese women concluded that "excess pounds are nothing more than a symptom of a personality out of kilter." On the basis of Rorschach inkblot tests, fat people were judged to be less well adjusted than others. See "The Obese Person," *Time* (March 1, 1943), 66, and "Fat Personality," *Newsweek* (November 17, 1952), 110. For the outline of this transformation I am indebted to Jessica Ruth Johnston, "The Double Bind: 'Eat and Stay Thin': Food as a Condensed Cultural Symbol in Advertising and the Overweight Stigma, 1890–1980," Master's thesis, California State University, 1983, esp. chap. 3.

59. Bruch, *Eating Disorders*, p. 224.

9. Modern Dieting

1. The word "diet," formerly a more general term for the regulation of food intake for a variety of purposes, has now come to mean the reduction of food intake to lower weight and slim the body. We commonly say, for example, "I am on a diet," but specify particular types of diets for health purposes—for example, salt-free diet, diabetic diet, low-cholesterol diet. See Margaret Ohlson, "Diet Therapy in the United States in the Past 200 Years," *Journal of the American Dietetic Association* 60 (November 1976), 490–497. Modern dieting has another characteristic that distinguishes it from its predecessors: in the twentieth century the diet is generally based on some quantitative system or unit of measurement that can be counted, such as exchange lists based on the food groups, or calories.

The best discussions of the nineteenth-century pattern of dieting are in Stephen Nissenbaum, *Sex, Diet, and Debility in Jacksonian America* (Westport, Conn., 1980), chap. 6, note 33; James C. Whorton, *Crusaders for Fitness: The History of American Health Reformers* (Princeton, 1982); Harvey Green, *Fit for America: Health, Fitness, Sport and American Society* (New York, 1986). On the American romance with dieting in the nineteenth and twentieth centuries see Hillel Schwartz, *Never Satisfied: A Cultural History of Diets, Fantasies and Fat* (New York, 1986).

For my initial understanding of twentieth-century trends I am indebted to two undergraduates whose work I advised: Janet Beth Abrams, "The Thinning of America: The Emergence of the Ideal of Slenderness in American Popular Culture, 1870–1930," B.A. thesis, Harvard University, 1983, and Lisa Norling, "The Origins of Popular Dieting in America," Independent Study paper, Cornell University, 1985. Also useful was Jessica Ruth Johnston, "The Double Bind: 'Eat and Stay Thin': Food as a Condensed Cultural Symbol in Advertising and the Overweight Stigma, 1890–1980," Master's thesis, California State University, 1983. Two additional feminist works deal with modern dieting and the cultural imperative for slimness in women: Kim Chernin, *The Obsession: Re-*

flections on the Tyranny of Slenderness (New York, 1981), and Ann Scott Beller, *Fat and Thin: A Natural History of Obesity* (New York, 1977).

2. For a historical study of concepts of beauty in the United States see Lois Banner, *American Beauty* (New York, 1983). In *France, 1848–1945*, vol. 2, *Intellect, Taste and Anxiety* (New York, 1977), Theodore Zeldin noted the triumph of the thin woman over the fat woman in the twentieth century (p. 440).

3. See Wendell C. Phillips, "Introduction," in *Your Weight and How to Control It*, ed. Morris Fishbein (New York, 1927), p. xiii. Fishbein includes papers from the 1926 Adult Weight Conference. Quoted also in Clarence W. Lieb, *Eat, Drink and Be Slender: What Every Overweight Person Should Know and Do* (New York, 1929), p. vi.

4. Morris Fishbein, "The Craze for Reducing," in Fishbein, *Your Weight*, pp. 22–27.

5. There is no complete catalog of twentieth-century diet techniques, although Schwartz, *Never Satisfied*, provides much useful and suggestive information. For references to some of the different popular regimens in this period see Arthur J. Cramp, "Obesity Cures," *Journal of the American Dietetic Association* 1: 3 (1925), 141–142; W. C. Martin, "Pathological Consideration of Weight Reduction," *New York Physician* 11 (September 1938), 24–25; "Obesity Cures," Bureau of Investigation, American Medical Association (Chicago, 1929); James Harvey Young, *The Medical Messiahs: A Social History of Health Quackery in Twentieth Century America* (Princeton, 1967).

6. Typical of the journalistic and medical warnings against unsupervised dieting are Fishbein, "Craze for Reducing," p. 27; Jane Foster, "Dieting Daughters," *Hygeia* (February 1937), 141–143; Martin, "Pathological Considerations," pp. 24–27; Walter H. Eddy, "Significance of Little Things in Reducing Diets," *New York Physician* 11 (September 1938), 28–34; Lieb, *Eat, Drink and Be Slender*, p. vi. A short story for girls by Margaret Taylor MacDonald, "The Reducing Club," *St. Nicholas Magazine* (February 1923), 352–358, described unsupervised dieting in a girl's boarding school and intervention by the headmistress and the school doctor. The September 1938 issue of *New York Physician* was devoted to a symposium on obesity that included a broad discussion of the doctor's role in dieting.

7. My rendering of the standardization of weight in this period is based on William Bennett and Joel Gurin, *The Dieter's Dilemma: Eating Less and Weighing More* (New York, 1982), esp. chap. 5; Abrams, "Thinning of America," chap. 3; Schwartz, *Never Satisfied*, chap. 6. Daniel Boorstin, *The Democratic Experience* (New York, 1973), pp. 189–193, discusses the new "language of numbers."

8. Bennett and Gurin, *Dieter's Dilemma*, pp. 125, 131; Abrams, "Thinning of America," pp. 60–61.

9. Johnston, "Double Bind," pp. 33–34.

10. Bennett and Gurin, *Dieter's Dilemma*, p. 133; Abrams, "Thinning of America," p. 62.

11. Morris Fishbein, *An Hour on Health* (Philadelphia, 1929), p. 25; Lieb, *Eat, Drink and Be Slender*, p. v.

12. According to Schwartz, *Never Satisfied*, pp. 168–175, bathroom scales were first introduced at the turn of the century. In 1925 Detecto, one of a number of scale companies, claimed to have sold one million.

13. Bennett and Gurin, *Dieter's Dilemma*, p. 136.

14. Fishbein, *Your Weight*, p. 35.

15. On the history of pediatrics see Thomas E. Cone, Jr., *History of American Pediatrics* (Boston, 1979); Kathleen W. Jones, "Sentiment and Science: The Late 19th Century Pediatrician as Mother's Advisor," *Journal of Social History* 17 (1983), 79–86; John L. Morse, "Recollections and Reflections on Forty-five Years of Artificial Infant Feeding," *Journal of Pediatrics* 7 (September 1935), 303–307.

16. See for example S. A. Levinsohn, "A Child Who Will Not Eat," *Journal of the Medical Society of New Jersey* 30 (April 1933), 314–318; D. P. Arnold, "Why a Child Refuses to Eat," *New York State Medical Journal* 33 (January 1, 1933), 20–21; R. P. McLeod, "My Child Simply Won't Eat," *Hygeia* 17 (February 1939), 116–118; Joseph Brennemann, "Psychological Aspects of Nutrition in Childhood," *Journal of Pediatrics* 1 (August 1932), 145–171.

17. Brennemann, "Psychological Aspects," pp. 157–161. In 1932 Brennemann claimed that anorexia nervosa in children had become, in the past two decades, a "pediatric meal ticket." His suggestion that educated middle-class mothers were implicated in childhood eating problems was confirmed by Winona L. Morgan, *The Family Meets the Depression* (Minneapolis, 1939), pp. 30–32. Morgan reported that mothers who had studied home economics had more feeding problems with their children than those who had not.

18. On the scientific cooking movement see Laura Shapiro, *Perfection Salad: Women and Cooking at the Turn of the Century* (New York, 1986). On the history of home economics see Emma Seifert Wigley, "It Might Have Been Euthenics: The Lake Placid Conferences and the Home Economics Movement," *American Quarterly* 26 (March 1974), 79–96; Margaret Rossiter, *Women Scientists in America: Struggles and Strategies to 1940* (Baltimore, 1982), pp. 65–70. One of the most important early progenitors of the domestic science movement was Catharine Beecher, whose *Treatise of Domestic Economy* (New York, 1841) was a critical concordance for nineteenth-century homemakers. See Kathryn Kish Sklar, *Catharine Beecher: A Study in American Domesticity* (New York, 1976). On Ellen Swallow Richards, "founder" of home economics, see Janet Wilson James, "Ellen Swallow Richards," *Notable American Women* (Cambridge, Mass., 1971), vol. 2, pp. 143–146; Caroline Hunt, *The Life of Ellen Swallow Richards* (Boston, 1912). For samples of Richards' ideas consult her writings: *The Cost of Living* (New York, 1899); *The Cost of Shelter* (New York, 1905); *The Dietary Computer* (New York, 1902); "Domestic Science," *Outlook* (April 24, 1897), 1078–80; and "The Social Significance of the Home Economics Movement," *Journal of Home Economics* (April 1911), 117–125. Also useful is Alice Ravehill, *The Teaching of Domestic Science in the United States of America* (London, 1905), and articles on Martha Van Rensselaer, Isabel Bevier, and Mary Swartz Rose, in *Notable American Women*.

19. Lulu Hunt Peters, *Diet and Health with a Key to the Calories* (Chicago, 1918), p. i.

20. On the decline of live-in domestic service in the twentieth century see Faye E. Dudden, "Experts and Servants: The National Council on Household Employment and the Decline of Domestic Service in the Twentieth Century," *Journal of Social History* (December 1986), 269–289. In the absence of live-in domestics, eating was privatized to a new degree.

21. For information on Atwater's work see Charles E. Rosenberg, "Wilbur Olin Atwater," *Dictionary of Scientific Biography* (1970), vol. 1, pp. 325–326, and Shapiro, *Perfection Salad,* pp. 73–77.

22. The calorie was discovered during the study of animal heat and metabolism, a process begun by Antoine Lavoisier and Adair Crawford (in the eighteenth century) and Edward Frankland (1825–1899). According to Elmer Verner McCollum, *A History of Nutrition: The Sequence of Ideas in Nutrition Investigations* (Boston, 1957), Frankland was "the first to study foods for the quantitative energy values which they yielded on combustion" (p. 127). In the early twentieth century, a calorie was determined with an apparatus known as the bomb calorimeter, which had two chambers: the inner (containing dry food) and the outer (filled with water). The food was ignited with an electrical connection and burned. This generated heat, which was transferred to the water. When one pound of water was raised four degrees Fahrenheit, the amount of heat used was arbitrarily chosen as a unit of heat and called the calorie. In Munich, in the laboratory of Max Von Pettenkofer (1818–1901), allegedly the first professor of hygiene anywhere, Wilbur Atwater was exposed to the calorimeter and to a respiration apparatus large enough to accommodate a man. Together with Carl Voit, Von Pettenkofer conducted experiments that yielded the respiratory quotients of protein, carbohydrates, and fat when metabolized in the body (McCollum, *History of Nutrition,* chap. 10). On the eighteenth-century history of energy metabolism see Everett Mendelsohn, *Heat and Life: The Development of the Theory of Animal Heat* (Cambridge, Mass., 1964).

23. Sarah Tyson Rorer (1849–1937) was nutrition editor of the *Ladies' Home Journal*; see Emma Seifrit Weigley, *Sarah Tyson Rorer* (Philadelphia, 1977). Mary Swartz Rose, a professor of nutrition at Teacher's College, Columbia University, authored a popular guide, *Feeding the Family* (New York, 1916), and often wrote for women's magazines. In *Perfection Salad* Shapiro observes that home economists often saw food as an adversary, as something that conflicted with the delicacy and gentility of the preparer. In other words, Shapiro is suggesting that home economics continued the tradition of the "lifeless palate" that was born in the Victorian era.

24. The movement to reduce infant and child mortality began in the latter part of the nineteenth century, but public commitment to child welfare expanded in the twentieth century as the Progressives made improvement of child mortality rates a national priority. In 1908, the world's first public bureau devoted exclusively to the health of children was established in New York City; in 1912, the United States Children's Bureau was established. On Progressive activities in this area see "Child Health," in Robert Bremner, ed., *Children and Youth in America* (Cambridge, Mass., 1971), vol. 2, pp. 812–815; John Duffy, *A History of Public Health in New York City, 1866–1966* (New York, 1968); James Leiby, *A History of Social Welfare and Social Work in the United States* (New York, 1978).

Milk stations and depots were established by municipalities and wealthy philanthropists, as medicine uncovered the connection between bad milk and child health. See Bremner, "Child Health," pp. 811–812; Kathleen W. Jones, "Sentiment and Science: The Late Nineteenth Century Pediatrician as Mother's Advisor," *Journal of Social History* 17 (Fall 1983), 80–96; Patricia Melvin, "Milk to Motherhood: The New York Milk Committee and the Beginning of Well-Child Programs," *Mid America* 65 (1983), 111–134; George Rosen, "The First Neighborhood Health Center Movement—Its Rise and Fall," *American Journal of Public Health* 61 (1971), 1620–35; Manfred J. Wasserman, "Henry L. Coit and the Certified Milk Movement in the Development of Modern Pediatrics," *Bulletin of the History of Medicine* 46 (1972), 359–390. On weighing in the schools see Luther H. Gulick and Leonard P. Ayres, *Medical Inspection of Schools* (New York, 1913); "A Pair of Scales in Every School," *Ladies' Home Journal* 36 (September 1919), 125; Elizabeth Irwin, "What the Child's Weight Tells," *Delineator* 97 (December 1920), 29.

25. Rose, *Feeding the Family*, p. ii.

26. "On Growing Fat," *Atlantic Monthly* (March 1907), 430–431.

27. In *Eating and Drinking* (New York, 1871), George M. Beard complained that many Americans still had Puritan ideas about subduing the appetite. He rejected the idea of satiety as "a conviction of sin" (p. v).

28. Overweight was associated with promiscuity and infanticide in female criminals. See Caesar Lombroso and William Ferrero, *The Female Offender* (New York, 1899). Among juvenile delinquents overweight was associated with girls, underweight with boys.

29. For the history of couture fashion I rely on Michael Batterberry and Ariane Batterberry, *Mirror Mirror: A Social History of Fashion* (New York, 1977); Diana DeMarly, *The History of Haute Couture, 1850–1950* (New York, 1980); Jo Ann Olian, *The House of Worth: The Gilded Age, 1860–1918* (New York, 1982). Abrams, "Thinning of America," chap. 2, first provided me with the basic progression of events described here. Charles Frederick Worth is credited with having transformed the craft of dressmaking into the art of haute couture. He was the first to present a collection of dresses that could be ordered by individual customers and the first to sign his work with labels (Olian, *House of Worth*, p. 1).

30. DeMarly, *History of Haute Couture*, pp. 81–83; Batterberry and Batterberry, *Mirror Mirror*, pp. 286–297. For Poiret see *The Autobiography of Paul Poiret* (Philadelphia, 1931). On Chanel see Edmonde Charles-Roux, *Chanel: Her Life, Her World, and the Woman behind the Legend She Herself Created* (New York, 1975). Banner, *American Beauty*, pp. 214, 218, reports the use of depilatories by 1918.

31. P. Rostaine, "How to Get Thin," *Medical Press and Circular* 149 (December 23, 1914), 643–644. Rostaine, clinical director of the Faculty of Medicine in Paris, approved of the emphasis on slenderness because of the connection between fat and high mortality.

32. On the ready-to-wear industry and its "leveling" consequences see Stuart Ewen and Elizabeth Ewen, *Channels of Desire: Mass Images and the Shaping of American Consciousness* (New York, 1982), esp. pt. 4; Claudia

Kidwell and Margaret C. Christman, *Suiting Everyone: The Democratization of Clothing in America* (Washington, D.C., 1974); Margaret Walsh, "The Democratization of Fashion: The Emergence of the Women's Dress Pattern Industry," *Journal of American History* 66 (September 1979); Boorstin, *Democratic Experience,* pp. 100, 188–189. In *Democracy and Social Ethics* (New York, 1902), Jane Addams portrayed clothing as a great leveler: "Have we worked out our democracy further in regard to clothes than anything else?" (p. 36).

33. *Vogue* (January 1, 1923), 63.

34. Banner, *American Beauty,* p. 262; Ewen and Ewen, *Channels of Desire,* pp. 193–198. On women and the late-nineteenth-century and early-twentieth-century department store see William R. Leach, "Transformations in a Culture of Consumption: Women and Department Stores, 1890–1925," *Journal of American History* 71 (September 1984), 319–342; Susan Porter Benson, *Counter Culture: Saleswomen, Managers, and Customers in American Department Stores, 1890–1940* (Champaign, Ill., 1986); Elaine S. Abelson, "'When Ladies Go A-Thieving': The Department Store, Shoplifting, and the Contradictions of Consumerism, 1870–1914," Ph.D. diss., New York University, 1986.

35. Quoted in "'San-gri-na': Another Fake Cure," *Journal of the American Medical Association* 83: 21 (1924), 1703.

36. Banner, *American Beauty,* p. 287; Anne Hollander, *Seeing through Clothes* (New York, 1975). Hollander argues not so much that the camera distorts reality as that photographs are read differently than three-dimensional bodies.

37. Peters, *Diet and Health,* p. 11. Peters' book, which between 1918 and 1922 went through seventeen editions, was dedicated to Herbert Hoover, then head of the effort for recovery in Europe. In 1924, and in 1925, it was number one on the nation's nonfiction best-seller list. See Alice Payne Hackett and James Henry Burke, *Eighty Years of Best Sellers, 1895–1975* (New York, 1977), pp. 97, 99.

38. Peters, *Diet and Health,* pp. 24, 39.

39. Ibid., pp. 12, 104, 110.

40. Ibid., pp. 12–13, 109.

41. Ibid., pp. 85, 94.

42. Ibid., pp. 85, 93, 94.

43. The foremost critic of calorie counting as a diet technique is Dr. William Bennett. See note 7 above and William Bennett, "Dieting: Ideology versus Physiology," *Psychiatric Clinics of North America* 7 (June 1984), 321–334, and idem, "Dietary Treatments of Obesity," unpublished.

44. Banner, *American Beauty,* pp. 214–216, makes this point.

45. "On Her Dressing Table," *Vogue* (April 24, 1902), 413, and ibid. (July 1, 1918), 78; Helena Rubenstein, *The Art of Feminine Beauty* (New York, 1930), p. 133.

46. Mary Douglas, *Purity and Danger* (London, 1970). An important discussion of the body in relation to social theory is that of Bryan Turner, *The Body and Society: Explorations in Social Theory* (Oxford, 1984). Turner argues for the relationship between dietary management and capitalist society's need for increasing social control of bodies. Michael Featherstone, "The Body in

Consumer Culture," *Theory, Culture and Society* 1: 2 (1982), 18–33, hypothesizes that contemporary patterns of dieting and body maintenance are regarded as vehicles to release the temptations of the flesh (rather than as a defense against them).

47. On women in the 1920s see Mary Ryan, *Womanhood in America from Colonial Times to the Present,* 2nd ed. (New York, 1975), pp. 151–182; William Chafe, *The American Woman: Her Changing Social, Economic, and Political Roles, 1920–1970* (New York, 1972); Paula S. Fass, *The Damned and the Beautiful: American Youth in the 1920s* (New York, 1977); Ewen and Ewen, *Channels of Desire,* esp. pt. 3.

48. On the primacy of nineteenth-century women's relationships with one another, see Carroll Smith-Rosenberg, "The Female World of Love and Ritual: Relations between Women in Nineteenth Century America," *Signs* 1 (Autumn 1975), 1–29; and Martha Vicinus, *Independent Women: Work and Community for Single Women, 1850–1920* (Chicago, 1985). On the sexuality of nineteenth-century women see Peter Cominos, "Late Victorian Sexual Respectability and the Social System," *International Review of Social History* 8 (1963), 18–48, 216–251; Carl Degler, "What Ought to Be, and What Was: Woman's Sexuality in the Nineteenth Century," *American Historical Review* 79 (December 1974), 1467–90; John S. Haller and Robin M. Haller, *The Physician and Sexuality in Victorian America* (Urbana, Ill., 1974); Nancy Cott, "Passionlessness: An Interpretation of Victorian Sexual Ideology, 1790–1850," *Signs* 4 (Winter 1978), 219–236.

49. On the history of birth control in the United States see Linda Gordon, *Women's Bodies, Women's Rights* (New York, 1976); Daniel Scott Smith, "The Dating of the American Sexual Revolution: Evidence and Interpretation," in *The American Family in Social-Historical Perspective,* ed. Michael Gordon (New York, 1974), pp. 328–332.

50. On Kellerman see the portraits in *Bookman* 47 (May 1918), 314–315; *Cosmopolitan* (June 1910), 86; *Harper's Weekly* (January 27, 1912), 19. See also Banner, *American Beauty,* pp. 207, 267, 341. According to Robert Grau, *Forty Years Observation of Music and Drama* (New York, 1909), Kellerman's success was based on the "extraordinary sensationalism" of her publicity (p. 40).

51. See the review of "Daughter of the Gods," *New York Times Film Reviews* 9 (October 9, 1916), 1. James R. McGovern, "The American Woman's Pre–World War I Freedom in Manners and Morals," *Journal of American History* 55 (September 1968), 315–333, suggests that the sexual revolution occurred before 1920.

52. Annette Kellerman, *Physical Beauty* (New York, 1918), p. 24.

53. Ibid., p. 50.

54. Physical culturists such as Bernarr A. McFadden, editor of the monthly *Physical Culture* magazine, promoted strength, fitness, and sexuality. In particular, McFadden viewed intercourse as a healthy, recreative function, not simply a procreative technique. See Green, *Fit for America,* pp. 245–251, for an excellent discussion of the physical culture movement.

55. Annette Kellerman, "Why and How Girls Should Swim," *Ladies' Home*

Journal 27 (August 1910), 11. Green, *Fit for America,* makes the point that "health and sex were intimately linked" in the physical culture movement and that publications such as *Physical Culture* catered to middle-class males by displaying nubile young women in revealing outfits (pp. 245–251).

56. On the history of beauty pageants see Banner, *American Beauty,* pp. 249–270, and Kellerman, *Physical Beauty,* p. 17.

57. Elaine Tyler May, *Great Expectations: Marriage and Divorce in Post Victorian America* (Chicago, 1980); Michael Gordon, "From an Unfortunate Necessity to a Cult of Mutual Orgasm: Sex in Marital Education Literature, 1830–1940," in James Henslin, ed., *Studies in the Sociology of Sex* (New York, 1971), pp. 53–80.

58. Kellerman, *Physical Beauty,* p. 15.

59. Ibid., p. 16.

60. Ewen and Ewen, *Channels of Desire,* pp. 100–101.

61. Kellerman, *Physical Beauty,* p. 16.

62. See Mary Ryan, "The Projection of a New Womanhood: The Movie Moderns in the 1920s," in *Our American Sisters: Women in American Life and Thought,* ed. Jean E. Friedman and William G. Shade, 2nd ed. (Boston, 1976), pp. 366–384, for a discussion of early films and the rise of sexual allure; and Ewen and Ewen, *Channels of Desire,* pp. 97–99, for a description of Theda Bara and her personification of the "Vamp."

63. In *Advertising the American Dream* (Berkeley, 1985), Roland Marchand argues that advertising campaigns of the 1920s and 1930s made beauty a "duty" (pp. 176–179).

64. The emphasis on personal appearance translated into a preoccupation with having certain material goods, especially the accoutrements of current fashion. On working-class girls see Addams, *Democracy and Social Ethics,* pp. 34–36. In "Ladies Go A-Thieving" Abelson ties middle-class women's escalating consumer desires to the origins of kleptomania.

65. Harlow Brooks, "The Price of a Boyish Form," in Fishbein, *Your Weight,* p. 32.

66. On women in the 1930s and 1940s, see Ryan, *Womanhood,* pp. 183–198; Chafe, *The American Woman;* Winifred Wandersee Bolin, "The Economics of Middle Income Family Life: Working Women during the Great Depression," *Journal of American History* 65 (June 1978), 60–74; Susan Ware, *Holding Their Own: American Women in the 1930s* (Boston, 1982); Susan Hartman, *The Home Front and Beyond: American Women in the 1940s* (Boston, 1982); D'Ann Campbell, *Women at War with America: Private Lives in a Patriotic Era* (Cambridge, Mass., 1984). It is interesting to note how views of female body configuration have changed since the 1930s. Images of women in the Depression era, captured by Works Progress Administration photographers, seemed horrific at the time because the women were so gaunt and thin. Today their bodies would not be an issue; in fact, they look rather like those of contemporary fashion models.

67. Schwartz, *Never Satisfied,* p. 269, writes that American anxieties about overweight and obesity settled in the 1940s and 1950s on adolescents; in the 1960s, on grade-schoolers; and in the 1970s, on toddlers, infants, and newborns.

68. On the improvement in child mortality in this period, see Cone, *American Pediatrics,* pp. 159–160, 171–179, 202. According to Cone, the most significant decline in childhood tuberculosis and child mortality occurred after 1925.

69. Bird T. Baldwin, "Use and Abuse of Weight-Height-Age Tables as Indexes of Health and Nutrition," *Journal of the American Medical Association* 92 (1924), 1–4.

70. Kathryn McHale, "Comparative Psychology of the Overweight Child," Ph.D. diss., Columbia University, 1926, p. 89.

71. In the 1930s Bruch was the first to emphasize the importance of emotional problems within the families of fat children over any endocrinologic or glandular abnormality. Among a number of articles written in this period the best-known is Hilde Bruch and Grace Touraine, "Obesity in Childhood, V: The Family Frame of Obese Children," *Psychomatic Medicine* 2 (1940), 141–206. Related articles by Bruch were published in the *American Journal of the Diseases of Children, Journal of Pediatrics, American Journal of Orthopsychiatry, American Journal of Psychiatry,* and *Nervous Child.* Bruch's thinking on the subject of obesity and the problems it creates were synthesized in her *Importance of Overweight* (New York, 1957); Benjamin Spock, *The Common Sense Book of Baby and Child Care* (New York, 1945), pp. 359–360.

72. Literature typical of the late 1930s and the 1940s includes Mildred H. Bryan, "Don't Let Your Child Get Fat!" *Hygeia* 15 (1937), 801–803; G. D. Schultz, "Forget That Clean-Plate Bogey!" *Better Homes and Gardens* 21 (September 1942), 24; J. H. Kenyon, "Don't Let Your Child Get Fat," *Good Housekeeping* 121 (October 1945), 62. On adolescents see Regina J. Woody, "Reducing the Adolescent," *Hygeia* 19 (1941), 476–482; F. W. Schultz, "What to Do about the Fat Child at Puberty," *Journal of Pediatrics* 19 (1941), 376–381; Lulu Graves, "Should the Teens Diet?" *Parents' Magazine* 15 (April 1940), 76.

73. Louise Paine Benjamin, "I Have Three Growing Daughters," *Ladies' Home Journal* 57 (June 1940), 74. Benjamin had her three daughters, all under fifteen years of age, doing posture exercises in order to guard against "protruding derrières and tummy bulges." See also the monthly "Sub-Deb" column of *Ladies' Home Journal* for expressions of concern about beauty and overweight.

74. See for example a market research study conducted for *Photoplay* magazine, *The Age Factor in Selling and Advertising: A Study in a New Phase of Advertising* (Chicago, 1922), frontispiece and pp. 9, 43–44, 96.

75. Fass, *The Damned and the Beautiful,* p. 124 and chaps. 3 and 4.

76. *The Age Factor,* p. 18; Ewen and Ewen, *Channels of Desire,* p. 94.

77. James A. Gilbert, *A Cycle of Outrage: America's Reaction to Juvenile Delinquency in the 1950s* (New York, 1986), pp. 204–207.

78. Helen Valentine, "Seventeen Says Hello," *Seventeen* (September 1944), 33.

79. The material cited is from "You'll Eat It Up at Noon," *Seventeen* (September 1946), 21–22; Irma M. Phorylles, "The Lost Waistline" ibid. (March 1948), 124; "Overweight?" ibid. (August 1948), 184. On drugs in dieting see Johnston, "Double Bind," p. 55. See *New Republic* (August 1937) on the

"miracle drug" (alpha-dinitrophenol); *Time* (August 23, 1943) on "Weight Reducing Made Easy" (dextroamphetamine); *Newsweek* (September 15, 1947) on benzedrine.

80. Phorylles, "Lost Waistline," p. 124.

81. "Fattest Girl in the Class," *Seventeen* (January 1948), 21–22.

82. In the "Psychology of Dieting," *Ladies' Home Journal* (January 1965), 66, the editors explained: "Everybody knows that it is bad to be overweight, that it is unattractive, is a social and psychological handicap and even a threat to health. Still, this is not reason enough to reduce. You must know what difference it will make if you change your weight."

83. *USA Today,* August 11, 1986.

84. Jeffrey Zaslow, "Fourth Grade Girls These Days Ponder Weighty Matters," *Wall Street Journal,* February 11, 1986; "Dieting: The Losing Game," *Time* (January 20, 1986), 54. Both the *Wall Street Journal* and *Time* reported results from a University of California study. Dieting peaks, however, at the onset of middle age. See Jeremy Schlosberg, "The Demographics of Dieting," *American Demographics* 9 (July 1987), 35–37, 61–62.

85. Bennett and Gurin, *Dieter's Dilemma,* is the best statement about the ineffectiveness of dieting. See also *USA Today,* August 11, 1986, and *Time* (January 1, 1986), 54. Over 37 percent of all adults are dieting at any given time. According to the Calorie Control Council, an association of diet food producers, most people on diets cut out high-calorie foods (81 percent); increase exercise (78.5 percent); use special low-calorie foods (67 percent); or skip meals (31.5 percent).

86. Founded in 1961, the National Glandular Society in 1972 became the American Society of Bariatric Physicians.

87. Banner, *American Beauty,* pp. 283–285, points out that in the 1950s the asexual adolescent and the voluptuous beauty both held sway. In teen magazines, such as *Seventeen,* and on television the ideal for adolescent girls was the ingenue epitomized in petite women such as Sandra Dee and Debbie Reynolds.

88. See, as an example, David M. Garner et al., "Cultural Expectations of Thinness in Women," *Psychological Reports* 47 (1980), 483–491.

89. Quoted in Rita Freedman, *Beauty Bound* (New York, 1986), p. 150.

90. See "Coming on Strong: The New Ideal of Beauty," *Time* (August 30, 1982), 72–77, for a comprehensive overview of the ways in which American women are reshaping their bodies. Freedman, *Beauty Bound,* chap. 7, deals with the psychological impact of the "obsession with food and fitness."

91. On the move from countercuisine to a lighter diet see Warren Belasco, "Lite Economics: Less Food, More Profit," *Radical History Review* 28–30 (September 1984), 254–278. For a journalistic report on the shift in American diet, see *U.S. News and World Report* 96 (April 30, 1984), 20. Hilde Bruch was attuned to the role of food faddism in American culture; see her "The Allure of Food Cults and Nutrition Quackery," *Journal of the American Dietetic Association* 57 (October 1970), 316–320.

92. Freedman, *Beauty Bound,* pp. 166–167.

93. These two selections are taken from Hilde Bruch, *Conversations with*

Anorexics (New York, forthcoming), pp. 127, 140–141. Bruch was very sensitive to the competitive aspects of anorexic behavior and the ways in which this could operate in an inpatient therapeutic setting.

94. W. Stewart Agras and Helena C. Kraemer, "The Treatment of Anorexia Nervosa: Do Different Treatments Have Different Outcomes?" *Psychiatric Annals* 13 (December 1983), 929.

95. See P. Eveleth and J. Tanner, *Worldwide Variation in Human Growth* (New York, 1976); Bengt-olov Ljung et al., "The Secular Trend in Physical Growth in Sweden," *Annals of Human Biology* 1: 3 (1974), 245–256; R. E. Muuss, "Adolescent Development and the Secular Trend," *Adolescence* 5 (1970), 267–284.

96. George I. Szmukler and Digby Tantam, "Anorexia Nervosa: Starvation Dependence," *British Journal of Medical Psychology* 57 (1984), 303–310; D. M. Garner and P. E. Garfinkel, "Sociocultural Factors in the Development of Anorexia Nervosa," *Psychological Medicine* 10 (1980), 647–656; D. M. Garner et al., "Cultural Expectations of Thinness in Women," *Psychological Reports* 47 (1980), 483–491.

Afterword

1. See R. E. Kendell et al., "The Epidemiology of Anorexia Nervosa," *Psychological Medicine* 3 (1973), 200–203; David B. Herzog and Paul M. Copeland, "Eating Disorders," *New England Journal of Medicine* 313: 5 (1985), 295–303; Jane Y. Yu, "Eating Disorders," *Vital Signs* (September 1986), Cornell University Health Services, p. 2.

2. On post–World War II prosperity see William Chafe, *The Unfinished Journey: America since World War II* (New York, 1986). Chafe does not deal with the consequences of affluence for the American diet. The postwar American diet is the subject of a forthcoming study by Warren Belasco.

3. For an astute discussion of how we eat today, see Sidney Mintz, *Sweetness and Power: The Place of Sugar in Modern History* (New York, 1985), pp. 187–215. I am indebted to Mintz for his suggestions about segmentation of the market and the desocialization of eating. On the mass marketing of food as well as the distribution of the "roving palate," see Warren Belasco, "Lite Economics: Less Food, More Profit," *Radical History Review* 28–30 (September 1984) 254–278, and idem, "Ethnic Fast Foods: The Corporate Melting Pot," *Food and Foodways* 2 (November 1987), 1–30; also Wilbur Zelinsky, "You Are What You Eat," *American Demographics* 9 (July 1987), 31–33, 56–58. On contemporary fashions in food, the *New York Times* is a particularly instructive source. See Barbara Ehrenreich, "The Cult of Food in a World of Hunger," *New York Times*, January 17, 1985, for a suggestive analysis of the relationship between exercise and the new eating patterns.

4. Daniel Bell, *The Cultural Contradictions of Capitalism* (New York, 1976).

5. Hilde Bruch, *Eating Disorders: Obesity, Anorexia Nervosa, and the Person Within* (New York, 1973), p. 3. Some anthropologists would disagree.

See for example Marvin Harris, *Good to Eat: Riddles of Food and Culture* (New York, 1985).

6. *New Yorker* (July 21, 1986), 71.

7. The connection between eating habits and identity is captured in popular discourse about food and life-style. See for example "What's Your Food Status? Because the Way You Live Has a Lot to Do with the Way You Eat," *Mademoiselle* (September 1985), 224–226; "Food as Well as Clothes, Today, Make the Man—As a Matter of Life and Style," *Vogue* (June 1985), 271–273.

8. "Severe Growing Pains for Fast Food," *Business Week* (March 22, 1985), 255; on the ways in which eating was transformed by the automobile before World War II see Warren Belasco, *America on the Road: From Autocamp to Motel, 1910–1945* (Cambridge, Mass., 1979); Mintz, *Sweetness and Power*, pp. 213, 294–305; Claude Fischler, "Food Habits, Social Change, and the Nature/Culture Dilemma," *Social Science Information* 19: 6 (1980), 937–953; Bruce Cost, "Grazing Meals," *New York Times Magazine* (September 7, 1986), 95–96. Although both grazing (sometimes called modular eating) and vagabond eating appear to be atavistic behaviors, harking back to a time when eating was done on a catch-as-catch-can basis, the mobile eater of potential interest to the contemporary food and restaurant world is a creature of abundance rather than scarcity. This is a critical difference.

9. Greg Foster and Susan Howerin, "The Quest for Perfection: An Interview with a Former Bulimic," *Iris: A Journal about Women* [Charlottesville, Va.], no. 12 (1986), 21.

10. Before they even arrive on campus, during their senior year in high school and the summer before entering college, many girls begin to talk about the "freshman 10 or 15." This is the weight gain predicted as a result of eating starchy institutional food and participating in late-night food forays with friends. It has been reported in "Bulimia: The Binge-Purge Syndrome," an instructional video produced by Carle Medical Communications (1986), and in my own conversations with college students. I use the term "individualized" to capture the desocialized, noninteractive quality of student eating patterns; the substance of what they eat is actually very predictable and is marked by a high degree of conformity.

11. A Yale undergraduate quoted in Elizabeth Greene, "Support Groups Forming for Students with Eating Disorders," *Chronicle of Higher Education* (March 5, 1986), 1, 30. Parental control of eating is obviously a very real issue among anorectics still in high school and living at home. The personal diary of a woman who was anorexic in high school reveals that she deliberately slept late but left the house on weekend mornings in order to "be out . . . by lunch time." Weekday dinners always presented problems because of parental monitoring; therefore, the rest of the day had to be compensatory—that is, no food at all. The diarist, Jeanne X, wrote in August 1968:

Day of complete fast (except evening meal) . . . and God! Did I ever eat an evening meal! That's why I'm forcing myself to stay up late so I can lose (or use up) the excess . . . I'm still constipated too. My stomach is out a mile. I've got a few new pimples, I should get my friend soon (it's been almost 2 months). You can see I'm in spectacular shape. I've got one week until . . . [the] slumber party—Boy! This week is going to be devoted to Project Jeanne. And I mean a *real starvation* diet. (Italics added.)

12. See K. A. Halmi, J. R. Falk, and E. Schwartz, "Binge-Eating and Vomiting: A Survey of a College Population," *Psychological Medicine* 11 (1981), 697–706; R. L. Pyle et al., "The Incidence of Bulimia in Freshman College Students," *International Journal of Eating Disorders* 2: 3 (1983), 75–86; R. S. Stangler and A. M. Printz, "DSM-III: Psychiatric Diagnosis in a University Population," *American Journal of Psychiatry* 137 (1980), 937–940; Shoshana Nevo, "Bulimic Symptoms: Prevalence and Ethnic Differences among College Women," *International Journal of Eating Disorders* 4 (May 1985), 151–168; "College Life: When Food Is the Enemy," *Newsweek on Campus* (March 1987), 18–19.

13. Anne Charlton, "Smoking and Weight Control in Teenagers," *Public Health* 98 (1984), 277–281. Both Joan Austoker (Britain) and Allan Brandt (United States) confirm that the goal of weight control is influential in causing the high incidence of smoking in teenage girls.

14. This situation was first noted by Orlando Wayne Wooley and Susan Wooley, "The Beverly Hills Eating Disorder: The Mass Marketing of Anorexia Nervosa," *International Journal of Eating Disorders* 1 (Spring 1982), 57–68.

15. D. M. Schwartz, M. G. Thompson, and C. L. Johnson, "Anorexia Nervosa and Bulimia: The Socio-Cultural Context," *International Journal of Eating Disorders* 1 (Spring 1982), 20–36; Ruth Striegel-Moore, Lisa R. Silberstein, and Judith Rodin, "Toward an Understanding of Risk Factors in Bulimia," *American Psychologist* 41 (March 1986), 256. The mimetic quality of contemporary anorexia nervosa was of course observed by Bruch. A recent study suggests that the behavior is spreading to other age groups: according to Marianne Rosenzweig and Jean Spruill, "Twenty Years after Twiggy: A Retrospective Investigation of Bulimic-Like Behavior," *International Journal of Eating Disorders* 6 (January 1987), 57–65, significantly more adult women engage in bulimic behavior today than in their high school or college years.

16. Carol Gilligan, *In a Different Voice: Psychological Theory and Women's Development* (Cambridge, Mass., 1982).

17. I am grateful to Susan Bordo for this point about the difference beween male and female eaters in television ads. Susan Bordo, "How Television Teaches Women to Hate Their Hungers," *Mirror Images* [newsletter of Anorexia/Bulimia Support, Inc., Syracuse, N.Y.] 4 (Winter 1986), 1, 8–9.

18. Mirra Komarovsky, *Women in College: Shaping New Feminine Identities* (New York, 1985), pp. 89–92, 225–300.

19. *Ms.* (September 1986), n.p. The condom is called Mentor.

20. Ellen Goodman, *Close to Home* (New York, 1979).

21. In *Theories of Adolescence* (New York, 1962) R. E. Muuss wrote, "Societies in a period of rapid transition create a particularly difficult adolescent period; the adolescent has not only the society's problem to adjust to but his [or her] own as well" (p. 164). See also Paul B. Baltes, Hayne W. Reese, and Lewis P. Lipsitt, "Life Span Developmental Psychology," *Annual Review of Psy-*

chology 31 (1980), 76–79; J. R. Nesselroade and Paul B. Baltes, "Adolescent Personality Development and Historical Change: 1970–1972," *Monographs of Society for Research in Child Development* 39 (May 1974), ser. 154.

22. My view of this issue complements ideas presented in Robert Bellah et al., *Habits of the Heart: Individualism and Commitment in American Life* (New York, 1986).

23. These data are synthesized in Urie Bronfenbrenner, "Alienation and the Four Worlds of Childhood," *Phi Delta Kappan* (February 1986), 434.

Acknowledgments

In 1982–83, as a fellow at the Charles Warren Center for Studies in American History, Harvard University, I first began systematic study in the history of medicine. At the outset—in fact, throughout my writing and research—I profited greatly from conversations with Allan Brandt, Barbara Sicherman, and Nancy Tomes. In addition to introducing me to the literature, they acted as a sounding board at critical junctures. They also assured me, with confidence and clarity, that I *could* write a history of anorexia nervosa and that my background in the social history of religion was an asset rather than a liability. Each, in his or her own way, provided me with special friendship as well as intellectual sustenance. My commitment to a book on this subject solidified in an extended conversation with Nancy Tomes, while sitting on a mountainside at the 1982 Berkshire Conference of Women Historians in Canaan, New York.

During my term at Harvard and over the intervening years, I also received encouragement from Barbara Gutmann Rosenkrantz, who invited me to participate in a study group associated with the Department of the History of Science at Harvard and generously shared her wide knowledge. M. Jeanne Peterson gave me invaluable preliminary advice about British medicine and provided a critical reading of the manuscript at a later phase. Regina Morantz-Sanchez was a receptive listener when my medical vocabulary was still very limited. At an important point in the work Gerald Grob made astute suggestions. Interactions with Charles E. Rosenberg and Diana Long around the seminar table at the

Francis Clark Wood Institute (Philadelphia) were worthwhile and provocative. In short, many people within the history-of-medicine community provided me with sound counsel and direction.

A number of others deserve special thanks. William I. Bennett, M.D., fulfilled my ideal of the accessible physician, willing and able to move adroitly back and forth between "cutting-edge" medical science and historical questions; both formally and informally, he gave knowledgeable advice and asked stimulating questions. Ellen Bassuk, M.D., gave generously of her psychiatric knowledge. I also enjoyed the intellectual colleagueship of Caroline Walker Bynum. Fortunately, the Sixth Annual Berkshire Conference on the History of Women, in June 1984, and our mutual interest in the dynamics of fasting and female piety, brought us together; this relationship provided me with a comparative perspective that helped to highlight the distinctive features of the anorexic experience in the nineteenth century. In the process of writing and revising, I have been sustained by the unfailing receptivity and encouragement of Faye Dudden and Susan Ware. Both have been willing, at different times and in different capacities, to read lengthy, undisciplined drafts and have responded with good critical judgment and enthusiasm, even when the work was still very rough. Bernard Weisberger, who twenty years ago inspired my love for nineteenth-century sources, made a series of excellent suggestions about the integrity of the narrative.

In 1984–85, a Rockefeller Foundation Humanities Fellowship freed me from teaching responsibilities. I received further assistance along the way from the National Endowment for the Humanities Travel to Collections Grant and from faculty research funds in Cornell University's College of Arts and Sciences and the New York State College of Human Ecology. The Department of Human Development and Family Studies at Cornell made it possible for me to obtain a basic medical education in eating disorders. In a summer course given by the Division of Continuing Education at Harvard Medical School, I joined physicians and mental health practitioners in learning about diagnoses and treatment strategies for eating disorders.

Cornell University has been important for more than financial support, ultimately providing me with a responsive interdisciplinary environment that stretched my thinking about my subject. I am indebted to many at Cornell who are not historians: Sandra and Daryl Bem, in particular, asked many penetrating questions that helped me clarify the relationship between history and psychology. In addition, Urie Bronfenbrenner, Howard Feinstein, Sander Gilman, the late Rose Goldsen, Davydd Greenwood, David Holmberg, Mary Katzenstein, David Lyons, Kathryn March, Dorothy Nelkin, and Harry Shaw supplied insightful suggestions and reactions. Among my fellow historians, Robert Harris, Jr., I. V. Hull, R. Laurence Moore, and Mary Beth Norton either read or listened to various pieces of research and responded with perceptive comments. And I learned a great deal from Steven Kaplan, who expanded my knowledge of the world of scholarship about food. Many of the ideas presented here first surfaced in presentations at Cornell, in the Women's Studies Sex and Gender study group; the Food and Foodways Seminar series; the 1983 Summer Institute on Medicine and the Professions; the colloquium series of the Graduate Program in the History and Philosophy of Science; and the History of Psychiatry Section, Cornell Medical Center, New York City.

I enjoyed lively visits to Women's Studies and Women's History programs, where interest in the subject of anorexia nervosa is deep and often passionate. Lecture invitations from, among others, Joyce Antler and Judith Ebel Tsipis (Brandeis), Ann Lane (Colgate), Linda Gordon and Judith Walzer Leavitt (University of Wisconsin), Patricia King and Barbara Haber (Schlesinger Library, Radcliffe), Marilyn Hoder-Salmon (Florida Atlantic University), the late Janet Wilson James (Boston College), Sally McMurry (Pennsylvania State University), Susan Reverby (Wellesley), and Kay Warren (Princeton) provided me with important opportunities to distill my thinking at different stages of my research and writing.

Librarians and archivists have played a significant role in my research. Profound thanks are due the entire reference staff of the John M. Olin Library at Cornell, who offered knowledgeable assistance throughout this project. I am particularly grateful to Ann Carson, Julie Copenhagen, Robert Kibee, Nancy Skipper, Carolyn Spicer, and Susan Szasz, who handled my frequent requests with professional aplomb as well as personal interest. At the Francis J. Countway Library, Harvard Medical School, I had the able and enthusiastic assistance of Richard J. Wolfe, Garland Librarian. During a valuable research trip to the Wellcome Institute for the History of Medicine in London, I was advised by R. J. Palmer and William Shupach. And I am indebted to JoAnn Miller of Basic Books, who made available to me Hilde Bruch's posthumous manuscript, *Conversations with Anorexics* (New York, forthcoming).

My understanding of anorexia nervosa as a clinical diagnosis was enhanced by the opportunity to use clinical case materials in a number of different hospital archives. Leonard Kerlan and Alexander Lucas of the Mayo Clinic, Rochester, Minnesota, kindly provided access to their well-managed records. I was fortunate also to be extended privileges as a Visiting Research Fellow at McLean Hospital, Belmont, Massachusetts; my thanks go to Terry Bragg, archivist, for his informed help and to James Hudson for sharing his view of strategies for treating eating disorders. John W. Goethe and John H. Houck allowed me to use nineteenth-century patient records from the Institute for Living, Hartford, Connecticut. A search for unpublished clinical material in London and environs was assisted by Julia Shephard of the Wellcome Institute and G. M. Pentelow at the King's College Medical School. Jonathan Peppler, district archivist at London Hospital, provided stalwart, good-humored support in getting me to case materials that really were physically inaccessible.

The preparation of this manuscript was consistently eased by the competence of Roberta Ludgate, with whom I have worked for nearly a decade. Probably more than anyone else, Roberta pushed me into the computer age. At Cornell, Jo Balog and Janice Wright handled a vast amount of correspondence related to this manuscript, and Theresa Windhausen provided backup support for my administrative responsibilities as director of the Women's Studies Program. For brief periods Amanda Bryans, Lisa Ginet, Eve Saltzman, and Carol Smith delivered reliable bibliographic assistance.

At Harvard University Press, I am grateful to Aida Donald for her early interest and solid support of this endeavor; to Vivian

Wheeler for the astute manner in which she polished my prose; and to Claire Silvers, Elizabeth Suttell, and Gayle Treadwell for their competence and good ideas.

I have a few debts that are personal rather than professional. Through the generosity of Courtney Cazden, I was able to live comfortably, in easy access to major libraries, during my fellowship year at the Warren Center. Having a hospitable home away from home meant more to me than anyone can imagine. In the process of writing this book, I have not always been easy to be with and my preoccupation with writing translated into a high degree of self-absorption. For their moral support I want to express my gratitude to a circle of accepting and affectionate family and friends: Adam Brumberg and Sarah Bowman, Marshall Blake, Paul and Ellen Grebinger, Helen and Tom Johnson, Midge and Joel Kerlan, Ron Lopez, Steven and Marjorie Moore, Millie O'Connell, Amy Opperman and Randy Cash, and David Yeh and Rachel Weitzman-Yeh. Finally, I am grateful to my husband, David Brumberg, for his integrity, his sound instincts as a historian, his good-humored patience with me, and his love.

Index

Bulimia: and anorexia nervosa, 11–12; Jane Fonda and, 18; publicity on, 19–20; college eating patterns and, 262, 264; among blacks, 284n14. *See also* Eating disorders
Burrows, George Man, 309–10n7
Butler, Josephine, 184
Bynum, Caroline Walker, 2, 44–45, 294n1; *Holy Feast and Holy Fast*, 45
Byron, Lord, 43, 182, 183, 333n53; *Childe Harold*, 183

Cacositis (aversion to food), 58
Calories, 237, 241, 248, 252
Campbell, J. A., 107
Capitalism, 3, 34, 260, 270
Carlini, Benedetta, 296n10
Carpenter, Karen, 15
Catherine of Siena, Saint, 2, 41, 42, 44–45, 183, 184, 301n38
Catholicism: and fasting, 41–46, 47–49, 62–63; and Mollie Fancher case, 84
Chanel, Gabrielle, 239, 240
Charcot, Jean-Martin, 144, 165
Chernin, Kim, 29–30, 33, 34
Children: as anorectics, 228, 335n1, 343n17; weight problems, 235, 237, 249–250; dieting in 20th century, 253
Chipley, William Stout, 105–110
Chlorosis, 172, 173–174, 176
Christian Science, 75, 76
Cigarette smoking, 264
Clarke, Edward H., 151; *Sex in Education*, 151
Class, social: of anorectics, 9, 12–13, 27, 113, 220, 330–31n21; and 19th-century medicine, 102, 111; and asylums, 105, 109, 113, 145; and slenderness ideal, 185–187. *See also* Middle-class families; Working class
Clinical Society of London, 114–115; Gull's address to, 118–125
Clothing: ready-to-wear, 239–240; standard sizing, 240–241. *See also* Fashion
Clouston, T. S., 151
Clow, Fred Ellsworth, 218–219
Clymer, Meredith, 85
College women: incidence of anorexia nervosa, 9, 10, 12, 220; disapproval of early medical men, 151; increasing

numbers in 20th century, 244, 251; incidence of eating disorders, 258, 262–265; parental food monitoring, 352–53n11
Columba of Rieti, Saint, 41
Commercials. *See* Advertising
Competitiveness, as symptom of anorexia nervosa, 5, 256, 280–81n9
Constituency of anorexia nervosa, 14, 220, 271; social class, 9, 12–13, 27, 113, 128, 330n21; geographic aspects, 13, 27; in black population, 284n14
Consumerism, 251, 260, 270, 271
Control issues of anorectics, 16, 28. *See also* Appetite Control; Parents of anorectics
Conversion hysteria, 214
Copeland, Paul M., 24
Coppague, Helen, 306–07n103
Cornaro, Luigi, 55
Corner, George, 207
Cosmetics industry, 231, 243
Cottage hospitals, 323n14, for care of anorectics, 145, 156, 159–162
Counseling Centers of America, 22
Cultural model for anorexia nervosa, 31–38, 46, 142, 164–188, 270–271

Darwin, Erasmus, 54, 58
Davies, Henry Harris, 68
De Berdt Hovell, Dennis, 155–156
Deceptiveness, attributed to food-refusing women, 49, 60, 62, 66, 67, 71, 73, 84; of anorectics, 16; of Mollie Fancher, 85, 89; adolescent, 170. *See also* Fraudulence; Secret eating
Deecke, Theodore, 96
Democritus, 54
Depression (psychological), anorexia nervosa and, 143, 157, 303–31n21. *See also* Melancholia
Depression, Great, 249
Diagnosis of anorexia nervosa: lack of standardization, 11–12, 120, 162–163, 174; increasing likelihood of, 13–14, 43, 258; earliest, 101, 110; differential, 101–102, 120–121, 125; Gull and, 111–112, 115–125, 148–149; and sitophobia, 112. *See also* Symptomatology of anorexia nervosa